Functionalized Polysulfones

Synthesis, Characterization, and Applications

Functionalized Polysulfones

Synthesis, Characterization, and Applications

Edited by
Silvia Ioan

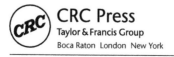

CRC Press
Taylor & Francis Group
Boca Raton London New York

CRC Press is an imprint of the
Taylor & Francis Group, an **informa** business

CRC Press
Taylor & Francis Group
6000 Broken Sound Parkway NW, Suite 300
Boca Raton, FL 33487-2742

First issued in paperback 2017

ISBN-13: 978-1-4822-5554-6 (hbk)
ISBN-13: 978-1-138-74929-0 (pbk)

Visit the Taylor & Francis Web site at
http://www.taylorandfrancis.com

and the CRC Press Web site at
http://www.crcpress.com

Dedication

This book is dedicated to the 65th anniversary of the "Petru Poni" Institute of Macromolecular Chemistry—Romanian Academy, Iasi, Romania

Contents

Preface

The term *functionalized polysulfones* applies to a large number of organic materials. Over the past decades, considerable attention has been devoted to the investigation of new applications of polysulfones and functionalized polysulfones, mainly due to some of their specific properties. This book focuses on polysulfones and their derivatives, which are widely used as new functional materials in biochemical, industrial, and medical fields, owing to their structural and physical characteristics such as good optical properties, high thermal and chemical stability, mechanical strength, resistance to extreme pH values, and low creep. The functional groups, which modify the hydrophilicity of polysulfones, are of special interest for biomedical applications, antimicrobial action, solubility characteristics, water permeability, and separation. In addition, the functional groups are an intrinsic requirement for affinity, ion exchange, and other special membranes. In this book, the bioapplications of polysulfones are presented, in two categories: blood-contacting devices (e.g., as membranes for hemodialysis, hemodiafiltration and hemofiltration and cell- or tissue-contacting devices (e.g., bioreactors made by hollow-fiber membrane, nerve generation through polysulfone semipermeable hollow membrane). Surface wettability and hydrophilicity trends, as well as the morphological characteristics of some modified polysulfones, are analyzed for semipermeable membrane purposes. Some chapters furnish an introduction to chelating units on the modified polysulfone structure to obtain potential applications, such as surface coatings on metals and glasses, adhesives, high-temperature lubricants, electrical insulators, semiconductors, and the reduction of heavy-metal pollution in ecosystems.

This book contains recent scientific information and contributes significantly to the basic knowledge of students and researchers working in the field of polymeric materials, including physicists, chemists, engineers, bioengineers, and biologists.

Silvia Ioan
"Petru Poni" Institute of Macromolecular Chemistry
Romanian Academy

Editor

Dr. Silvia Ioan, PhD, is a senior scientific researcher in the Department of Chemical Physics at the "Petru Poni" Institute of Macromolecular Chemistry, Iasi, Romania, of the Romanian Academy since 1966. She obtained her PhD in physical sciences from 1980 at the University of Bucharest, Romania. Her scientific contributions include interdisciplinary research for theoretical and experimental substantiations of the processes and technologies at nano-, micro-, and macroscales. Dr. Ioan's research has focused on realizing multifunctional materials through the participation of some polymers with special architectures and includes studies concerning the improvement of some properties for predetermined goals as theoretical assessment of physical characteristics to obtain synthetic papers and cardboards with different destinations, polymers used in the purification of polluted water, polymers as nonconductive and conductive materials, polymers as fire-retardant materials, polymer as superior optical materials, biocompatible polymers, theoretical study on the ultrahigh molecular weight polymers, and so on. In 48 years of work, Dr. Ioan has published approximately 300 scientific papers, books, or book chapters. Dr. Ioan is the PhD supervisor in chemistry at the doctoral school of the Institute of Macromolecular Chemistry—Romanian Academy, is expert reviewer of prestigious scientific journals, and was awarded the Nicolae Teclu prize by the Romanian Academy of Science in 1972.

Editor

Contributors

Raluca Marinica Albu
"Petru Poni" Institute
    of Macromolecular Chemistry
Romanian Academy
Iasi, Romania

Ecaterina Avram
"Petru Poni" Institute
    of Macromolecular Chemistry
Romanian Academy
Iasi, Romania

Luminita-Ioana Buruiana
"Petru Poni" Institute
    of Macromolecular Chemistry
Romanian Academy
Iasi, Romania

Anca Filimon
"Petru Poni" Institute
    of Macromolecular Chemistry
Romanian Academy
Iasi, Romania

1 General Introduction

Silvia Ioan

This book provides a wide range of information concerning recent advances in functionalized polysulfone compounds, based on an interdisciplinary approach of the synthesis process, computerized structures used to evidence specific properties, adaptation of various structures for specific applications, and thermodynamic aspects. After a basic introduction to each specific domain, the authors, who are specialists in the areas outlined, explore topics that include molecular technologies, thermodynamic aspects, nano or biomaterials—involving biocompatibility and antimicrobial properties—formation of metal nanoparticles in polysulfonic matrices, metal film deposition on polysulfone surfaces, polysulfone compounds with chelating groups, and specific electro-optical properties, all discussed in the context of possible new applications.

This book brings together investigations of some actively engaged researchers in various fields, mentioned in an extensive list of references. Organized into 10 chapters, this book explores the preparation, characterization, and specific applications of new functionalized polysulfones, covering the following topics:

- Obtaining of polysulfones with pendant functional groups
- Mathematical models and numeric simulation of the specific interactions in solutions of modified polysulfones
- Structure–property relationships of functionalized polysulfones
- Phosphorus-containing polysulfones for high-performance applications in advanced technologies
- Origin of dielectric response and conductivity of some functionalized polysulfones
- Functionalized polysulfone–metal complexes
- Biocompatibility of polysulfone compounds
- Antimicrobial activity of polysulfone structures
- Potential biomedical applications of functionalized polysulfones

Combining different properties of functionalized polysulfones with the technologies for obtaining complex structures for specific applications, this book clearly demonstrates the importance of these materials in electrotechnical domains, biotechnology, biomedicine, and environmental remediation. In addition, it offers recent scientific information and can significantly enrich the basic knowledge of students and researchers working in the field of polymeric materials: physicists, chemists, engineers, bioengineers, and biologists.

Thus, this book:

- Presents a broad, interdisciplinary view of the field of functionalized polysulfones.
- Discusses interactions and molecular assemblies of polysulfones under the influence of external factors, involved in bioactive membrane technologies.
- Covers a wide range of topics, from basic chemistry, biology, and physics to the integration of these subjects into biomedicine, optoelectronics, and environmental technologies.
- Includes contributions from experts in these fields.
- Suggests future applications on how thermodynamic theories and computer analyses regarding structural properties and contributions of substructures to different properties—optoelectronic, biocompatibility, antimicrobial activity—contribute to the diversification of application domain of complex polysulfone structures.
- Provides comprehensive material suited to practitioners, researchers, and students.

2 Aromatic Linear Polysulfones with Pendant Functional Groups

Ecaterina Avram and Anca Filimon

CONTENTS

2.1 INTRODUCTION

Polymer-analogous reactions represent a general method for obtaining macromolecular compounds with desirable functional groups in the side chain, which can be used as reagents or catalysts in various macromolecular organic or inorganic syntheses. The method consists of introducing functional groups into the polymer main chain and has the advantage of not being conditioned by the synthesis of a particular monomer [1].

In recent years, separation membranes have become essential materials not only for industries but also in daily human life [2–4]. Thus, they have been used in many practical applications [5–14], including in producing potable water from seawater by reverse osmosis, recovering valuable solution constituents by electrolysis, cleaning industrial effluents, and so on. Membranes have also been used to separate, remove, purify, or partially recover individual components of gas mixtures, such as hydrogen, helium, carbon monoxide, carbon dioxide, oxygen, nitrogen, argon, methane, and other light hydrocarbons. The membranes required for such applications are prepared from high-performance polymers such as polyimide, poly(amide-imide), polyphosphazene, and polysulfone. The separation ability of a membrane is dependent, in particular, on its composition [15–23] and morphology [24,25]. Membranes with controlled morphology can be used both in the separation process and in chemical conversion, supplying highly ordered and confined geometries for chemical reactions [26,27]. Even though such characteristics are continuously studied, reliable data in the field of pore design and preparation are still scarce. The most often investigated and applied methods in the organic–inorganic membrane preparation are sol-gel [28–31], demixing processes [18,32,33], phase inversion (by forming a polymeric ultra-thin layer [13,34–38]), and the dry–wet spinning technique [39–41].

Superior thermal, chemical, and mechanical properties of polysulfones determine a number of advantages in many applications such as filtration membranes [42–46], coatings [47–49] composites [50–52], microelectronic devices [53,54], thin-film technology [55,56], biomaterials [57], and fuel cells [58–61]. However, despite tremendous progress in their synthesis and applications, these materials have some limitations related to stress cracking with certain solvents, poor tracking resistance, and weathering properties. The introduction of functional groups into polysulfones not only overcomes these limitations but also extends the range of potential applications of these high-performance materials through the specific properties gained, and thus provides wider scope.

Therefore, the chemical modification of some polymers with aromatic rings by chloromethylation reaction is one of the most important methods for obtaining polymers with chloromethylene groups, which are precursors in the synthesis of other polymers with desirable functional groups [62]. This is explained by the high reactivity of the $-CH_2Cl$ chloromethyl group linked to the aromatic rings, which gives it the ability to transform into another functional group. Starting polymers can be synthetic or natural. Among the synthetic ones, the most used are polystyrene, aromatic polysulfones, and styrene-divinylbenzene copolymers.

From the considerations mentioned above, polymers from the aromatic polysulfones class—used in the fields of materials science, biology, and polymer science and have been the basis of numerous applications—have imposed themselves on

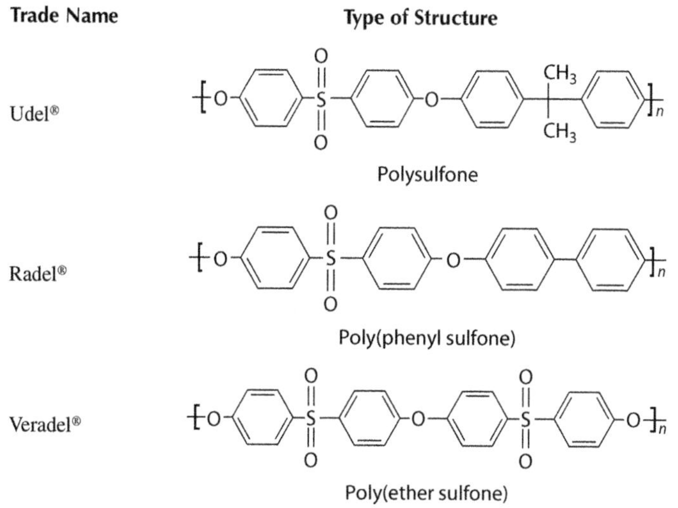

Trade Name   Type of Structure

Udel®

Polysulfone

Radel®

Poly(phenyl sulfone)

Veradel®

Poly(ether sulfone)

FIGURE 2.1 Commercially available polysulfones.

the world market (Figure 2.1). In addition, amorphous thermoplastic polymers are technopolymer materials [63] with high performance, present strong transparence and rigidity, have high glass transition temperatures and good thermal stability, possess high hydrolytic resistance against attack of acid or base, can be easily workable, and have good film-forming properties.

This chapter covers the novel chemical approaches applied for the functionalization of polysulfones. Although many functionalization methods are available, they usually require careful control of reaction conditions. In order to avoid side reactions which lead to backbone degradation, judicious synthesis conditions must be selected. This chapter aims to illustrate the possibilities offered by the chemical modification of aromatic polysulfones.

2.2 POLYSULFONES WITH PENDANT CHLOROMETHYL GROUPS

Polysulfones are produced by polycondensation and are known as membranes with good thermo-oxidation stability and resistance to sudden changes in the pH. Chemical modification by introduction of a chloromethyl group causes a change in the hydrophobic–hydrophilic balance of the macromolecular chain, causing an increase in the membrane permeability.

Polycondensed polysulfone commercialized under the name of Udel® P-3500, the IUPAC name of which is poly[oxy-1,4-phenylsulfonyl-1,4-phenyleneoxy-1,4-phenylene (1-methylethylidene)-1,4-phenylene] aromatic polysulfone, was chloromethylated with a chloromethylation agent—a Lewis-type acid catalyst—and a good solvent for the starting polysulfone, which allowed obtaining a soluble polymer with chloromethylenic groups. Initially, chlorination ethers, such as 1,4-bis(chloromethoxy)butane and 1-chloromethoxi-4-chlorobutane, were used as chloromethylation agents [64]. The reaction was performed at room temperature, using chlorinated hydrocarbons as solvent and stannic tetrachloride ($SnCl_4$) as catalyst. The reaction conditions applied determined the introduction of a single chloromethylene group along the structural unit.

Daly [62] has obtained soluble chloromethylated polysulfone (CMPSF) with two chloromethyl groups along the structural unit, using monochloromethyl methyl ether as the chloromethylation agent. As solvents, most often, alkyl chloride derivatives (chloroform, dichloroethane, trichloroethane, etc.) were used. In their study Daly et al. [63] observed the efficiency of a Lewis-type catalyst in the course of the reaction and established the following descending series: $SnCl_4 > ZnCl_2 > AlCl_3 > TiCl_4 > SnCl_2 > FeCl_3$.

Warshawsky et al. [65,66] have synthesized halomethylated polysulfones (chloromethylation and bromomethylation), using halomethyl octyl ether as the halomethylation agent and stannic tetrahalides as the catalyst.

The major inconvenience of these methods is the high toxicity of chlorinated ethers, an inconvenience that can be avoided by using a mixture of paraformaldehyde with an equimolar amount of trimethylchlorosilane as the halomethylation agent, stannic tetrachloride as the catalyst, and chloroform as the solvent [67–69]. The reaction proceeds as shown in Schemes 2.1 and 2.2.

Under the action of stannic tetrachloride, paraformaldehyde generates active formaldehyde, which reacts with the trimethylchlorosilane forming chloromethyltrimethyl silyl ether with a structure similar to that of monochloromethyl methyl ether. This is the chloromethylation agent and it has the advantage of being formed *in situ*, so that the toxicity of the entire process is greatly reduced and the degradation products are less toxic than those of a conventional chloromethylation agent.

The chloromethylation reaction is an electrophilic substitution at the aromatic rings of bisether of bisfenol, and not the arylsulfonic cycle, which confirms that the disabling aromatic rings are determined by the sulfone group. It is possible that, in the course of the chloromethylation reaction, cross-linking might take place with the formation of methylene linkages between the main macromolecular chains, leading to insoluble CMPSF (Scheme 2.3) [70].

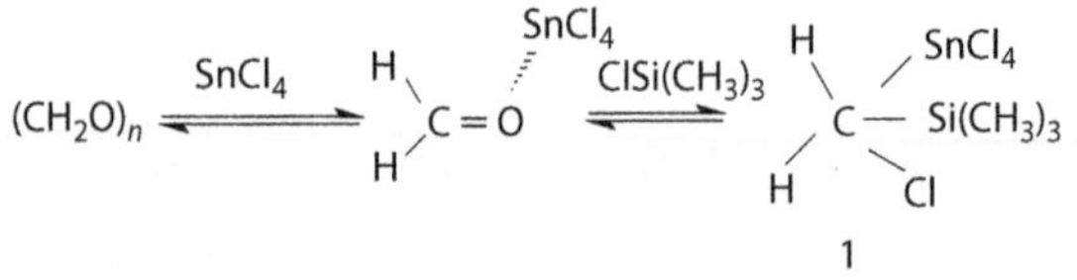

SCHEME 2.1 Training reactive species in the chloromethylation reaction.

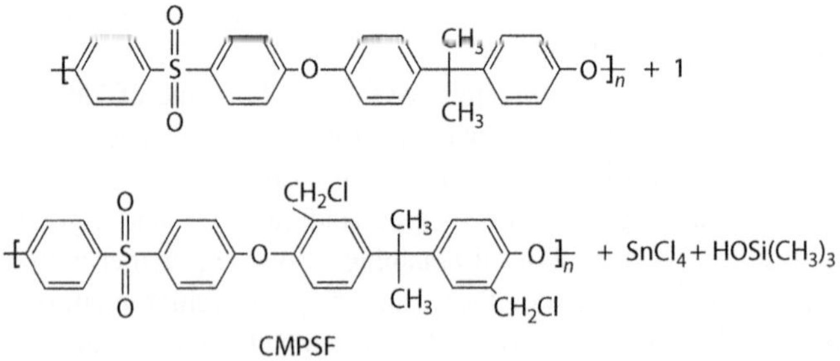

SCHEME 2.2 Chloromethylation reaction of polysulfones.

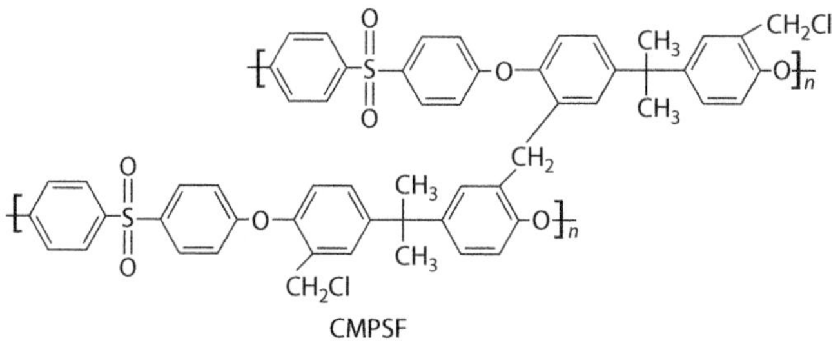

SCHEME 2.3　Training of methylenic bridges during of the chloromethylation reaction.

It has been established that an excess of chloromethylation agent, a molar ratio of 1:20, between the structural unit of polysulfone and monochloromethyl methyl ether and a small amount of catalyst (0.1 mmol $SnCl_4$) prevent the formation of methylene bridges between macromolecular chains [63,68].

The total chlorine content of CMPSFs was determined by the modified Schöninger method [71] and the degree of substitution (DS) was calculated using the following equation:

$$DS = \frac{M_{PSF} \times m_{Cl}}{(M_{Cl} \times 100)\,(M_{CH_2Cl} \times m_{Cl})} \tag{2.1}$$

where:
　M_{PSF} is the molecular weight of the PSF structural unit
　M_{Cl} is the atomic weight of chlorine
　M_{CH_2Cl} is the molecular weight of $-CH_2Cl$ group
　m_{Cl} is chlorine concentration, analytically determined

To prevent secondary reactions, certain working conditions must be respected, as can be observed in Table 2.1.

It has been found that increasing the catalyst amount and the polymer concentration by 5% may favor the cross-linking of CMPSF. Therefore, to obtain soluble CMPSFs with high content of chloromethylene groups, the following conditions are required:

1. An increase in the reaction time (Figure 2.2), as well as a high molar ratio between the structural unit and the chloromethylation agent.
2. Under the same reaction conditions, if a small quantity of catalyst is utilized, a chloromethylated polymer with a DS equal to 1.97 is obtained.

In comparison with the polystyrene chloromethylation conditions, soluble CMPSF can be achieved at a low dilution (less than 2%) of the polymer in chloroform, and using $SnCl_4$ as the catalyst does not favor the formation of the chloromethylene linkages between macromolecular chains, which would lead to insoluble CMPSF [65].

The chloromethylation degree was calculated from the chlorine content of the CMPSF, whereas the number average molecular weight and polydispersity (M_w/M_n) of the CMPSF were determined by gel permeation chromatography with

TABLE 2.1

Conditions of Chloromethylation Reaction, Including Concentration of Polymers in CH₃Cl, Molar Ratio of Polymer Structural Unit: Me₃ClSi:(CH₂O)ₙ, and Reaction Time and Characteristics of Chloromethylated Polysulfones, Including Content of Chlorine and Degree of Substitution

Code	C (%)	Molar ratio	SnCl₄ (mol g⁻¹)	Time (h)	CMPSF Cl (%)	DS	Observations
CMPSF$_R$-1.69	5	1:3:3	0.45	24	11.47	1.69	Cross-linked, white
CMPSF$_R$-1.16	2	1:3:3	0.45	24	8.23	1.16	Cross-linked, white
CMPSF-0.41	2	1:3:3	0.18	5	3.16	0.41	Soluble, white
CMPSF-0.62	2	1:3:3	0.18	15	4.65	0.62	Soluble, white
CMPSF-0.77	2	1:3:3	0.18	28	5.70	0.77	Soluble, white
CMPSF-1.26	2	1:3:3	0.18	80	8.85	1.26	Soluble, white
CMPSF-1.68	2	1:10:10	0.18	1200	11.35	1.68	Soluble, white
CMPSF-1.97	2	1:10:10	0.10	140	12.97	1.97	Soluble, white

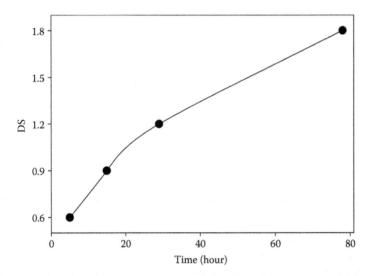

FIGURE 2.2 Influence of the reaction time on the substitution degree of CMPSFs.

a GPC-PL-EMD.950 instrument (Perkin Elmer Diamond, Shelton, CT, USA) from Polymer Laboratories, using standard polystyrene (Table 2.2).

It has been found that, through the chloromethylation reaction, the polydispersity of the resulting polysulfone does not change significantly, as it does in the case of polystyrene chloromethylation [67] (see Table 2.2).

A slight increase in the molecular weight with the DS can be observed; therefore, no chain scission takes place during the substitution reaction. The DS for one structural unit varies from 0.48 to 1.84. Therefore, the obtained CMPSFs have at least

TABLE 2.2

Characteristics[a] of the Studied Chloromethylated Polysulfones

Code	Cl (%)	DS	M_{SU}[b]	$\overline{M}_n$	M_w/M_n
PSF	0.18	0.00	442.00	18,619	2.636
CMPSF-0.48	3.16	0.48	465.27	17,350	2.742
CMPSF-0.49	3.25	0.49	465.93	17,556	2.734
CMPSF-0.87	5.70	0.87	483.97	18,766	2.874
CMPSF-1.25	8.23	1.25	502.60	19,840	2.951
CMPSF-1.74	11.47	1.74	526.46	20,523	2.863
CMPSF-1.84	12.12	1.84	531.95	21,502	2.960

[a] Characteristics include chlorine content, molar substitution degree, molecular weight of structural unit, number molecular weight average, and molecular weight distribution.

[b] Calculated on the basis of chlorine content found in the sample composition.

one $-CH_2Cl$ group per ether sulfone structural unit to approximately two groups per structural unit, and the DS increased with the reaction time. The reaction time was from 5 to 140 hours. For each DS, the samples are denoted as CMPSF-0.48 to CMPSF-1.84. All products were insoluble in water, methyl, ethyl, butyl alcohol, and acetone and totally soluble in chloroform, dichloroethane, N,N-dimethylacetamide, dimethyl-sulfoxide, dioxane, benzene, and N,N-dimethylformamide, even for high DS [72,73].

The introduction of the $-CH_2Cl$ groups has been evidenced in the infrared (IR) spectra by the presence of C—Cl bands at 760 cm^{-1}; $-CH_2Cl$ signal at $d = 4.45$ ppm was recorded in ^{1}H-NMR spectra on a JEOL spectrometer at 80 MHz with CDCl$_3$ as the solvent (Figure 2.3).

Thermogravimetric curves (TG and DTG) were recorded on a Paulik-Paulik-Erdey-type derivatograph MOM, Budapest, under the following conditions: heating rate of 12°C min^{-1}, temperature range of 20°C–600°C, sample weight of 50 mg, in air flow of 30 cm^3 min^{-1} [73].

Several isothermal experiments were also performed at 250°C. The experiments on evolution of volatile products during the degradation (TVA experiments) were performed in a continuously evacuated system under the following conditions: heating rate of 5 min^{-1}, 20°C–500°C temperature range, 0.2 g sample weight, 10^{-3}–10^{-4} torr initial pressure. Gas and liquid products were collected in traps at liquid nitrogen temperature; the *cold* fraction was deposited near the outlet of the oven on the cold wall of the reaction vessel and the residue remained in the sample pan. The gas, liquid, and the cold fraction and residue result as thermal decomposition products. The IR spectra of the polymer samples, cold fraction, and residue resulting from the TVA experiments were recorded on a SpecordM 80 IR spectrometer; the samples were deposited in thin layers onto KBr tablets.

A new thermo-oxidative or thermal decomposition step was observed at low temperatures and became well defined with increasing degrees of substitution. It has been noted that although for the CMPSF with a low DS (DS < 0.5) the decomposition mechanism of the PSF was perturbed or changed, for a higher DS, thermal instability

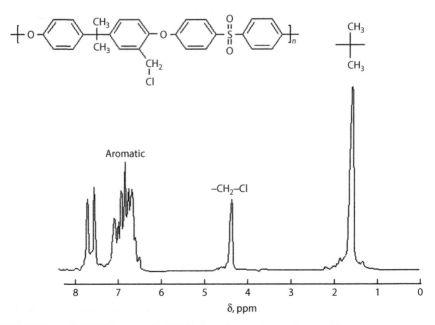

FIGURE 2.3 ^{1}H-NMR spectra in CDCl$_3$ for chloromethylated polysulfones.

occurred and a particular way of degradation developed. The thermal characteristics of this first thermogravimetric step significantly changed when DS > 1.6. For a low DS, the steps occurring from 200°C to 400°C were not very well separated. The variation of the characteristic temperature and weight loss with the DS can be established on the basis of the data presented in Table 2.3.

CMPSFs exhibit a supplementary thermal and thermo-oxidative decomposition step, occurring at low temperatures, in comparison with unmodified PSF. Weight losses, characteristic temperatures, and overall kinetic parameters have a particular variation with an increase in DS. It can be supposed that the particular decomposition step of CMPSFs occurs by both the elimination of functional groups and a cross-linking reaction.

2.3 POLYSULFONES WITH PENDANT QUATERNARY AMMONIUM GROUPS

2.3.1 QUATERNIZATION REACTION OF CMPSFs WITH ALIPHATIC TERTIARY AMINES

Recently, it has been reported that quaternary ammonium-functionalized polysulfones have been used as membranes with novel properties. In this context, in order to extend the study on the quaternization reaction of CMPSFs and to obtain polymers with possible applications as disinfectant agents, the reactions of the above-mentioned polymers with tertiary amines—which, besides the two methyl substituents at tertiary nitrogen atom, contain an alkyl substituent with a number of two, C$_2$, four, C$_4$, or eight, C$_8$, carbon atoms—were investigated. The quaternization reactions

TABLE 2.3

Thermogravimetric Data for Polysulfone and Chloromethylated Polysulfones

Code	Temperature Range 250–340°C					Temperature Range 340–440°C				Temperature Range 440–550°C				$W_{450°C}$	Δw (%) (I + II)	CH_2Cl (%)
	T_i	$T_{5\%}$	T_m	T_f	Δw	T_i	T_m	T_f	Δw	T_i	T_m	T_f	Δw			
PSF	–	–	–	–	–	–	–	–	–	403	518	554	51	1	–	–
CMPSF-0.49	–	–	–	–	–	362	451	471	28.0	471	506	537	42.5	18.5	28	5.21
CMPSF-0.87	267	276	308	329	7.6	329	412	437	34.4	–	–	–	–	51.4	42.0	8.89
CMPSF-1.25	279	306	336	367	19.6	367	–	432	24.6	–	–	–	–	54.5	44.2	12.31
CMPSF-1.74	280	293	329	346	15.2	346	361	379	11.3	–	–	–	–	60	26.5	16.36
CMPSF-1.84	237	264	322	343	8.3	343	422	448	18.3	–	–	–	–	24	26.6	17.14

Notes: T_i, $T_{5\%}$, T_m, and T_f (°C) are temperatures corresponding to those initial, onset 5% weight loss, to the maximum rate of weight loss, and the end of the process, respectively; Δw (%) percentage of weight loss; $W_{450°C}$ is weight loss at 450°C; Δw (%) I + II is the weight loss corresponding to the two decomposition steps occurring in 250°C–440°C temperature range; CH_2Cl (%) represents percentage of CH_2Cl groups in the structural unit of the chloromethylated polysulfones.

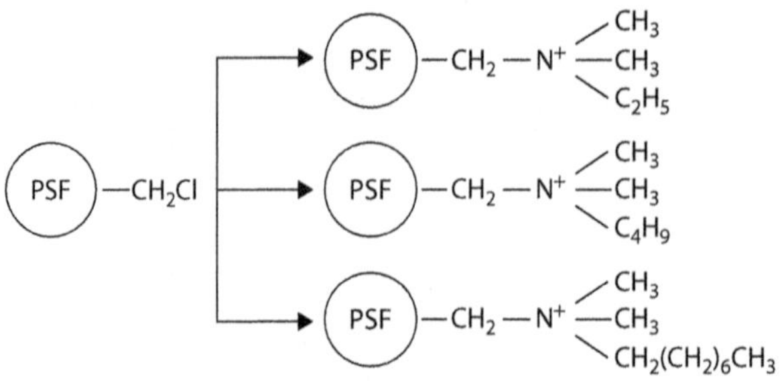

SCHEME 2.4 The reaction of chloromethylated polysulfone with N,N-dimethyl alkylamine.

for obtaining polysulfones functionalized with N,N-dimethylethylamine (P1), N,N-dimethylbutylamine (P2), and N,N-dimethyloctylamine (P3) were carried out as shown in Scheme 2.4.

2.3.1.1 Reaction Conditions and Factors Influencing the Quaternization of CMPSFs with N,N-Dimethyl Alkylamine

The objective of the research on the synthesis of quaternary polymers P1–P3 has been to obtain polymers with a larger number of quaternary ammonium groups on the polysulfone backbone [74–77]. The literature indicates that the starting polymer used is CMPSF, with a chlorine content of 23.70% [74]. It is known that the reaction between a tertiary amine and a halogenated derivative is a bimolecular nucleophilic substitution (SN2) and the reaction rate increases in parallel and not proportionally with the solvent dielectric constant, ε. Therefore, N,N-dimethylformamide, which is an aprotic polar solvent with the dielectric constant, $\varepsilon = 36.7$, at 25°C was selected as the reaction medium. The polymer concentration in DMF was of 10%, N,N-dimethylformamide being a good solvent for a starting polymer and a quaternary polymer [78–80].

In the present research, the CMPSF concentration in DMF was maintained constant, to investigate the influence of temperature and of the chloromethylated structural unit:amine molar ratio on the molar transformation degree, β. Occasionally, samples (2 mL) were taken for determining the chlorine content by potentiometric titration with 0.02 N AgNO$_3$ aqueous solutions, using an automatic TitraLab® Radimeter 840 (Copenhagen, Denmark). Chlorine ions were formed after the reaction of CMPSF with N,N-dimethyl alkylamine (Scheme 2.4), when the chlorine bound covalently turned into chlorine ions and quantitatively represents the degree of transformation, β, which is calculated using Equation 2.2

$$\beta = \frac{x}{b}100 \qquad (2.2)$$

where:

x represents the ionic chlorine concentration (Cl$^-$, mol L^{-1}), determined analytically at time t

b is the initial concentration of chlorine from the reaction mixture, expressed in mol L^{-1}

TABLE 2.4

Comparative Data on Transformation Molar Degree as a Function of the Reaction Temperature for Quaternized Polysulfones (P1–P3), in DMF at CMPSF: *N*,*N*′-Dimethyl Alkylamine Molar Ratio of 1:2

	Transformation Molar Degree, β (%)								
	Quaternization Temperature								
Reaction	30°C			40°C			50°C		
Time (min)	DMEA	DMBA	DMOA	DMEA	DMBA	DMOA	DMEA	DMBA	DMOA
15	14.86	14.39	14.13	24.62	23.15	22.74	43.16	39.40	37.10
30	31.72	29.00	26.27	45.70	44.50	44.36	64.18	53.85	59.45
45	39.45	38.40	37.00	61.56	60.15	59.23	76.40	76.19	70.90
60	45.59	45.34	46.78	63.40	65.68	63.91	83.50	82.75	80.60
75	54.44	53.54	53.29	73.87	72.62	69.36	89.90	90.26	88.72
90	59.20	57.42	55.45	78.08	77.25	76.00	98.13	97.20	96.78

From the comparative analysis of the data presented in Table 2.4, it can be concluded that, for every amine, an increase in temperature determines an increase in the conversion molar degree for the same reaction time.

It has been observed that for a molar ratio of chloromethyl structural unit:tertiary amine of 1:2, after 90 min at 50°C temperature, the molar conversion degree exceeds 95%, regardless of the nature of the amine, whereas at 30°C, it records values between 55% and 62% [71–75].

Regardless of temperature, for the quaternization of the CMPSF with those three amines, the molar conversion degrees have similar values, which leads to the conclusion that the size of the alkyl chain, with a number of carbon atoms C_2, C_4, and C_8, does not influence spectacularly the reactivity of *N*,*N*-dimethyl alkylamine.

Figure 2.4 illustrates the manner in which the chloromethylated structural unit: *N*,*N*-dimethyl alkylamine molar ratio influences the transformation degree. Results indicate that the optimal ratio of quaternization is 1:3; at lower molar ratios, of 1:1 or 1:2, after 90 min, the molar conversion degree is relatively low, between 65% and 80%, whereas at higher ratios, of 1:6 or 1:10, the value of β is slightly increased, which does not justify the high consumption of amine.

2.3.1.2 Chemical and Physical Characterization of Polysulfones with *N*,*N*-Dimethyl Alkylamine

For a more complete analysis of the P1–P3 polymers and for confirming the results attained previously, these polymers were synthesized under the optimal conditions, removed from the reaction medium by precipitation in ethylic ether, and dried in vacuum at room temperature. Then, they were purified by dissolution in methanol and by reprecipitation in ethylic ether—the operation was performed twice. Finally, the polymers with quaternary ammonium groups were dried under vacuum over P_2O_5, and the ionic chlorine, Cl_i, and nitrogen contents were determined analytically (Table 2.5).

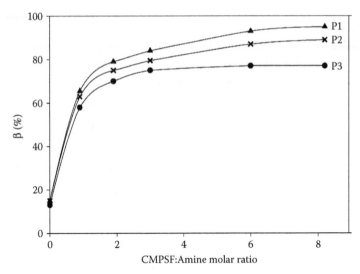

FIGURE 2.4 Influence of CMPSF:*N,N*-dimethyl alkylamine molar ratio on quaterniza-tion degree, β, for: (▲) P1 (CMPSF + DMEA); (×) P2 (CMPSF + DMBA); and (●) P3 (CMPSF + DMOA). Reaction occurs in DMF, at 40°C for 8 hours.

TABLE 2.5
Chemical Composition of P1–P3 Polysulfones

Polymer	Chlorine Content (%)		Nitrogen Content (%)		DS[a] (%)
	Calculated	Found	Calculated	Found	
P1	7.74	7.98	2.95	2.86	98.39
P2	7.05	7.44	2.78	2.66	95.91
P3	6.35	6.83	2.50	2.23	89.39

[a] Degree of substitution calculated as a function of nitrogen content.

The following reaction conditions were applied:

- CMPSF obtained from Udel® P-3500 polysulfone with a chlorine content of 23.70%
- DMF as reaction medium, a polymer concentration in solvent of 10%, a chloromethylene structural unit:*N,N*-dimethyl alkylamine molar ratio of 1:3, a temperature of 50°C, and a reaction time of 8 hours

The obtained polysulfones with quaternary ammonium groups were presented in the form of white powder, with solubility values displayed in Table 2.6 [81,82].

It is noteworthy that these polymers have a different solubility from that of other quaternary polymers, because they are insoluble in water at room temperature and soluble in some halogenated derivatives, which can be explained by the strong

TABLE 2.6
Quaternized Polysulfones Solubility at Ambient Temperature

Number	Solvent	Solubility[a]	Nr	Solvent/Mixed Solvents	Solubility[a]
1	Water	+	10	Dioxane	−
2	Methyl alcohol	+	11	Dioxane:DMF (1:1,v/v)	±
3	Ethyl alcohol	+	12	Dioxane:DMF (2:1, v/v)	−
4	Butyl alcohol	+	13	Benzene	−
5	Acetone	−	14	Dichloromethane	+
6	Methyl ethyl cetone	−	15	Chloroform	+
7	N,N-dimethylformamide (DMF)	+	16	Carbon tetrachloride	−
8	N,N-dimethylacetamide (DMAc)	+	17	Dichloroethane	−
9	Dimethyl sulfoxide (DMSO)	±	18	Tetrachloroethane	+

[a] +, slightly soluble; ±, hardly soluble (but soluble over 30°C); −, insoluble.

hydrophobic character of the polysulfone chain compared to the hydrophilic one of quaternary ammonium groups [83,84].

Figure 2.5 presents the viscometric behavior of polysulfone solutions with quaternary ammonium groups, P1–P3, in methanol. As can be observed from Figure 2.5, P1–P3 show an increase of the reduced viscosity, η_{sp}/c, with the decrease in polymer concentration—a behavior typical of polyelectrolytes. The curves reflect the expansion of the macromolecular coil, as a result of the electrostatic repulsion between charges of the same type [85].

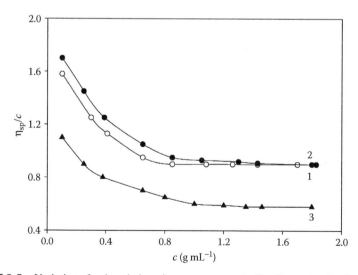

FIGURE 2.5 Variation of reduced viscosity versus concentration for quaternized polymers: (○) (CMPSF + DMEA)—1; (●) (CMPSF + DMBA)—2; and (▲) (CMPSF + DMOA)—3, at 25°C.

2.3.2 Polysulfones with Viologen Pendant Groups

The compounds from the bipyridyl class have attracted wide attention due to their interesting structure susceptible of numerous applications in various fields. A special class of compounds consists in the N-monosubstituted salts of 4,4'-bipyridyl and its derivatives, including a wide range of products, starting from low-molecular complexes with different metals to macromolecular compounds. This variety of bipyridyl compounds has known to be a real development, due to their exceptional electrochromism properties, which allowed them to be used as the main component in the rendering process of the electrochromic memory and as semiconductor electrodes. Some of them present interest in the study of nonconventional energy as electron transfer agents in systems designed for the achievement of water photolysis using solar energy or other types of irradiation. They are used as polymerization catalysts and curing agents for various resins. The applicability domain is not limited to such uses; the bipyridyl compounds also represent a subject on the biological field [86–91].

Owing to its structure, the 4,4'-bipyridyl [92–96] forms mono or diquaternary ammonium chloride salts (Scheme 2.5) with different substituents on the nitrogen atoms. Initially, these were called *viologen*, because under the influence of external factors (humidity, UV rays, electric field, etc.) they change their color, becoming violet.

Viologen compounds have attracted researchers' attention, and are used for electron transport, as redox catalysts, and in xerography. Besides the diquaternary ammonium salts of 4,4'-bipyridyl, monoquaternary ammonium salts are important [12,13]. The 4,4'-bipyridinium compounds represent a complex part in the field of heterocyclic compounds chemistry, and new chemical reactions thereof are being discovered. Their ability to participate at the 1,3-dipolar cycloaddition reactions proved to be of great interest [97–101] not only theoretically but also from the synthesis viewpoint of a number of heterocyclic compounds with nitrogen, which is difficult to achieve by other synthetic methods. The wide variety of bipyridinium salts is important in polymer chemistry, as well as those of complex compounds which present the electron donor character. The polymers incorporating viologen units have properties that make possible their use for obtaining light/electric field-sensitive materials, as redox polymers or polymers with antimicrobial and herbicidal activities [102]. Polymers with pendant viologen groups can be synthesized either by monomer polymerization [103–107] or by polymer-analogous reactions [108–110], the latter being more accessible, cheaper, and, therefore, widely used at the moment.

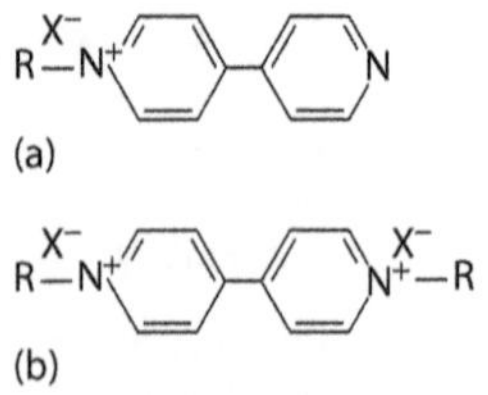

(a)

(b)

SCHEME 2.5   Structures of (a) mono and (b) diquaternary 4,4'-bipyridinium salts.

2.3.2.1   Synthesis of Polysulfones with Pendant Viologen Groups by Polymer-Analogous Reactions

Polymer-analogous reactions are a common method for obtaining polymers with pendant functional groups, being in fact an application of the reactions from organic chemistry to macromolecular chains. The method consists of introducing pendant functional groups onto the polymer main chain and has the advantage that it is not conditioned by the synthesis of a particular monomer. Such a functionalized polymer acts chemically similar to low-molecular-weight analogous compounds [111]. Therefore, the chemical reactions on polymers involve the following:

- The existence of a linear or branched polymer, with or without functional groups P-F, which can be converted by a chemical reaction into a polymer with other functional groups P–F
- The presence of a low-molecular-weight reactant, which will react with the functional group F—linked to the polymer—leading to another functional group F
- A solvent—in the case of linear polymers or a reaction medium—for cross-linked polymers

As regards the chemical reactions of linear polymers [112], the initial polymer is like a macromolecular chain, coiled as a bundle, which in the presence of the solvent may or may not alter its conformation. The solvent has an important role in the chemical modification of polymers, because it may cause the expansion or compression of a macromolecular coil. When a solvent is good thermodynamically, it makes the polymer expand the main macromolecular chain and thus, the small-molecule compound can become accessible to functional groups on the whole macromolecular chain, the reaction occurring with high speed [36]. If a poor solvent is used, the macromolecular coil remains compact, so that the access of the small-molecule compound to the functional groups is limited and, therefore, the reaction rate is low. Newly formed functional groups are found on the macromolecular chain in the most accessible place, but are not evenly distributed, as would be in the case of the polymerization or copolymerization of monomers with functional groups.

2.3.2.2   Quaternization Reaction of CMPSF with 4,4′-Bipyridyl and Its N-Monoquaternary Salts

Literature [92,93] reflects the intense interest in investigating viologen polymers obtained through the nucleophilic substitution reaction (SN2) of CMPSF with 4,4′-bipyridyl and N-monoquaternary salts of 4,4′-bipyridyl. Polysulfone membranes are known to have good thermo-oxidative stability, high flexibility, and good resistance to sudden pH changes. Also, the chemical modification of polysulfones, such as chlorometylation, sulfonation, or quaternization, leads to functionalized membranes to be used as resins, ion exchange fibers, or films with selective permeability.

Low-molecular viologen polymers have been reported to have interesting electrochemical properties. With a view to cumulating the properties of polysulfones with those of viologen compounds, the quaternization of CMPSFs with 4,4′-bipyridyl and their N-monoquaternary derivatives (Table 2.7) has been considered, synthesizing polysulfones with viologen groups in the side chain (Scheme 2.6).

In the research carried out by Druta et al., CMPSF with chlorine content of 8.78% was used for the reactions, which corresponds to a molar DS with $-CH_2Cl$ groups of 1.34, using N,N-dimethylformamide as the reaction medium [113].

The quaternization molar degree was determined by potentiometric titration of Cl^- ions with an aqueous solution of 0.02 N AgNO$_3$ and was calculated using Equation 2.2. Chlorine ions were formed from the reaction between chloromethylene groups of CMPSF and tertiary nitrogen of 4,4'-bipyridyl or its derivatives. Figure 2.6 illustrates the influence of temperature on the molar degree of the transformation of CMPSF with 4,4'-bipyridyl.

In this sense, the polymer concentration in the solvent was 5%, and the chloromethylated structural unit:4,4'-bipyridyl molar ratio 1:5. Considering that 4,4'-bipyridyl is a bifunctional compound, a high excess of bipyridyl was necessary to prevent the intrachain cross-linking reaction.

It was observed that at a reaction temperature of 85°C, after 180 min, the degree of conversion was 0.88, compared with 0.41, 0.50, and 0.73 when the reaction temperatures were 70°C, 75°C, and 80°C, respectively.

Analyzing the influence of temperature on β, for the reaction of CMPSF with N-benzyl-4,4'-bipyridinium chloride (Figure 2.7), it was found that after 14 hours at 85°C, β was 0.58, compared with 0.36 at 75°C. N,N-Dimethylformamide was used as the solvent and the chloromethylated structural unit:Bpy-CB molar ratio was 1:1.2. As a result of the transquaternization reaction, which occurred both on CMPSFs and chloromethylated polystyrene, a weak cross-linked product was obtained [114].

The IR spectrum of PSF-bipyridynium-chloride (PSF-Bpy-CB) benzene reveals a band characteristic of pirydinium quaternary nitrogen at a wavelength of 1640 cm^{-1}. Also, the band at 1240 cm^{-1}, assigned to the $-CH_2Cl$ group, linked to an aromatic ring, is significantly reduced. This proves that the obtained polymer has bipyridinium quaternary chloride groups, as well as unreacted chloromethylene groups.

In addition, for the reaction of CMPSF with 4,4'-bipyridyl, N-benzyl-4,4'-bipyridinium chloride, and N-propyl-4,4'-bipyridinium chloride (PSF-Bpy-CP), the effect of reaction time on the conversion molar degree was observed. The reactions occurred in N,N-dimethylformamide at a temperature of 85°C, using a chloromethylated structural unit:low-molecular-compound molar ratio of 1:2. After analyzing the experimental data, it was found that the tertiary nitrogen of 4,4'-bipyridyl was more reactive than the tertiary nitrogen of monoquaternary bipyridinium chloride. Thus, after 2 hours, the conversion molar degree of PSF-4,4'-bipyridyl was 0.72, compared with 0.10 and 0.18 for PSF-Bpy-CB and PSF-Bpy-CP, respectively. Also, the reactivity of the tertiary nitrogen of the two different monoquaternary salts was different.

Consequently, in the reaction of CMPSF with N-propyl-4,4'-bipyridinium chloride and N-benzyl-4,4'-bipyridinium chloride, after 4 hours, quaternized polysulfones with conversion molar degrees of 0.28 and 0.20, respectively, were obtained. This was possible due to the nucleophilicity of the tertiary nitrogen ($>N-$) from the monoquaternary compounds, which increases with the increase of inductive effect

TABLE 2.7

Characteristics of Monoquaternary Derivatives of 4,4′-Bipyridyl

R	X−	IR(KBr) (cm⁻¹)	¹H-NMR (δ-ppm)	Elemental Analysis[a]		
				C (%)	H (%)	N (%)	Cl (%)
$CH_2-C_6H_5$	Cl	3050 ($v_{CH,aromatic}$) 2800–3000 (v_{CH2}) 1640 ($v_C=C; v_C=N$)	D_2O (s; 2H; CH_2-) 5.9 (s; 5H; C_6H_5) 7.6 (m; 8H; $C_5H_4N^+$; C_5H_4N) 7.9–9.3	72.23/72.15	5.31/5.03	9.91/9.69	12.55/2.27
$CH_2-CH_2-CH_3$	Cl	3030 ($v_{C-H,aromatic}$) 2880–2970 (v_{alchil}) 1650 ($v_C=C; v_C=N$)	D_2O (>N⁺; $-CH_2$) 4.7 (t; 3H; CH_3) 1.1 (m; 2H; $-CH_2CH_3$) 2.2 (m; 8H; NC_6H_4) 7.7–9.3	66.54/66.34	6.40/6.12	11.94/11.57	15.12/14.94

[a] Represent values calculated/found.

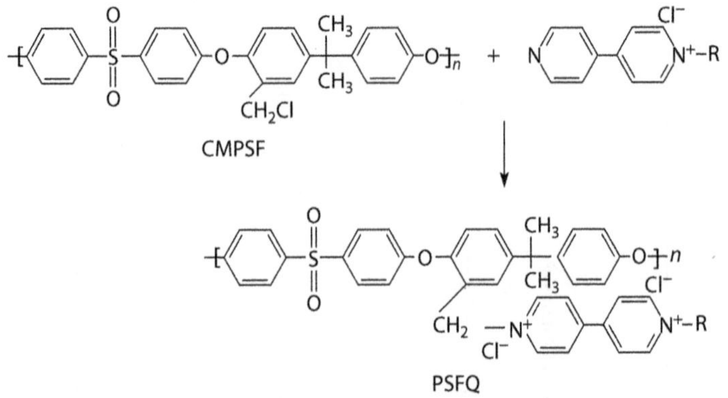

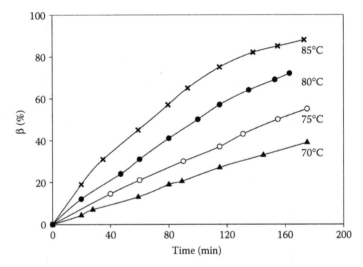

SCHEME 2.6 Synthesis of polysulfones with bipyridinium pendant groups.

FIGURE 2.6 Variation of the transformation molar degree versus reaction time for chloro-methylated polysulfones with 4,4'-bipyridyl, in molar ratio of 1:5 at different temperatures.

(+I) of the substituent from the quaternary nitrogen. Thus, the inductive effect of the alkyl radical (+I) is higher than that of the aryl–alkyl radical.

2.3.2.3 Kinetic Behavior of the Reaction between CMPSF with 4,4'-Bipyridyl and N-Benzyl-4,4'-Bipyridinium Chloride

The formation of a transition state in a bimolecular nucleophilic substitution is favored by a more polar solvent, which dissolves the developed charge. In particular, for the quaternization reaction of a compound model of polysulfone (Scheme 2.7) with a tertiary amine in dimethyl sulfoxide (DMSO), the kinetic behavior is represented by a line passing through the origin, as shown in Figure 2.8 [41].

In the kinetic study of the reaction between CMPSF and 4,4'-bipyridyl, a molar ratio of 1:5 was used, so that the excess amine prevented the cross-linking reaction

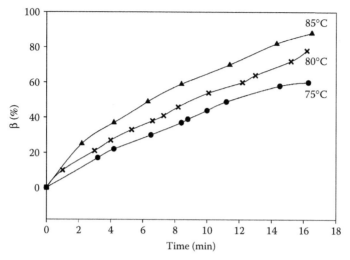

FIGURE 2.7 Variation of the transformation molar degree versus reaction time for chloromethylated polysulfones with 4,4′-Bpy-CB, in molar ratio of 1:2 at different temperatures.

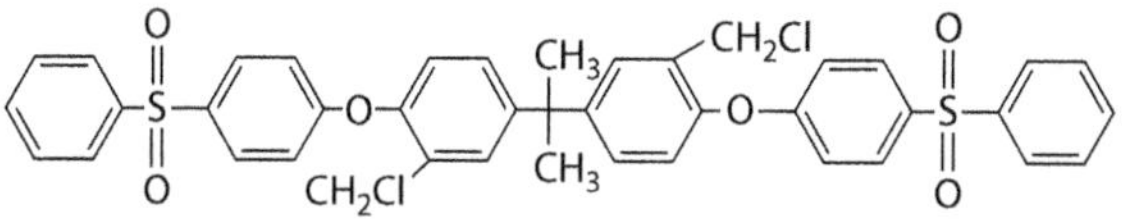

SCHEME 2.7 The compound model of polysulfone.

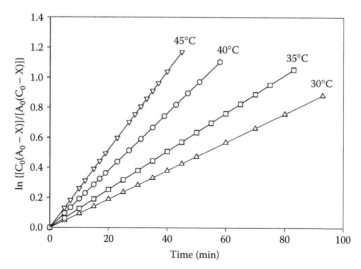

FIGURE 2.8 Kinetic representation of the quaternization reaction of model compound of the polysulfone with N,N-dimethyl-2-hydroxyethylamine in DMSO at different temperatures.

of the quaternized polymer. Figures 2.9 and 2.10 present the kinetic behavior of the reaction between CMPSF with 4,4′-bipyridyl and N-benzyl-4,4′-bipyridinium chloride, in DMSO. It can be seen from Figure 2.9 that the reaction of the CMPSF with 4,4′-bipyridyl in DMSO is characterized by a slight self-break, which appears at a conversion degree of $\beta = 15\%$, whereas the quaternization of CMPSF with N-benzyl-4,4′-bipyridyl in DMSO occurs with a sensitive self-acceleration at $\beta = 12\%$ (Figure 2.10).

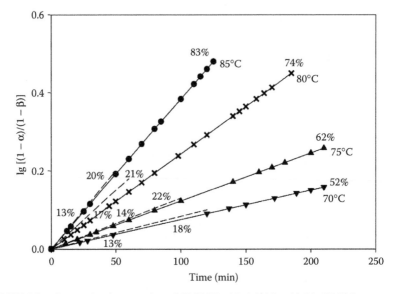

FIGURE 2.9 Quaternization reaction of CMPSF with 4,4′-bipyridyl in DMSO.

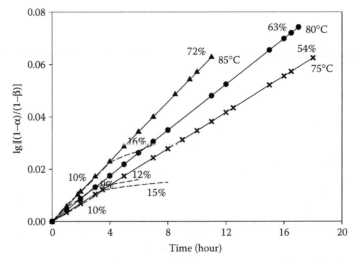

FIGURE 2.10 Quaternization reaction of CMPSF with N-benzyl-4,4′-bipyridinium chloride in DMSO.

TABLE 2.8
Kinetic Parameters of the Quaternization Reaction of CMPSFs

Nr.	Solvent	T (°C)	a (mol L^{-1})	b (mol L^{-1})	a/b	$k_1 \times 10^3$ (L mol^{-1} s^{-1})	$k_2 \times 10^3$ (L mol^{-1} s^{-1})	k_1/k_2
			Quaternization with 4,4′-bipyridyl					
1	DMSO	70	0.07429	0.01486	5.00	0.474	0.451	0.96
2	DMSO	75	0.07429	0.01486	5.00	0.783	0.728	0.93
3	DMSO	80	0.07429	0.01486	5.00	2.071	1.960	0.94
4	DMSO	85	0.07429	0.01486	5.00	2.650	2.552	0.96
			Quaternization with N-benzyl-4,4′-bipyridinium					
1	DMSO	75	0.06965	0.01393	5.00	0.293	0.854	2.91
2	DMSO	80	0.06965	0.01393	5.00	0.535	1.461	2.73
3	DMSO	85	0.06965	0.01393	5.00	0.863	2.071	2.40

The kinetic conditions, rate constants, k_1 and k_2, calculated using Equations 2.3 and 2.4, as well as the k_2/k_1 ratio values—which represent the kinetic behavior of the quaternization reaction of CMPSF with 4,4′-bipyridyl and N-benzyl-4,4′-bipyridinium chloride—are listed in Table 2.8.

$$k = \frac{1}{(a-b)t} \ln \frac{b(a-x)}{a(b-x)} = \frac{2.303}{(a-b)t} \log \frac{1-\alpha}{1-\beta} \tag{2.3}$$

where:

$\alpha = x/a$ represents the molar ratio of reacted amine at time t

b represents the molar ratio of CMPSF at time t

$$k = \frac{2.303}{(a-b)(t-\tau)} \left(\log \frac{1-\alpha}{1-\beta} - \log \frac{1-\lambda/a}{1-\lambda/b} \right) \tag{2.4}$$

where:

τ represents the time at the intersection of lines, expressed in seconds

λ represents the chloride ions concentration, Cl$^-$ (mol L^{-1}) at time τ

The activation energy values, E_a, and frequency factors, A, for the quaternization reactions are calculated according to the Arrhenius equation (Equation 2.5), using experimental data (see Table 2.9).

$$k = A \exp - \left(\frac{E_a}{RT} \right) \tag{2.5}$$

where:

k is the constant rate

R is the gas constant

T is the absolute temperature

TABLE 2.9

Values of Activation Energy (kcal mol⁻¹) and Frequency Factor (L mol⁻¹s⁻¹) for Quaternization Reaction of CMPSFs

Tertiary Amine	E_a	Log A
4,4'-bipyridyl	(k_1) 18.82	11.59
	(k_2) 17.89	12.18
N-benzyl-4,4'-bipyridinium chloride	(k_1) 16.65	10.39
	(k_2) 12.12	9.30

The values of k are given by the relation

$$k = \log A - \left(\frac{E_a}{2.303RT} \right) \tag{2.6}$$

The activation energy is determined from the slope of the line obtained by the log k versus $1/T$ plot and is calculated using Equation 2.7.

$$tg\alpha = \frac{E_a}{2.303R} \tag{2.7}$$

The kinetic behavior of the reaction between CMPSF and the compounds mentioned above depends on the activation energy value, which is confirmed by the values listed in Table 2.9. Thus, the quaternization of CMPSF with 4,4'-bipyridyl has activation energy values very close to those of the two-stage reaction, characterized by constants k_1 and k_2. The reaction with N-benzyl-4,4'-biprydinium has activation energy values slightly lower for the second stage of the reaction, which occurs at $\beta = 12\%$.

After the kinetic study of the quaternization reactions of CMPSF with tertiary amine, the following may be concluded:

- The quaternization of compound models of polysulfone with chloromethylene groups follows normal second-order kinetics, represented by a straight line passing through the origin, regardless of the solvent nature.
- The quaternization of CMPSF follows second-order kinetics, which reveals the self-acceleration phenomenon, occurring at certain values of β.
- It is believed that the major factor influencing the kinetic behavior of the polymer quaternization reaction is the polymer–solvent interaction—which is subjected to changes in the course of the reaction—leading to the conformational modification of the macromolecular chain of the newly formed quaternary polymer, as well as to different solvation of the polymer chain, which can be favorable or unfavorable to the reaction rate [115,116].

Changing of the macromolecular chain conformation is described below. Thus, the initial polymer is a statistical coil, more or less expanded, depending on its interaction with the solvent. If through the introduction of quaternary ammonium groups, the solvent becomes *good* for the obtained polymer, the macromolecular chain extends and the reactant's access to the small-molecular functional groups ($-CH_2Cl$) can normally proceed at the beginning of the reaction, or steric hindrance can occur because of the quaternary groups already established on the chain. It is justified that they should occur at values of $\beta \approx 50\%$, when statistically, unreacted structural units are in the vicinity of the already-reacted structural units. When the solvent becomes *poor* for the formed polymer (i.e., quaternary polymer), the macromolecular coil is shrinked, whereas for the flexible polymer, a separation of functional groups appears. Quaternary ammonium groups are oriented within the chain, and the initial ones ($-CH_2Cl$ or amine) are oriented to the outside of the macromolecular chain, making easier the access of a low-molecular reactant to them and causing the self-acceleration phenomenon. As in the case of CMPSF, which is a rigid polymer, both self-accelerating and self-breaking phenomena occur, this leads to the idea that the *solvent cage* created around the obtained quaternary ammonium polymer has an important role in the kinetic behavior of the quaternization reactions of macromolecular compounds.

2.3.3 SYNTHESIS AND CHARACTERIZATION OF PHOSPHORUS-CONTAINING POLYSULFONE

The chemical modification of the reactive groups present on the polymers is a useful way to prepare new polymers with specialized functional groups for various applications [117]. This modification can be easily achieved by the reaction of simple chemicals with a reactive pendant group, such as vinyl, carbonyl, oxiirane, and halomethyl, present on the polymer. Among these reactive groups, the chloromethyl group is especially useful, as it can be readily modified by a substitution reaction with various nucleophilic reactants. Therefore, polymers with chloromethyl pendant groups are often used as starting materials for obtaining new functional polymers, such as amino, azomethyne, siloxane, or carboxylic groups [68,118–120]. By grafting poly(ethylene glycol) on CMPSF, a hydrophilic but water insoluble membrane can be obtained with enhanced porosity and resistance to protein absorption [121–123]. A PSF modified with different phosphorus compounds could be blended with a bisphenol A-based epoxy resin to obtain a material with improved toughness and glass transition temperature, as well as flame retardancy of the thermosetting resin [124]. Wu et al. [125] synthesized and modified poly(epichlorohydrine) to be used for preparing flame-retardant polyurethanes.

In this context, phosphorus-modified polysulfone (PSF-DOPO) was prepared by the reaction of CMPSF with 9,10-dihydro-oxa-10-phosphophenanthrene-10-oxide, as shown in Scheme 2.8 [126].

The substitution of chlorine with the bulky cyclic phosphorus compound was carried out at elevated temperature using a large excess of phosphorus reactant. The reactive P-H group interacted with $-CH_2Cl$ group of CMPSF. The occurrence of HCl evolved from the reaction proved the substitution and could also offer kinetic data about the process. HCl was capped and analytically measured versus time in

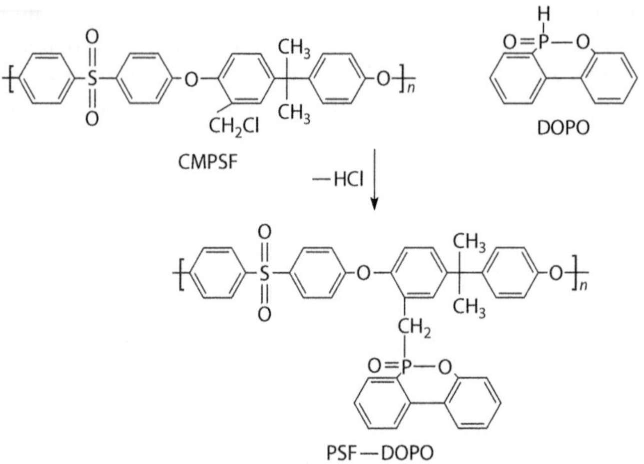

SCHEME 2.8 The reaction of chloromethylated polysulfone with 9,10-dihydro-oxa-10-phosphophenanthrene-10-oxide.

TABLE 2.10
Reaction-Rate Constants for Phosphorus-Modified Polysulfones with Different Substitution Degrees

Sample	DS	k (L mol^{-1}min^{-1})
PSF-DOPO-0.62	0.62	3.02
PSF-DOPO-0.74	0.74	3.10
PSF-DOPO-1.30	1.30	3.60

this reaction using CMPSF with different DS. Table 2.10 presents the reaction-rate constants obtained at 170°C for phosphorus-modified polysulfone with different DS. One can observe that the substitution of the chloromethylated group is enhanced when a greater number of groups are present.

The structure of a phosphorus-modified polysulfone (e.g., PSF-DOPO, Scheme 2.8) was identified by Fourier transform infrared (FTIR) spectroscopy and ^{1}H-^{13}C NMR spectroscopy. Figure 2.11a presents the FTIR spectra of PSF-DOPO in comparison with those of the phosphorus compound in the 4000–2000 cm^{-1} range. Of note is the disappearance of the absorption band for P–H at 2436 cm^{-1} in the phosphorus-modified PSF spectrum. Figure 2.11b presents the FTIR spectra of PSF-DOPO in comparison with those of CMPSF in the range 1700–600 cm^{-1}. Some difficulties in appreciating these spectra reside in the superposition of the absorption bands in the 1000–1300 cm^{-1} range. However, it is evident that the absorption bands assigned to C—Cl group at 691 and 716 cm^{-1} were replaced with a strong absorption band specific to aliphatic–phosphorus group, placed at 907.5 cm^{-1}. The absorption band in the range 1296–1241 cm^{-1} was larger

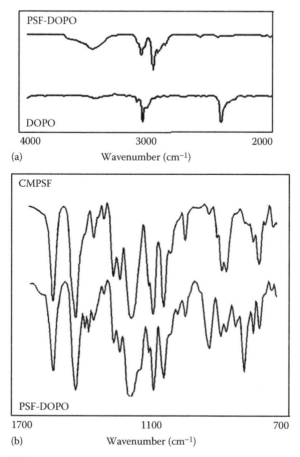

FIGURE 2.11 FTIR spectra for: (a) PSF-DOPO and DOPO in 4000–2000 cm^{-1} range and (b) PSF-DOPO and CMPSF in the range 1700–600 cm^{-1}.

for PSF-DOPO than that for CMPSF, suggesting a superposition of P=O and P—O—Ar stretching, respectively.

Furthermore, the success in substituting the chlorine from —CH$_2$Cl group with DOPO was demonstrated by ^{1}H-^{13}C NMR analysis. The characteristic peaks associated to the protons of —CH$_2$Cl group situated at 4.64 ppm in the CMPSF spectrum disappeared in the PSF-DOPO spectrum. The characteristic peak associated to the protons of —CH$_2$DOPO group was shifted to 3.5 ppm. Phosphorus-modified polysulfones were soluble in the same polar solvents as CMPSF, according to Table 2.11.

The solubility decreases with the increase of the DS. The inherent viscosity of phosphorus-modified polysulfone ranged between 0.44 and 0.47 dL g^{-1} (Table 2.12).

The values were lower than those of CMPSF with a similar DS, due to the presence of DOPO groups in the structure of phosphorus-modified polysulfone, which determined steric hindrance and did not allow a strong packing of the macromolecular chains.

TABLE 2.11

Solubility of CMPSF and Phosphorus-Modified Polysulfones with Different Substitution Degrees

Polymer	NMP	DMAc	DMF	CHCl$_3$	Dioxane	Acetone	Methyl Alcohol	Toluene
CMPSF	+	+	+	+	+	−	−	−
PSF-DOPO-0.62	+	+	+	+	+	−	−	−
PSF-DOPO-0.74	+	±	+	+	±	−	−	−
PSF-DOPO-1.30	+	−	+	±	±	−	−	−

DMAc, dimethylacetamide; DMF, N,N-methylformamide; NMP, N-methylpyrrolidone.
+, soluble; ±, partial soluble; −, insoluble.

TABLE 2.12

Inherent Viscosity for Functionalized Polysulfones, CMPSF, and PSF-DOPO, with Different Substitution Degrees

Polymer	DS	η_{inh} (dL g^{-1})
PSF	0.00	0.72
CMPSF	0.56	0.60
	0.90	0.64
	1.53	0.68
PSF-DOPO	0.62	0.474
	0.74	0.45
	1.30	0.44

2.4   CONCLUSIONS

Functionalized polysulfones will continue to be in demand as they are endowed with various superior properties, such as chemical, mechanical, and thermal resistance, which extend the range of their potential applications.

The introduction of quaternary ammonium groups into polysulfones can be accomplished by the polymerization of functional monomers or by the postfunctionalization of commercially available polymers. The functional monomer route can precisely control the amount of functional groups and their location along the polymer backbone by varying the monomer feed. However, as the synthesis of monomers is expensive and laborious the postfunctionalization method is widely employed for the synthesis of quaternized polysulfones. To conclude, the halomethylation is the most frequently applied method that can be further used for obtaining other functional polysulfones with various structures. In addition, the selection of a mild and efficient synthetic route is an important issue in the preparation of functionalized polysulfones.

ACKNOWLEDGMENT

This work was supported by a grant of the Romanian National Authority for Scientific Research, CNCS—UEFISCDI (project number PN-II-RU-TE-2012-3-143).

REFERENCES

1. Scherrington, D. C. and Mark, H. F. *Encyclopedia of Polymer Science and Engineering.* Wiley, New York, 1988.
2. Twardowski, Z. J. Dialyzer Reuse Part II: Advantages and disadvantages. *Semin. Dial.*, 19 (3), 217–226, 2006.
3. Isla, A., Gacon, A. R., Maynar, J., Arzuaga, A., Coral, E., Martin, A., Solinis, M. A., and Munoz, J. L. P. *In vitro* and *in vivo* evaluation of enoxaparin removal by continuous renal replacement therapies with acrylonitrile and polysulfone membranes. *Clin. Therap.*, 27 (9), 1444–1451, 2005.
4. Choi, Y. J., Hwang, E. H., and Hwang, T. S. Preparation and property of SBS ion exchange membrane via post-sulfonation. *Korean Chem. Eng. Res.*, 48 (6), 731–736, 2010.
5. Camachu-Zuniga, C., Ruiz-Trevino, F. A., Henandez-Lopez, S., Zolotukhin, M. G., Maurer, F. H. J., and Gonzales-Montiel, A. Aromatic polysulfone copolymers for gas separation membrane applications. *J. Membr. Sci.*, 340 (1–2), 221–226, 2009.
6. Garganciuc, D., Batranescu, G., Nechifor, G., and Olteanu, M. Functionalization of polymers, such as polysulfone and polyphenylenoxide for the development of affinity membranes. *Mat. Plast.*, 45 (1), 29–33, 2008.
7. Hamciuc, C. and Hamciuc, E. Sulphonated aromatic polymer. *Mat. Plast.*, 3, 204–218, 2006.
8. Kim, D. S., Robertson, G. P., and Guiver, M. D. Comb-shaped poly(arylene ether sulfone)s as proton exchange membranes. *Macromolecules*, 41 (6), 2126–2134, 2008.
9. Ahn, J., Chung, W. J., Pinnau, I., and Guiver, M. D. Polysulfone/silica nanoparticle mixed-matrix membranes for gas separation. *J. Membr. Sci.*, 314 (1), 123–133, 2008.
10. Fu, Y. Z., Manthiram, A., and Guiver, M. D. Blend membranes based on sulfonated poly(ether ether ketone) and polysulfone bearing benzimidazole side groups for DMFCs. *Electrochem. Solid State Lett.*, 10 (4), B70–B73, 2007.
11. Liu, B., Robertson, G. P., Kim, D. S., Guiver, M. D., Hu, W., and Jiang, Z. Aromatic polyether ketones with pendant sulfonic acid phenyl groups prepared by a mild sulfonation method for proton exchange membranes (PEM)s. *Macromolecules*, 40 (5), 1934–1944, 2007.
12. Gao, Y., Robertson, G. P., Guiver, M. D., Wang, G., Jian, X., Mikhailenko, S. D., Li, X., and Kaliaguine, S. Sulfonated co-poly(phthalazinone ether ketone nitrile)s as proton exchange membrane materials. *J. Membr. Sci.*, 278 (1), 26–34, 2006.
13. Li, Z., Ding, J., Robertson, G. P., and Guiver, M. D. A novel bisphenol monomer with grafting capability and the resulting poly(arylene ether sulfone)s. *Macromolecules*, 39 (20), 6990–6996, 2006.
14. Sun, Y. M., Wu, S., Lee, H. C., Jung, G. B., Guiver, M. D., Gao, Y., Liu, Y. L., and Lai, J. Y. Sulfonated poly(phthalazinone ether ketone) for proton exchange membranes in direct methanol fuel cells. *J. Membr. Sci.*, 265 (1), 108–114, 2005.
15. Arthanareeswaran, G., Thanikaivelan, P., and Raajenthiren, M. Preparation and characterization of poly(methylmethacrylate) and sulfonated poly(etheretherketone) blend ultrafiltration membranes for protein separation applications. *Mater. Sci. Eng. C*, 29 (1), 246–252, 2009.
16. Wu, H., Fang, X., Zhang, X. F., Jiang, Z. Y., Li, B., and Ma, X. C. Cellulose acetatepoly(N-vinyl-2-pyrrolidone) blend membrane for pervaporation separation of methanol/MTBEmixtures. *Sep. Purif. Technol.*, 64 (2), 183–191, 2008.

17. Nara, S. and Oyama, T. H. Effects of partial miscibility on the structure and properties of novel high performance blends composed of poly(p-phenylene sulfide) and poly-(phenylsulfone). *Polym. J.*, 46 (1), 568–575, 2014.

18. Mohammadi, T., Kikhavandi, T., and Moghebeli, M. Synthesis and characterization of poly(ether-block-amide) membranes. *Macromol. Symp.*, 264 (1), 127–134, 2008.

19. Mansourizadeh, A. and Azad, A. J. Preparation of blend polyethersulfone/cellulose acetate/polyethylene glycol asymmetric membranes for oil–water separation. *J. Polym. Res.*, 21 (1), 375–384, 2014.

20. Wang, B., Huangfu, F., and Liu, W. Preparation of polysulfonebenzylthiourea reactive ultrafiltration plate membranes and their rejection properties for heavy toxic metal cations. *J. Appl. Polym. Sci.*, 108 (6), 4014–4022, 2008.

21. Yoshikawa, M., Izumi, J., Ooi, T., Kitao, T., Guiver, M. D., and Robertson, G. P. Carboxylated polysulfone membranes having a chiral recognition site induced by an alternative molecular imprinting technique. *Polym. Bull.*, 40 (1), 517–524, 1998.

22. Quiclet-Sire, B., Wilczewska, A., and Zarda, S. Z. A practical process for polymer supported synthesis. *Tetrah. Lett.*, 41 (6), 5673–5677, 2000.

23. Arad-Yellina, R., Firerb, M., Kahanaa, N., and Greenc, B. S. Functionalized polysulfone as a novel and useful carrier for immunization and antibody detection. *React. Funct. Polym.*, 54 (1), 5–16, 2003.

24. Yave, W. and Quijada, R. Preparation and characterization of porous microfiltration membranes by using tailor-made propylene/1-octadecene copolymers. *Desalination*, 228 (1), 150–158, 2008.

25. Rahimpour, A. and Maidaeni, S. S. Polyethersulfone (PES)/cellulose acetate phthalate (CAP) blend ultrafiltration membranes: Preparation, morphology, performance and anti-fouling properties. *J. Membr. Sci.*, 305(1–2), 299–3001, 2007.

26. Fontanova, E., Donato, L., Drioli, E., Lopez, L., Favia, P., and D'Aagostino, R. Heterogenization of polyoxometalates on the surface of plasma-modified polymeric membranes. *Chem. Mater.*, 18 (6), 1561–1568, 2006.

27. Carraro, M., Gardan, M., Scorrano, G., Drioli, E., Fontananova, E., and Bonchio, M. Solvent-free, heterogeneous photooxygenation of hydrocarbons by Hyflon® membranes embedding a fluorous-tagged decatungstate: The importance of being fluorous. *Adv. Synth. Catal.*, 345 (4), 1119–1126, 2003.

28. Wijaya, S., Duke, M. C., and Da Costa, J. C. D. Carbonised template silica membranes for desalination. *Desalination*, 236 (1–3), 291–298, 2009.

29. Battersby, S., Tasaki, T., Smart, S., Ladewig, B., Liu, S. M., Duke, M. C., Rudolph, V., and Da Costa, J. C. D. Performance of cobalt silica membranes in gas mixture separation. *J. Membr. Sci.*, 329 (1–2), 91–98, 2009.

30. Taurozzi, J. S., Arul, A., Bosak, V. Z., Burban, A. B., Voice, T. C., Bruening, M. L., and Tarabara, V. V. Effect of filler incorporation route on the properties of polysulfone–silver nanocomposite membranes of different porosities. *J. Membr. Sci.*, 325 (1), 58–68, 2008.

31. Ficai (Manzu), D., Ficai, A., Voicu, G., Vasile, B. S., Guran, A., and Andronescu, E. Polysulfone based membranes with desired pores characteristics. *Mat. Plast.*, 47 (1), 24–27, 2010.

32. Han, M. J., Bummer, P. M., Jay, M., and Bhattacharyya, D. Phase transitions of polysulfone solution during coagulation. *Polymer*, 36 (24), 4711–4714, 1995.

33. Zhou, J., Zhang, H., Wang, H., and Du, Q. Effect of cooling baths on EVOH microporous membrane structures in thermally induced phase separation. *J. Membr. Sci.*, 343 (1), 104–109, 2009.

34. Qtaishat, M., Khayet, M., and Matsuura, T. Novel porous composite hydrophobic/hydrophilic polysulfone membranes for desalination by direct contact membrane distillation. *J. Membr. Sci.*, 341 (1–2), 139–148, 2009.

35. Li, S., Gao, Y., Bai, H., Zhang, L., Qu, P., and Bai, L. Preparation and characteristics of polysulfone dialysis composite membrane modified with nanocrystalline cellulose. *BioResources*, 6 (2), 1670–1680, 2011.

36. Wu, H., Zhao, Y., Nie, M., and Jiang, Z., Molecularly imprinted organic-inorganic hybrid membranes for selective separation of phenylalanine isomers and its properties. *Sep. Purif. Technol.*, 68 (1), 97–104, 2009.

37. Yi, Z., Xu, Y., Zhu, L., Dong, H., and Zhu, B. Hydrophilic modification of peak porous membranes *via* aqueous surface-initiated atom transfer radical polymerization. *Chin. J. Polym. Sci.*, 27 (5), 695–702, 2009.

38. Chwojnowski, A., Wojciechowski, C., Dudziński, K., and Lukowska, E. Polysulphone and polyethersulphone hollow fiber membranes with developed inner surface as material for bio medical applications. *Biocybern. Biomed. Eng.*, 29 (3), 47–59, 2009.

39. Hodge, P. and Scherrington, D. C. *Polymer Supported Reactions in Organic Synthesis.* Wiley, New York, 1980.

40. Olabisi, O. *Handbook of Thermoplastics.* Marcel Dekker Inc., New York, 1997.

41. Daly, W. H. and Wu, S. J. *New Monomers and Polymers.* Plenum Press, New York, 1984.

42. Du, R. H. and Zhao, J. S. Properties of poly (*N,N*-dimethylaminoethyl methacrylate)/ polysulfone positively charged composite nanofiltration membrane. *J. Membr. Sci.*, 239 (1), 183–188, 2004.

43. Liu, J. Q., Xu, Z. L., Li, X. H., Zhang, Y., Zhou, Y., Wang, Z. X., and Wang, X. J. An improved process to prepare high separation performance PA/PVDF hollow fiber composite nanofiltration membranes. *Sep. Purif. Technol.*, 58 (1), 53–60, 2007.

44. Ohya, H., Shiki, S., and Kawakami, H. Fabrication study of polysulfone hollow-fiber microfiltration membranes: Optimal dope viscosity for nucleation and growth. *J. Membr. Sci.*, 326 (2), 293–302, 2009.

45. Sikder, J., Pereira, C., Palchoudhury, S., Vohra, K., Basumatary, D., and Pal, P. Synthesis and characterization of cellulose acetate-polysulfone blend microfiltration membrane for separation of microbial cells from lactic acid fermentation broth. *Desalination*, 249 (1), 802–808, 2009.

46. Nady, N., Franssen, M. C. R., Zuilhof, H., Eldin, M. S. M., Boom, R., and Schroen, K. Modification methods for poly(arylsulfone) membranes: A mini-review focusing on surface modification. *Desalination*, 275 (1), 1–9, 2011.

47. Klein, E., Eichholz, E., and Yeager, D. H. Affinity membranes prepared from hydrophilic coatings on microporous polysulfone hollow fibres. *J. Membr. Sci.*, 90 (1), 69–80, 1994.

48. Sivaraman, K. M., Kellenberger, C., Pane, S., Ergeneman, O., Luehmann, T., and Luechinger, N. A. Porous polysulfone coatings for enhanced drug delivery. *Biomed. Microdevices*, 14 (2), 603–612, 2012.

49. Jarosiewicz, A. and Tomaszewska, M. Polysulfone coating with starch addition in CRF formulation. *Desalination*, 163 (1), 247–252, 2004.

50. Aerts, P., Van Hoof, E., Leysen, R., Vankelecom, I. F. J., and Jacobs, P. A. Polysulfone-aerosil composite membranes. Part 1. The influence of the addition of aerosil on the formation process and membrane morphology. *J. Membr. Sci.*, 176 (1), 63–73, 2000.

51. Sanchez, S., Pumera, M., Cabruja, E., and Fabregas, E. Carbon nanotube/polysulfone composite screen-printed electrochemical enzyme biosensors. *Analyst J.*, 132 (1), 142–147, 2007.

52. Wenz, L. M., Merritt, K., Brown, S. A., Moet, A., and Steffee, A. D. In vitro biocompatibility of polyetheretherketone and polysulfone composites. *J. Biomed. Mater. Res.*, 24 (1), 207–215, 1990.

53. Trisca-Rusu, C., Nechifor, A. C., Mihai, S., Parvu, C., Voicu, S. I., and Nechifor, G. Polysulfone-functionalized multiwalled carbon nanotubes composite membranes for potential sensing applications. *International Semiconductor Conference Proceedings*, IEEE, Bucharest, Romania, 12–14 October, Vol. 2, 285–288, 2009.

54. Von Kraemer, S., Puchner, M., Jannasch, P., Lundblad, A., and Lindbergh, G. Gas diffusion electrodes and membrane electrode assemblies based on a sulfonated polysulfone for high-temperature PEMFC. *J. Electrochem. Soc.*, 153 (6), A2077–A2084, 2006.

55. Agarwal, A. K. and Huang, R. Y. M. Studies on the enhancement of separation characteristics of sulfonated poly(phenylene oxide)/polysulfone thin film composite membranes for reverse osmosis applications. II. Effects of nitromethane and the chemical treatment combined with gamma-ray. *Angew. Makromol. Chem.*, 163 (1), 15–21, 1988.

56. Kuroiwa, T., Miyagishi, T., Ito, A., Matsuguchi, M., Sadaoka, Y., and Sakai, Y. A Thin film polysulfone based capacitive type relative humidity sensor. *Sens. Actuators. B*, 25 (1–3), 692–695, 1995.

57. Claes, L. Carbonfibre reinforced polysulfone—A new biomaterial. *Biomed. Tech.*, 34 (12), 315–319, 1989.

58. Karlsson, L. E. and Jannasch, P. Polysulfone ionomers for proton conducting fuel cell membranes sulfoalkylated polysulfones. *J. Membr. Sci.*, 230 (1), 61–70, 2004.

59. Lufrano, F., Gatto, I., Staiti, P., Antonucci, V., and Passalacqua, E. Sulfonated polysulfone ionomer membranes for fuel cells. *Solid State Ionics*, 145 (1), 47–51, 2001.

60. Lufrano, F., Squadrito, G., Patti, A., and Passalacqua, E. Sulfonated polysulfone as promising membranes for polymer electrolyte fuel cells. *J. Appl. Polym. Sci.*, 77 (6), 1250–1256, 2000.

61. Manea, C. and Mulder, M. Characterization of polymer blends of polyethersulfone/sulfonated polysulfone and polyethersulfone/sulfonated polyetheretherketone for direct methanol fuel cell applications. *J. Membr. Sci.*, 206 (1–2), 443–453, 2002.

62. Daly, W. H. Modification of condensation polymers. *J. Macromol. Sci. Chem.*, A22 (3), 713–728, 1985.

63. Daly, W. H., Chotiwana, S., and Nielsen, R. Chloromethylation of condensation polymers and oxi 1,4-phenilene backbone. *Polym. Prepr. Am. Chem. Soc. Div. Polym. Chem.*, 20 (1), 835–838, 1979.

64. Moulay, S. and Daly, W. H. Chemical reactions on redox polymer precursors. I. Chloromethylation and lithiation. *Eur. Polym. J.*, 33 (6), 929–935, 1997.

65. Warshawsky, A., Zahana, N., Deshe, A., Gottlieb, H.E., and Arad-Yellin, R. Halomethylated polysulfone: Reactive intermediates to neutral and ionic film-forming polymers. *J. Polym. Sci. Part A Polym. Chem.*, 28 (11), 2885–2905, 1990.

66. Warshawsky, A. and Deshe, A. Halomethyl octyl ethers: Convenient halomethylation reagents. *Polym. Sci. Polym. Chem.*, 23 (6), 1839–1841, 1985.

67. Avram, E. Polymers with pendent functional groups. *Polym. Plast. Technol. Eng.*, 40 (3), 275–281, 2001.

68. Avram, E., Butuc E., Luca, C., and Druta, I. Polymers with pendent functional groups. III. Polysulfones containing viologen group. *J. Macromol. Sci. Pure Appl. Chem.*, A34 (9), 1701–1714, 1997.

69. Mudryk, B., Rajaramanb, S., and Soundararajana, N. A practical synthesis of chloromethyl esters from acid chlorides and trioxane or paraformaldehyde promoted by zirconium tetrachloride. *Tetrah. Lett.*, 43 (36), 6317–6318, 2002.

70. Amoto, J. S., Karady, S., Sletzinger, M., and Weinstok, L. M. A new preparation of chloromethyl methyl ether free of bis[chloromethyl] ether. *Synthesis*, 12, 970–971, 1979.

71. Haslan, J., Hamilton, B., and Squirell, D. M. The determination of chlorine by the oxygen flask combustion method: A single unit for electrical ignition by remote control and potentiometric titration. *Analyst*, 85 (1), 556–561, 1960.

72. Vasile, C., Calugaru, M. E., Stoleriu, A., Mihai, E., and Sabliovschi, M. *Thermal Behaviour of Polymers*. Romanian Academy, Bucharest, Romania, 1983.

73. Avram, E., Brebu, M. A., Warshawsky, A., and Vasile, C. Polymers with pendent functional groups. V. Thermo-oxidative and thermal behavior of chloromethylated polysulfone. *Polym. Degrad. Stabil.*, 69 (2), 175–181, 2000.

74. Luca, C., Avram, E., and Petrariu, I. Quaternary ammonium polyelectrolytes. V. Amination studies of chloromethylated polystyrene with N,N-dimethylalkylamine. *J. Macromol. Sci. Chem.*, A25 (1), 375–361, 1988.

75. Avram, E., Neagu, V., and Luca, C. Obtaining the cationic polymers with quaternary ammonium groups. *Conference of Polymer Science*, Iasi, Romania, 1991.

76. Wang, C. Y., Li, N., Shin, D. W., Lee, S. Y., Kang, N. R., and Lee, Y. Polymer electrolyte membranes derived from new sulfone monomers with pendent sulfonic acid groups. *Macromolecules*, 44 (18), 7296–7306, 2011.

77. Lisa, G., Avram, E., Paduraru, G., Irimia, M., Hurduc, N., and Aelenei, N. Thermal behaviour of polystyrene, polysulfone and their substituted derivatives. *Polym. Degrad. Stabil.*, 82 (1), 73–79, 2003.

78. Acácio, A. M., Filho, F., and Gomes, A. S. Sulfonated bisphenol-A-polysulfone based composite PEMs containing tungstophosphoric acid and modified by electron beam irradiation. *Int. J. Hydrogen Energy*, 37 (7), 6228–6235, 2012.

79. Ioan, S., Albu, R. M., Avram, E., Stoica, I., and Ioanid, E. G. Surface characterization of quaternized polysulfone films and biocompatibility studies. *J. Appl. Polym. Sci.*, 121 (1), 127–137, 2011.

80. Vico, S., Palys, B., and Buess-Herman, C. Hydration of a polysulfone anion-exchange membrane studied by vibrational spectroscopy. *Langmuir*, 19 (8), 3282–3287, 2003.

81. Ioan, S., Filimon, A., and Avram, E. Conformational and viscometric behavior of quaternized polysulfone in dilute solution. *Polym. Eng. Sci.*, 46 (7), 827–836, 2006.

82. Filimon, A., Avram, E., and Ioan, S. Specific interactions in ternary system quaternized polysulfone/mixed solvent. *Polym. Eng. Sci.*, 49 (1), 17–25, 2009.

83. Huang, Y. and Xiao, C. Miscibility and mechanical properties of quaternized polysulfone/benzoyl guar gum blends. *Polymer*, 48 (1), 371–381, 2007.

84. Luca, C., Avram, E., and Neagu, V. *Chemical Transformation of Poly(Methyl Styrene)*. Polymer Chemistry and Physics Nowadays, Iasi, Romania, 1991.

85. Ghimici, L. and Avram, E. Viscometric behavior of quaternized polysulfones. *J. Appl. Polym. Sci.*, 90 (1), 465–469, 2003.

86. Näther, C., Riedel, J., and Jeß, I. 4,4'-Bipyridine dihydrate at 130 K. *Acta Crystallogr.*, 57 (1), 111–112, 2001.

87. Tenenbaum, L. E. Alkylpyridines and arylpyridines, In: *Pyridine and Its Derivatives*, Part Two, Klingsberg, E. ed., Wiley Interscience Inc., New York, Chap. V, pp. 155, 1961.

88. Micetich, R. G. Reaction of acethylenic triple bond, In: *Pyridine and Its Derivatives*, Supplement Part Two, Abramovich, R. A. ed., Wiley Interscience Inc., New York, Chap. V, pp. 347, 1974.

89. Zhang, L. -J., Shen, X. -C., and Liangc, H. 4,4'-Bipyridinium bis-(oxalato-κ2 O^1,O^2) cuprate(II): An ion-pair complex. *Acta Crystallogr. Sect. E Struct. Rep.*, 65 (11), 1276–1277, 2009.

90. Sliwa, W., Bachovska, B., and N. Zelichowicz. Chemistry of viologens. *Heterocycles*, 32 (11), 2241–2273, 1991.

91. Näther, C., Jeß, I., and Bolte, M. 4,4'-Bipyridylium di-μ-chlorotetrachlorodicuprate(II): A redetermination. *Acta Crystallogr. Sect. E Struct. Rep.*, 57 (2), 78–79, 2001.

92. Candan, M. M., Erouglu, S., Ŏzbey S., Kendi E., and Kantarci, Z. Structure and conformation of 4,4'-bipyridine. *Spectrosc. Lett.*, 32 (1), 35–45, 1999.

93. Bukowska-Strzyezewska, M. and Tosik, A. Structure of the 4,4'-bipyridyl clathrate of octaaquayttrium (III) chloride. *Acta Cryst.*, B38 (3), 950–951, 1982.

94. Galasso, V., De Alti, G., and Bigotto, A. MO calculations on the preferred conformation and electronic structure of phenylpyridines and bipyridines. *Tetrahedron*, 27 (5), 991–997, 1971.

95. McIntyre, E. F. and Hameka, H. F. Photochemistry. *J. Chem. Phys.*, 70 (6), 2215–2231, 1979.

96. Koivunen, M. E., Gee, S. J., Park, E. K., Lee, K., Schenker, M. B., and Hammock, B. D. Application of an enzyme-linked immunosorbent assay for the analysis of paraquat in human-exposure samples. *Arch. Environ. Contam. Toxicol.*, 48 (1), 184–190, 2005.

97. Monk, P. M. S. Electrochemistry and spectroelectrochemistry of bipyridilium redox species. PhD Thesis, University of Exeter, Devon, 1990.

98. Zugravescu, I. and Petrovanu, M. *Chemistry of N-ilides*, Bucharest, Romania, 1976.

99. Acheson, R. M. and Plunkett, A. O. Addition reactions of heterocyclic compounds. Part XVIII. The structures and reactions of adducts from pyridines, dimethyl-acetylenedicarboxylate, and carbon dioxide at low temperatures. *J. Chem. Soc.*, 513, 2676–2683, 1964.

100. Cookson, R. C. and Isaacs, N. S. The reaction between pyridazine and maleic anhydride. *Tetrahedron*, 19 (9), 1237–1242, 1963.

101. Ross, J. H. and Krieger, R. I. Synthesis and properties of paraquat (methyl viologen) and other herbicidal alkyl homologues. *Agric. Food Chem.*, 28 (5), 1026–1031, 1980.

102. Sliwa, W., Matusiak, G., and Postawka, A. 1,3-Dipolar cycloaddition reactions of 4,6-diazaphenanthrene 6-phenacylide. *Monatshefte für Chem. Chem. Monthly*, 124 (2), 161–165, 1993.

103. Kamojawa, H., Mizuno, H., Todo, Y., and Nanasawa, M. Syntheses of polymerizable viologens bearing a terminal vinyl group. *J. Polym. Sci. Polym. Chem. Ed.*, 17 (8), 3149–3157, 1979.

104. Nanbu, Y., Yamamoto, K., and Endo T. Selective formation of polymer-bound mono-meric and dimeric viologen cation radicals by choice of pendant group linkage. *J. Chem. Soc. Chem. Commun.*, 7 (1), 574–576, 1986.

105. Ageishi, K., Endo, T., and Okawara, J. M. Preparation of viologen polymers from alkyl-ene dipyridinium salts by cyanide ion. *Polym. Sci. Polym. Chem. Ed.*, 21 (1), 293–300, 1983.

106. Kitamura, M., Nambu, Y., and Endo, T. Synthesis and radical copolymerization of new type pyridinum monomer and redox behavior of its polymers. *J. Polym. Sci. Part A Polym. Chem.*, 28 (2), 345–352, 1990.

107. Sato, T., Nambu, Y., and Endo, T. Preparation of cellulose derivatives containing the viologen moiety. *J. Polym. Sci. Part C Polym. Lett.*, 26 (8), 341–345, 1988.

108. Endo, T., Kameyama, A., Nambu, Y., Kashi, Y., and Okawara, M. Synthesis of poly-ethers containing viologen moiety and their application to electron-transfer catalyst. *J. Polym. Sci. Part A Polym. Chem.*, 28 (9), 2509–2516, 1990.

109. Ergozhin, E. E., Tausarova, B. R., and Turbibekova, A. B. Synthesis of warwe-soluble cationic and amphoteric polyelectrolytes based on polysulfone. *Dokl. Nats. Akad. Nauk. Resp. Kaz.*, 1 (1), 39–48, 1993.

110. Flory, P. J. *Principles of Polymer Chemistry*, Cornell University Press, Ithaca, UT, 1953.

111. Merrifield, R. B. The role of the support in solid phase peptide synthesis. *Br. Polym. J.*, 16 (4), 173–178, 1984.

112. Druta, I. and Avram, E. *Transquaternized Reaction in Quaternary Ammonium Salts Field.* "Al. I. Cuza" Univesity Days, Iasi, Romania 1996.

113. Druta, I., Avram, E., and Cozan, V. Polymers with pendent functional groups. IV. The reaction of chloromethylated polystyrene with N-phenacyl-4,4′-bipyridinium bromides. *Eur. Polym. J.*, 36 (1), 221–224, 2000.

114. Luca, C., Barboiu, V., Avram, E., and Streba, E. Kinetic aspects of reactions on poly-mers containing amine and chloromethylene groups. *The 8th Conference on Physical Chemistry*, Bucharest, Romania, 25–27 September, 1996.

115. Zhang, A., Li, X., Nan, C., Hwang, K., and Lee, M. H. Facile modifications of a poly-imide *via* chloromethylation. I. Novel synthesis of a new photosensitive polyimide. *J. Polym. Sci. Part. A. Polym. Chem.*, 4 (1), 22–29, 2003.

116. Cozan, V. and Avram, E. Side chain thermotropic liquid crystalline polysulfone obtained from polysulfone UDEL by chemical modification. *Eur. Polym. J.*, 39 (1), 107–114, 2003.

117. Racles, C., Avram, E, Marcu, M., Cozan, V., and Cazacu, M. New siloxane ester modified polysulfones by phase transfer catalysis. *Polymer*, 41 (23), 8205–8021, 2000.

118. Guiver, M. D., Black, C. M., Tam, C. M., and Deslandes, Y. Functionalized polysulfone membranes by heterogeneous lithiation. *J. Appl. Polym. Sci.*, 48 (9), 1597–1606, 1993.

119. Park, Y. J., Acar, M. H., Akthakul, A., Kuhlmann, W., and Mayes, A. M. Polysulfone-graft-poly(ethylene glycol) graft copolymers for surface modification of polysulfone membranes. *Biomaterials*, 27 (6), 856–865, 2006.

120. Wavhal S. and Fisher, E. R. Hydrophilic modification of polyethersulfone membranes by low temperature plasma-induced graft polymerization. *J. Membr. Sci.*, 209 (1), 255–269, 2002.

121. Song, Q., Sheng, J., Wei, M., and Yuan, X. B. Surface modification of polysulfone membranes by low-temperature plasma-graft poly(ethylene glycol) onto polysulfone membranes. *J. Appl. Polym. Sci.*, 78 (3), 979–985, 2000.

122. Iwata, M., Ivanchenko, M. I., and Miyaki, Y. Preparation of anti-oil stained membrane by grafting polyethylene glycol macromer onto polysulfone membrane. *J. Appl. Polym. Sci.*, 54 (1), 125–128, 1994.

123. Perez, R., Sandler, J. K. W., Altstadt, V., Hoffmann, T., Pospiech, D., Ciesielski, M., Doring, M., Balabanovich, A. I., and Schartel, B. Novel phosphorus modified polysulfone as a combined flame retardant and toughness modifier for epoxy resins. *Polymer*, 48 (2), 778–790, 2007.

124. Hoffmann, T., Pospiech, D., Haußler, L., Komber, H., Voigt, D., Harnisch, C., Kollann, C., Ciesielski, M., Doring, M., Perez-Graterol R., Sandler, J., and Altstadt, V. Novel phosphorous-containing aromatic polyethers-synthesis and characterization. *Macromol. Chem. Phys.*, 206 (4), 423–431, 2005.

125. Wu, C. S., Liu, Y. L., and Chiu, Y. S. Preparation of phosphorous-containing poly(epichlorohydrin) and polyurethane from a novel synthesis route. *J. Appl. Polym. Sci.*, 85 (10), 2254–2259, 2002.

126. Petreus, O., Avram, E., and Serbezeanu, D. Synthesis and characterization of phosphorus-containing polysulfone. *Polym. Eng. Sci.*, 50 (1), 48–52, 2010.

3 Mathematical Models and Numeric Simulations of Specific Interactions in Solutions of Modified Polysulfones

Anca Filimon

CONTENTS

3.1   INTRODUCTION

Last decade saw a continuous miniaturization of mechanical, chemical, thermal, optical, and electronic devices in the engineering sciences, along with an increased ability to manipulate large biomolecular complexes and subcellular organelles in biological sciences. These developments have led us to the exciting era of nanoscience and nanotechnology. However, chemical, physical, and biological nanoscale systems pose fundamental challenges in theoretical modeling and numerical computation, due to their excessively large number of degrees of freedom [1].

In polymer science and engineering, the knowledge of the specific interactions of polymer–solvent systems, as well as the study of polymer associations in solution and solvent mixtures, represents a fundamental step in the processing of advanced materials. In this context, in recent years, the research directions on the characterization of polymers with complex structures (i.e., polysulfones, chloromethylated and quaternized polysulfones, etc.) in the solution have been oriented toward the preparation of a thermodynamically stable solution. In addition, the strength of the interactions between components is the key factor in polymer materials characterization. Attention was focused on the experimental investigations and theoretical approximations, using mathematical simulations for underlying the establishment of some properties prior to the synthesis process, and for elucidating some aspects concerning the behavior of macromolecular compounds in different fields [2,3].

As known, the statistical–mechanical approach permits to establish relationships that reflect the macroscopic behavior of substances in correlation with their atomic and/or molecular properties. Same principles when applied in polymer science get complicated, due to the higher number of degrees of freedom that influence or are influenced by intra- and intermolecular interactions. In this context, many existent mathematical models have focused on finding the structure–property relationships in order to predetermine some structures with specific applications. Proposed theories start from the knowledge of atomic coordinates (zero-order connectivity indices), types of atomic and molecular bonds (higher order connectivity indices), and structural variables of polymers, thus generating the scheme for the calculation of physical properties. It is also known that the molecular theory of polymer solutions can be developed in accordance with the statistical–mechanical theory, correlated with the equilibrium and nonequilibrium state theory of liquids, by introducing some specific parameters. Thus, the physical processes that occur as a result of excluded volume effects are described by means of mathematical models included in the so-called theory of the two parameters and, more recently, in the renormalized group theory. The properties of dilute solutions of polymers—such as weight average molecular weight, intrinsic viscosity, and second virial coefficient—are mainly expressed in terms of root-mean-square radii of gyration in unperturbed state, and according to the excluded volume parameter. Through their intermediary, the main problems of the theory have been focused on the relationships between solution properties and chemical structure. An accurate description of these aspects was, and still remains, a problem of interest from both theoretical and experimental viewpoints.

Consequently, based on these considerations, this chapter emphasizes the importance of mathematical models and numeric simulations in the predetermination of structure–property relationships, referring in particular to polysulfone (PSF) architectures in dilute solution and solvent mixtures.

3.2   TYPES OF INTERACTION IN POLYMERIC SYSTEMS: THEORETICAL CONSIDERATIONS

Control of polymeric structure is among the most important targets of modern macromolecular science. In particular, tailoring the position and strength of interaction forces within macromolecules by synthetic methods and, therefore, structural control on the final polymeric materials have become possible. Besides other interaction forces, hydrogen bonds appear as unique intermolecular forces, enabling the tuning of material properties via self-assembly processes, over a wide range of interaction strength values, ranging from a few kJ mol^{-1} to several tens of kJ mol^{-1}. In all cases, the weak and strong interactions can act as the central structural-directing forces for the organization of polymer chains, and thus for establishing the final properties of materials. Consequently, the high level of structural diversity of many systems, as well as their high level of directionality and specificity in recognition phenomena, is unbeaten in polymer chemistry. Their stability can be tuned over a wide range of strength values, and it is important for tuning the properties of the resulting materials, ranging from elastomeric to thermoplastic and even to highly cross-linked duroplastic structures and networks.

Starting from such considerations, the behavior of dilute polymer solutions, expressed by different parameters (the second virial coefficient, mean dimensions, and intrinsic viscosity), and influenced by temperature, solvent quality, and molecular weights domain, can be discussed through different excluded volume theories [4–6]. All these theories mutually differ by the mathematical methods and approximations used, but all of them relate the excluded volume effects to measurable quantities, by considering different possible interactions.

Development of adequate descriptions of the influence of the excluded volume effect on the properties of macromolecular chains in good solvents at infinite dilution was, and remains, an important problem in the theoretical study of polymer chemistry. Conformation of macromolecular chains in the solution is greatly influenced by the interactions between chain elements. These interactions are conveniently divided into two classes:

1. *Short-range interactions*, manifested as steric repulsion forces caused by the overlapping of the electron clouds, occur between the neighboring atoms or groups separated only by a small number of valence bonds, being dependent on the bond angles and internal rotation. The macromolecular chain in which these interactions are manifested is a *Gaussian chain* called *unperturbed* or *theta state*.
2. *Long-range interactions* result from the attractive and repulsive forces between segments widely separated in a chain (occasionally approaching one another due to molecular flexing) as well as between segments and solvent molecules. These are often termed *excluded volume effects*. They are,

therefore, identical in nature and in magnitude to van der Waals interactions between the parts of two different molecules. The macromolecular chains in which these interactions occur are called *perturbed chains*.

In the absence of both types of interactions, excluding the covalent bond forces, which establish the chain length, a long chain molecule obeys the Gaussian statistics. According to this assumption, the mean-square radius of gyration is defined by Equation 3.1.

$$\left\langle S^2 \right\rangle_{of} = \frac{l^2 N}{6} \tag{3.1}$$

where:
   N is the number of bonds
   l is the length of a statistic element
   of is the absence of both types of interactions

Short-range interactions introduce a serious change in the average dimensions of the chain, but they do not modify the proportionality between the mean-square radius of gyration and N, and, therefore, they do not disrupt the Gaussian character of the distribution function of chain segments. Besides the long-range interactions, the chain may be regarded as unperturbed, and the mean-square radius of gyration becomes

$$\left\langle S_\theta^2 \right\rangle = \sigma^2 \left\langle S_{of}^2 \right\rangle \tag{3.2}$$

where:
   σ is a structural parameter independent on N, called the *steric factor*, which represents a measure of chain flexibility in unperturbed state

Long-range interactions introduce the excluded volume effect, which can be described by Gaussian statistics and can be regarded as an osmotic swelling of the statistic coil, due to solvent–polymer interactions. As a result of both types of interactions, the mean-square gyration radius of the linear real chain in the diluted solution is given by

$$\left\langle S^2 \right\rangle = \alpha_s^2 \left\langle S_\theta^2 \right\rangle \tag{3.3}$$

where:

   α_s is the expansion factor dependent on N, which is a measure of n flexibility chain in perturbed state

A deficiency of the excluded volume theory lies in the fact that the approximate formulas are obtained frequently from first-order perturbation calculations, so that the required mathematical transformations are only permitted for infinite molecular weight. Therefore, on the one hand, these equations are no longer valid for coils with large expansion, and on the other hand, for the polymers with small molecular weights.

As far as the dependence of polymer properties (e.g., the second virial coefficient and Huggins coefficient) on molecular weight is involved, the theory of inter- and intramolecular contacts has proved to be a simple and efficient alternative to the excluded volume theory [7–10]. Thus, it may be stated that:

- *Intramolecular interactions* occur between polymer segments belonging to the same macromolecule. These interactions increase with improving the quality of the solvent, opposing to the scission of the macromolecular chain, due to increased polymer–solvent interactions.
- *Intermolecular interactions* occur between segments belonging to different chains. With increasing solvent quality, these segments are separated and tend toward maximum expansion, attained in the insulating state, so that the intermolecular interactions decrease with increasing polymer–solvent interactions.

This concept starts from the fact that the dimensions of dissolved polymer coils change upon dilution. Therefore, in addition to contacts between polymer segments belonging to different molecules, intramolecular intersegmental contacts are also produced as the solvent is added. The advantages of the model lie in the simple mathematical expressions and in the possibility to assign only the two necessary adjustable parameters to the intra- and intermolecular contributions. These contributions can be subsequently studied in their mutual dependence and their variation with the thermodynamic quality of the solvent.

3.3 THERMODYNAMIC MODELING OF POLYMER AND/OR POLYELECTROLYTES SOLUTIONS

Thermodynamics of polymers have posed much attention in the last years [11,12], when modeling of the phase equilibrium of polymeric systems is becoming increasingly important for many industrial processes and products. Therefore, the knowledge on the phase behavior of polymer solutions is essential for the development of several polymer processes, such as the recovery and separation of organic vapors using polymeric membranes, the production of paints and coatings [13,14], the impregnation of polymers, the encapsulation of pharmaceutical substances inside biodegradable polymer matrices [15] and in the preparation of polymer nanocomposites and films using solution casting methods [16–18]. Furthermore, the phase behavior of polymer–solvent mixtures is momentous in polymer synthesis, as many polymeric products are produced *in solution* with a solvent (or a mixture of solvents) and often with other low-molecular-weight compounds (plasticizers, etc.).

In the last two years, there has been an increase in publications on the interactions study for polymer–solvent systems [11,19–21]. However, the expansion of accurate thermodynamic models for polymer solutions is also vital in the design of advanced polymeric materials and separation processes that utilize polymer solutions. The available thermodynamic models for the prediction of polymer solution properties can be classified into two main categories: base and van der Waals models. Some models are based on the van der Waals theory [22], whereas several authors [23–26] further developed models according to the lattice pattern.

Consequently, the modeling of a polymer solution needs an accurate equation of state to predict the phase equilibrium of such systems with appropriate mixing rules. Cubic equations of state are extensively applied in engineering, for computing phase equilibrium and the thermodynamic properties of simple mixtures.

Solution properties are generally interpreted by classical and statistical thermodynamic concepts [4,5,27]. The classical thermodynamic state of a system is described in terms of the macroscopically different variables (temperature and pressure), assuming continuity of matter. Instead, statistical mechanics explains matter properties at atomic and molecular scale (where continuity can be assured) through thermodynamic functions, allowing the deduction of other thermodynamic parameters.

The straightforward thermodynamic description of polymer solutions starts in most cases from the well-known Flory–Huggins (FH) theory [28,29]. Thus, the thermodynamics of binary polymer–solvent systems is based on the well-known lattice model, which evidences the effect of the differences in molecular size between the polymer and solvent molecules on the entropy of mixing. Quantitative calculation of the entropy of mixing led to the introduction of a dimensionless value, the so-called FH interaction parameter, χ, for the thermodynamic description of polymer solutions.

For deducing the equations that link the thermodynamic parameters to the molecular constants, a particular model for representing the solutions is necessary. The simplest model is the reticular one, where the ideal solution is composed of substances whose molecules are identical in size and chemical structure. The reticular model can serve to represent binary systems with low and high contents of solvent when the solvate may be considered a polymer or monomer, with the hydrogenated unit representing the structural unit model; when interchanging the positions of different types of molecules, an increase of the thermodynamic probability occurs and, consequently, the system entropy increases. The size of mixing entropy depends on the solvate, which may be either a polymer (the units are linked to each other) or a monomer (units are employed); the solvent molecules can change their place with that of the monomer molecules or polymer chain units. Therefore, the change in the interactions upon mixing (enthalpy of mixing) governs miscibility. The interactions considered here are not only short-range ones but also van der Waals interactions (also known as *dispersions*), hydrogen bonding, and dipole–dipole interactions. Figure 3.1 illustrates the change in the two-dimensional rendering of the lattice. ε_{SS}, ε_{PP}, and ε_{PS} represent the solvent–solvent, polymer–polymer, and polymer–solvent interactions, respectively. Mixing of the solvent with the polymer modifies the overall interaction energy (Equation 3.4) through the rearrangement of contacts.

$$\Delta\varepsilon = \varepsilon_{PS} - \frac{\varepsilon_{PP} + \varepsilon_{SS}}{2} \tag{3.4}$$

Consequently, parameter χ, called the *Flory–Huggins parameter*, is defined as the product of the lattice coordinate z and the energy change reduced by

$$\chi = \frac{z\Delta\varepsilon}{k_B T} \tag{3.5}$$

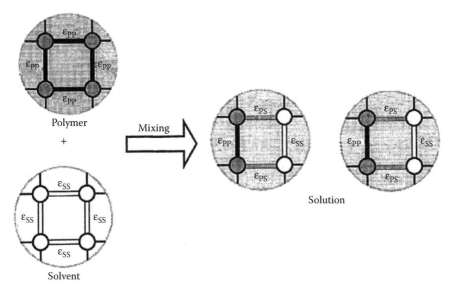

FIGURE 3.1   Schematic representations of the contacts produced by different types of interactions between nearest neighbors in macromolecular solutions, when a polymer chain is mixed with solvent molecules.

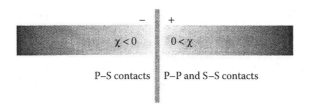

FIGURE 3.2   Variation of interaction parameter, χ: negative value promotes mixing of polymer with solvent, whereas positive value prefers polymer–polymer (P–P) and solvent–solvent (S–S) contacts to polymer–solvent (P–S) contacts.

A positive χ denotes that the polymer–solvent contacts are less favored compared with the polymer–polymer and solvent–solvent contacts (Figure 3.2). A negative value of χ means that polymer–solvent contacts are preferred, promoting the solvation of the polymer. In general, the magnitude of χ decreases with increasing temperature, because of (k_BT) in the denominator, but the pair of interactions also depends on the temperature in a manner characteristic to each polymer–solvent system.

Generally, for a spontaneous occurrence of any solution, the thermodynamics rules require that the Gibbs free energy change in the mixing process should be zero or negative. In a simplified description, the reduced molar Gibbs energy of mixing, $\Delta G_M/RT$, is given by the following equation:

$$\frac{\Delta G_M}{RT} = \left(x_1 \ln \varphi_1 + x_2 \ln \varphi_2 \right) + g\, x_1 \varphi_2 = \frac{\Delta G_M^C}{RT} + \frac{\Delta G_M^R}{RT} \tag{3.6}$$

where:

  R is the gas constant
  T is the temperature (K)
  x_i refer to mole fractions of components
  φ_i refer to volume fractions of components
  g is the P–S interaction parameter

The $(x_1 \ln \varphi_1 + x_2 \ln \varphi_2) = \Delta G_M^C / RT$ sum, of purely statistical origin, is called the *combinatorial part*, whereas the noncombinatorial part, $g x_1 \varphi_2 = \Delta G_M / RT$, constitutes the so-called reduced residual Gibbs energy of mixing.

Partial differentiation of $\Delta G_M / RT$ with respect to the number of moles of components, n_i, yields the reduced partial molar Gibbs energy of mixing of the solvent, $\Delta G_1 / RT$, and of the polymer, $\Delta G_2 / RT$, respectively, expressed in the following equations:

$$\frac{\Delta G_1}{RT} = \left\{ \ln(1 - \varphi_2) + \left[1 - \left(\frac{V_1}{V_2}\right)\right]\varphi_2 \right\} + \chi \varphi_2^2 = \frac{\Delta G_1^C}{RT} + \frac{\Delta G_1^R}{RT} \tag{3.7}$$

$$\frac{\Delta G_2}{RT} = \left\{ \ln(1 - \varphi_1) + \left[1 - \left(\frac{V_2}{V_1}\right)\right]\varphi_1 \right\} + \xi \left(\frac{V_2}{V_1}\right)\varphi_1^2 = \frac{\Delta G_2^C}{RT} + \frac{\Delta G_2^R}{RT} \tag{3.8}$$

where:

  V_i is the molar volume of components i
  χ and ξ are the FH parameters
  $\Delta G_i^C / RT$ and $\Delta G_i^R / RT$ are the combinatorial and the residual contributions of
    the reduced partial molar Gibbs energy of mixing of the components,
    respectively

Thus, the following expressions for the different interaction parameters are obtained, which demonstrate that their measure shows the deviations of a real polymer solution from the purely combinational behavior:

$$g = \frac{\Delta G_M^R}{RT x_1 \varphi_2} \tag{3.9}$$

$$\chi = \frac{\Delta G_1^R}{RT \varphi_2^2} \tag{3.10}$$

$$\xi = \frac{\Delta G_2^R}{RT(V_2/V_1)\varphi_1^2} \tag{3.11}$$

From phenomenological thermodynamics, one obtains the interrelation between these parameters, $g = f(\chi, \xi)$, $\chi = f(g)$, and $\xi = f(g)$ (Equations 3.12 through 3.14).

$$g = \varphi_2 \chi + (1 - \varphi_2)\xi \tag{3.12}$$

$$\chi = g - \left(1 - \varphi_2\right)\frac{\partial g}{\partial \varphi_2} \qquad (3.13)$$

$$\xi = g + \varphi_2 \frac{\partial g}{\partial \varphi_2} \qquad (3.14)$$

Rearrangement of Equation 3.7 leads to

$$\chi = \frac{\Delta G_1^R}{RT\varphi_2^2} = \left(\frac{\Delta G_1}{RT\varphi_2^2}\right) - \left(\frac{1}{\varphi_2^2}\right)\left\{\ln\left(1 - \varphi_2\right) + \left[1 - \left(\frac{V_1}{V_2}\right)\right]\varphi_2\right\} \qquad (3.15)$$

Because $\Delta G_1 = RT \ln a_1$, the interaction parameter, χ, is accessible from the calculated activity of solvent a_1, which represents the ratio between the partial vapor pressures of the solvent exceeding that of the solution and exceeding that of the pure solvent.

This parameter, which accounts for the specific interactions between polymer segments and solvent molecules, was at first considered to be independent on composition, but experiments have demonstrated the necessity of treating the FH parameter, χ, as being concentration dependent. For an analytical representation of the experimentally found concentration dependence, the following power series is normally adequate:

$$\chi = \chi_0 + \chi_1\varphi_2 + \chi_2\varphi_2^2 + \cdots \qquad (3.16)$$

Thus, the following three characteristics can be distinguished (Figure 3.3):

1. In the case of poor solvents, χ increases strongly with polymer concentration.
2. In the case of good solvents, χ seems to be independent on concentration.
3. In a few situations, mostly in the case of highly exothermal systems, χ decreases with concentration.

The interaction parameter, χ, measures the effect associated with the insertion of a solvent molecule between two polymer segments contacting each other. χ_0 is independent on the composition for sufficiently dilute solutions that can be described by binary intersegmental contacts.

The reduced molar Gibbs energy of mixing expressed in Equation 3.6 could be also written as follows:

$$\frac{\Delta G_M}{RT} = \left(x_1 \ln x_1 + x_2 \ln x_2\right) + \frac{\Delta G_M^E}{RT} = \frac{\Delta G_M^{\text{ideal}}}{RT} + \frac{\Delta G_M^E}{RT} \qquad (3.17)$$

where:
$\Delta G_M^E/RT$ is the reduced excess molar Gibbs energy of mixing

For the solvent, the partial reduced excess molar Gibbs energy will be as follows:

$$\frac{\Delta G_1}{RT} = \frac{\Delta G_1^{\text{ideal}}}{RT} + \frac{\Delta G_1^E}{RT} \qquad (3.18)$$

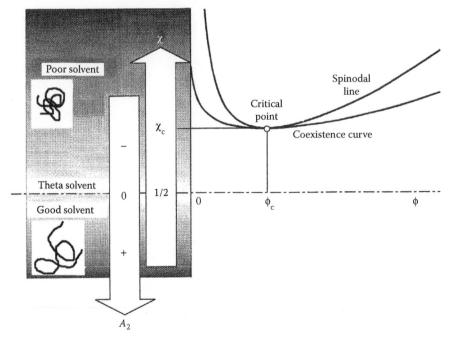

FIGURE 3.3 An illustration of variation of the second virial coefficient, A_2, and of interaction parameter, χ, as a function of solvent quality, together with the phase diagram. Chain conformation is influenced by the solvent.

where:

$$\Delta G_1^{ideal} = RT \ln x_1$$

This is related to osmotic pressure by the following equation:

$$\frac{\Delta G_1}{RT} = -\frac{\Pi V_1}{RT} = \frac{-c_2 V_1}{M} - c_2^2 V_1 A_2 \ldots \tag{3.19}$$

where:

    c_2 is the polymer concentration
    V_1 is the molar volume of the solvent
    A_2 is the second osmotic virial coefficient
    M is the average molecular weight of the polymer

Thus, in terms of the thermodynamic excess functions, one obtains for A_2 the following expression:

$$A_2 = \frac{-\Delta G_1^E}{RT c_2^2 V_1} \tag{3.20}$$

A_2, like χ_0, does not depend on c_2 and measures the effect of adding 1 mol of the solvent to the solution at any given constant composition within the concentration range of binary contacts. These contacts concern undivided solute molecules, considered invariable entities. The following relation between A_2 and χ_0 holds true:

$$A_2 = \frac{\left[(1/2) - \chi_0\right]}{\rho_2^2 V_1}$$

(3.21)

where:

ρ_2 is the polymer density ($\rho_2 = c_2/\varphi_2$)

Therefore, the polymer–solvent interactions could be discussed by studying A_2 and/or χ_0. These two parameters depend on solvent quality and temperature.

Despite the long-standing engagement in the thermodynamics of polymer solutions, our knowledge in some important areas is still rudimentary. One such example concerns the thermodynamic behavior of the polyelectrolyte solutions. This statement does not imply the absence of research on such systems; numerous studies have been performed on polyelectrolyte systems [20,30–32]. The difficulty with the reported knowledge lies in the fact that it refers to systems, which are, by nature, complex and contain a multitude of different components. For a more comprehensive understanding of the above-mentioned systems, it appears mandatory to dispose of reliable information concerning the thermodynamic behavior of the corresponding binary systems.

The thermodynamic description of polymer solutions starts in most cases from the FH theory. However, this approach was designed for solutions of linear chain-like macromolecules in low-molecular-weight solvents. In view of underlying the central assumption of combinatorial mixing as the reference behavior (placing the polymer segments on a lattice), this approach cannot be expected to hold true without fundamental changes for solutions of polyelectrolytes (because of their counterions), for globular proteins (because of their compact structure), or even for nonlinear-chain molecules (because of their molecular architecture). Such highly different characteristics of macromolecules constitute a considerable obstacle for a consistent modeling of ternary and multinary mixtures containing more than one type of polymer. In order to minimize artifacts due to systematic deviations of the individual approaches, it would be very helpful to apply a method that enables modeling of all binary subsystems with one and the same expression. Therefore, recent researches [19–21] suggest possibilities for a unified thermodynamic description encompassing solutions of all types of high-molecular-weight compounds. They attempt at a common mathematical representation of the solution behavior of polyelectrolytes and different types of macromolecular chains with different architecture.

The theoretical treatment rests on the laws of phenomenological thermodynamics. Thus, all specific contributions of systems are lumped together in the FH interaction parameter, χ, so that, for modeling polyelectrolyte systems, χ should be treated as depending on the composition, which normally requires two to three adjustable parameters. In an attempt to generalize and extend expression χ to cover different polymer architectures and to include charged macromolecules, Equation 3.7 can be rewritten as follows:

$$\frac{\Delta G_1}{RT} = a\varphi_2 + b\varphi_2^2 + c\varphi_2^2\left(1 - 2\varphi_2\right) + z\ln\left(1 - \varphi_2\right)$$

(3.22)

Quantitative modeling by means of a mathematical expression has considered the following requirements:

1. In view of the impracticality to use polymer segments defined in the usual manner for all types of polymers, factor $(1 - 1/N)$ is replaced by parameter a.
2. The second term of Equation 3.7 remains, but redefined as b; all parameters refer to the formation of binary contacts between the components established upon mixing of the pure substances (integral Gibbs energies).
3. A term quantified by parameter c is introduced, to account for extra effects (not covered by parameter b), resulting from the formation of triple contacts (polymer–polymer–solvent) or of other possible types of ternary heterocontacts (solvent–solvent–polymer).
4. Finally, the logarithmic term of the FH expression is modified; factor $(1 - \varphi_2)$ is replaced by the z specific constant of the system.

Parameters involved in Equation 3.21 are expressed by the following equations:

$$(a - z) = -\frac{V_1 \rho_2}{M} = -k \tag{3.23}$$

$$(b - z) = -V_1 A_2 \rho_2^2 = -l \tag{3.24}$$

Normally, the value of parameter k, introduced into Equation 3.23, is readily accessible from the known molar mass (M) and density of the polymer (ρ_2) plus the molar volume of the solvent. In contrast to k, the value of l (Equation 3.24) is normally not known experimentally, because of the lack of information on A_2. Insertion of a from Equation 3.23 into 3.22 leads to the following expression:

$$\frac{\Delta G_1}{RT} = (z - k)\varphi_2 + b\varphi_2^2 + c\varphi_2^2 (1 - 2\varphi_2) + z \ln(1 - \varphi_2) \tag{3.25}$$

Integration according to

$$\Delta G_M = -\frac{1}{1 - \varphi_2} \int_1^{\varphi_2} \Delta G_1 \varphi_2 \tag{3.26}$$

yields the reduced molar Gibbs energy of mixing as follows:

$$\frac{\Delta G_M}{RT} = z(1 - \varphi_2)\ln(1 - \varphi_2) + k\varphi_2 \ln \varphi_2 + b\varphi_2(1 - \varphi_2) - c(1 - \varphi_2)\varphi_2^2 \tag{3.27}$$

Compared with the classical FH theory, the present approach introduces two additional parameters: z and c. Parameter z modifies the contribution of the solvent to the FH combinatorial entropy of mixing. By analogy to the meaning of k, it can be interpreted as the inverse of the effective number of solvent segments. However, parameters z and k are no longer based on the volumes of the components, because this method would ignore possible contributions of the differences to the free volumes of the pure components and to their molecular shape. On the other hand, parameter c was introduced to account for the extra effects caused by the presence of an additional polymer molecule in the vicinity of a given solvent–polymer system. The analogous ternary interaction parameter for the presence of a further solvent molecule in the vicinity of a given solvent–polymer system can be neglected in the present context, but it may become important in special cases.

The above-discussed integral Gibbs energies of mixing need to be completed by the second derivative of Gibbs energies for the straightforward assessment of the phase state of polymer solutions. Equation 3.27 yields the following expression:

$$\frac{\partial\left(\Delta G_{M}/RT\right)}{\partial \varphi_2^2} = -2(b+c)+\frac{k}{\varphi_2}+\frac{z}{1-\varphi_2}+6c\varphi_2 \tag{3.28}$$

This enables the determination of the spinodal conditions from the requirement that the second derivative be zero at the border between metastable and unstable mixtures. The mathematical form of the expression resulting from the FH theory is regained by setting $z = 1$ and $c = 0$.

3.4 STATISTICAL THEORIES AND MATHEMATICAL APPROXIMATIONS FOR REAL POLYMERIC CHAINS: SHORT- AND LONG-RANGE INTERACTIONS

3.4.1 EXCLUDED VOLUME EFFECT

In real polymer chains, the effects of both the excluded volume and chain entanglements should be taken into account [33,34]. The concept of excluded volume is based on the fact that two polymer chain segments cannot occupy the same place in space; a segment excludes others by its own volume. This volume is a measure of the net interaction between two segments, with the solvent as a surrounding medium. Under specific conditions, determined by the nature of the polymer and solvent and by the temperature, this net interaction is zero. Flory has called the state satisfying such conditions as a *theta state*, which implies a *theta solvent* and a *theta temperature*. In this state, also called *unperturbed state*, a polymer molecule behaves like an ideal random flight chain.

Using a series of approximations [4,28], Flory has shown that the excluded volume leads to a significant increase of the average random coil dimensions and changes in the number of accessible conformers. Flory has also demonstrated that, in a thermodynamically *poor* solvent, the proper volume of chain segments could be balanced by their mutual attractions, leading to a pseudoideal state, highly similar to the Boyle point for real gases [33]. Typically, however, is the situation of a *good* solvent, where the effect of the excluded volume is large. Thus, solvents in which the net repulsive interactions between segments are large and the polymer coils are swollen with respect to their dimensions in a theta state are denoted as *good*. In these conditions, a positive volume effect appears. Thus, the excluded volume increases, passing from a bad solvent to a good one and, at a certain temperature (the theta temperature), it disappears.

Theta temperature, θ, is the most important thermodynamic parameter of polymer solutions. Around the θ temperature, the excluded volume is lower, and, therefore, the interactions are weak and can be treated in the Gaussian domain. The total energy of interaction between chains is given by Equation 3.29:

$$U = \sum_{i<j} V\left(r_{ij}\right) \tag{3.29}$$

where:

$V\left(r_{ij}\right)$ is the local potential and the formula $r_{ij} = r_i - r_j$ represents the connection vectors of monomers i and j

Fixman parameter, z, is defined by the following relation:

$$z = \left(\frac{2\pi}{3}\right)^{3/2} \frac{V}{a^3} N^{1/2} \tag{3.30}$$

The above equation expresses the energy of interaction between Gaussian chain segments, whose distance between the ends of the chain is R_0. In Equation 3.29, N and a are the number and length of the segments, respectively, and V is the excluded volume of the segments.

Theoretical investigations have established different equations, in which the second virial coefficient, A_2, and the expansion factor, α_s, depend on the short- and long-range interactions through the interpenetration function, $\Psi(z)$, defined by Equation 3.31.

$$\Psi(z) = \frac{A_2 M^2}{\left(4\pi^{3/2} N_A \left\langle s^2 \right\rangle^{3/2}\right)} \tag{3.31}$$

The equations belong to the so-called two-parameter theory [5,35]. Part of them became classical relations describing the excluded volume for linear, flexible uncharged polymers, and proved to be accurate in the small excluded volume regime. More theories and equations try to describe the static and large-scale properties of long-chain polymers in good solvents at infinite dilution. One can cite, for example, the lattice calculation of Domb and Barett [36,37], used over the whole range of excluded volume interactions, and/or the renormalization group theory of Douglas and Freed [38], which represents an approximate method for converting two-parameter calculations into three dimensions, to renormalize group expressions. Each theory has a limited applicability and validity, so that testing their reliability with experimental data on polymers in good solvents seems very attractive. Douglas and Freed [38] made a critical presentation of the existing theories *versus* experimental data and gave their interpretation over a large domain of the excluded volume.

The two-parameter theory of flexible polymers in dilute solution indicates that the expansion factor, α_s, and the interpenetration function, $\Psi(z)$, are universal functions of a single variable Z, defined as the excluded volume parameter.

$$Z = \left(\frac{1}{4\pi}\right)^{3/2} \left(\frac{B}{A^{3/2}}\right) M^{1/2} \tag{3.32}$$

where:

M is molecular weight of the polymer

$B = \beta/m^2$, β is the binary cluster integral for the interaction between repeating units, m is the molecular weight of the repeating unit of the polymer

$A = \langle S_0^2 \rangle / M$, $\langle S_0^2 \rangle$ is the unperturbed mean-square radius of gyration

Interpenetration is defined by the following:

$$\Psi(z) = \frac{A_2 M^2}{\left(4\pi^{3/2} N_A \langle S^2 \rangle^{3/2}\right)} \tag{3.33}$$

where:

N_A is Avogadro's number

$\langle S^2 \rangle$ represents the perturbed mean-square radius of gyration

Combination of different approximations permits the discussion of Z and $\Psi(z)$ calculated on the basis of different theoretical and approximate expressions established for α_s and $\Psi(z)$ [35] as follows:

- The original Flory theory of α_s and the original Flory–Krigbaum–Orofino theory of $\Psi(z)$ (combination F, o):

$$\alpha_s^5 - \alpha_s^3 = 2.60z \tag{3.34}$$

$$\Psi(z) = (2.30)^{-1} \ln(1 + 2.30Z) \tag{3.35}$$

- The modified Flory theory of α_s and the modified Flory–Krigbaum–Orofino theory of $\Psi(z)$ (combination F, m):

$$\alpha_s^5 - \alpha_s^3 = 1.276z \tag{3.36}$$

$$\Psi(z) = (5.73)^{-1} \ln(1 + 5.73Z) \tag{3.37}$$

- The Yamakawa–Tanaka theory of α_s and the Kurata–Yamakawa theory of $\Psi(z)$ (combination Y):

$$\alpha_s^2 = 0.541 + 0.459(1 + 6.04z)^{0.46} \tag{3.38}$$

$$\Psi(z) = 0.541[1 - (1 + 3.903Z)]^{-0.4683} \tag{3.39}$$

where:

$Z = z/\alpha_s^3$

- The Domb–Barrett expression [36] of α_s (obtained by interpolating computer data of self-avoiding lattice chains and two-parameter perturbation theory expansion in the small excluded volume regime):

$$\alpha_s^2 = 1.53 Z^{2/5}, \quad Z \gg 1 \tag{3.40}$$

- Huber–Stockmayer equations (derived from Equations 3.38 and 3.39):

$$\alpha_s^2 = 0.541 + 0.459\left(1 + 4.53 K z\right)^{0.45} \tag{3.41}$$

$$\Psi(z) = 0.638\left[1 + 1.3623 Q\left(\frac{z}{\alpha_s^3}\right)\right]^{-0.468} \tag{3.42}$$

where:
K and Q are functions of the contour length

- The renormalized two-parameter theory (RTP theory) of Douglas and Freed [38] of α_s and $\Psi(z)$:

$$\alpha_s^3 = \left(\frac{1 + 32z}{3}\right)^{3/8} (1 - 1.130\lambda_1)^{3/2}, \quad Z \le 0.15 \tag{3.43}$$

$$\alpha_s^3 = 2.26 z^{0.558}, \quad Z \ge 0.75 \tag{3.44}$$

$$\Psi(z) = 0.207\lambda_2 + 0.062\lambda_2^2 \tag{3.45}$$

where:

$$\lambda_1 = \frac{(32z/3)}{(1 + 32z/3)} \tag{3.46}$$

$$\lambda_2 = \frac{6.441z}{(1 + 6.44z)} \tag{3.47}$$

On the other hand, the renormalized group theory [39,40] evidences a strong coupling between the hydrodynamic interactions and the excluded volume, by examining the dependencies of α_H/α_s, α_η^3/α_s^3, and $\alpha_\eta^3/\alpha_s^2\alpha_H$ ratios on the excluded volume parameter, Z. Similar to the interpenetration function, $\Psi(z)$, Douglas and Freed define the *hydrodynamic penetration function* as a universal function of Z only within the nonfree-draining limit:

$$\Pi(z) = \left(\frac{A_2 M}{[\eta]}\right) = \left[2^{1/2}\left(\frac{2\pi}{6}\right)^{3/2}\left(\frac{N_A}{\Phi_0}\right)\frac{\Psi\alpha_s^3}{\alpha_\eta^3}\right] \tag{3.48}$$

which, in the RTP theory, turns to the following:

$$\Pi(z) = 3.64\left(0.207\lambda_2 + 0.062\lambda_2^2\right)\left(1 - 0.130\lambda_2\right)^{3/2}\left(1 - 0.276\lambda_2\right)^{-1} \tag{3.49}$$

where:

λ_2 is derived from Equation 3.47

α_η is expressed by

$$\alpha_\eta^3 = \frac{[\eta]}{[\eta]_\theta} = \left(\frac{\Phi}{\Phi_0}\right)\alpha_s^3 \tag{3.50}$$

where:

Φ is Flory viscosity factor and the subscript "0" refers to the unperturbed chain

In-field theoretic of renormalization group study of polyelectrolytes has been difficult to realize, due to their long-range Coulomb interactions. In addition, screening, complex-formation, counterion condensation and salt, and the comparable length scales of their interactions permit a comparison between theory and the experimental difficulties. Neutral polymers, on the other hand, have been successfully described by scaling ideas and renormalization group theories [32]. Literature proposed a new approach to the renormalization group theory applied to the study of screened charged chains, the so-called Debye–Huckel chains (DH) [41,42]. The formalism is developed considering that, at the range of the interaction, the Debye screening length represents an important and new parameter, independent on system size. This is fundamentally different from the systems usually studied in conventional statistical mechanics with short-range interactions, where the size of the system, or volume, is the only relevant macroscopic length-scale parameter upon which all extensive quantities depend by this volume.

3.4.2 Unperturbed Dimensions of PSF Chains

Under theta conditions, only short-range interactions are present. The molecules of polymeric chains obey the Gaussian statistics and may be regarded as being unperturbed. Literature [43,44] has pointed out investigations of the root-mean-square radius gyration in unperturbed state by different methods. In particular [45], the conformational properties of PSF and chloromethylated polysulfones (CMPSF) with different substitution degree (DS) (Scheme 3.1) in solutions of N,N-dimethylformamide (DMF) were evaluated from the modification of coil density (ρ—Equations 3.51 or 3.52) and gyration radius (R_g—Equation 3.53) at concentration values over both dilute and large domains (Figures 3.4 and 3.5).

$$\rho = \frac{c}{\eta_{sp}}\left(1.25 + 0.5\sqrt{56.4\eta_{sp} + 6.25}\right) \tag{3.51}$$

or

$$\rho = \frac{c*}{0.77^3}\left\{1 + \frac{[\eta] - [\eta]_\theta}{[\eta]_\theta}\left[1 - \exp\left(-\frac{c}{c*}\right)\right]\right\} \tag{3.52}$$

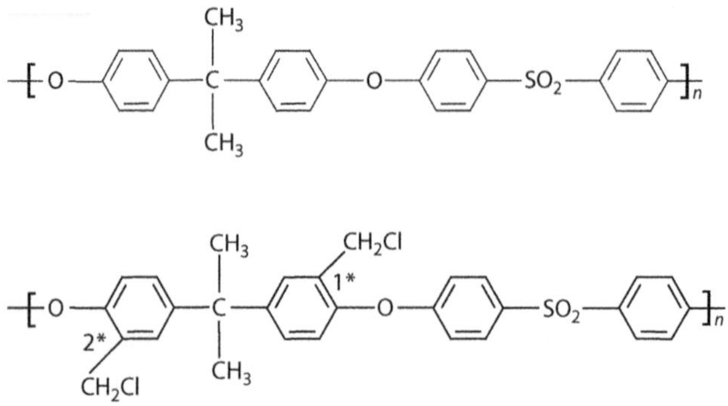

SCHEME 3.1 Chemical structures of the monomer unit of polysulfone (PSF) and chloromethylated polysulfone (CMPSF) with different substitution degrees (DS) (for CMPSF with DS < 1, the chloromethylation reaction of PSF may occur in position 1*, whereas for CMPSF with DS > 1, the chloromethylation reaction occurs in positions 1* and 2*).

$$R_g^3 = \frac{3M[\eta]}{3\phi\left\{1+\left[([\eta]-[\eta]_\theta)/[\eta]_\theta\right]\left[1-\exp(-[c/c^*])\right]\right\}} \qquad (3.53)$$

where:

η_{sp} is the specific viscosity

c is the polymer concentration

c^* is the critical concentration at which the polymer coils begin to overlap each other, defined by Equation 3.54

$[\eta]_\theta$ is the intrinsic viscosity in the unperturbed state, defined by Equation 3.55:

$$c^* = \frac{0.77}{[\eta]} \qquad (3.54)$$

$$[\eta]_\theta = \frac{[\eta]\left[1-\exp(-[c/c^*])\right]}{(0.77^3\rho/c^*)-\exp(-[c/c^*])} \qquad (3.55)$$

Polymer coil density increased with increasing polymer concentration, whereas at a critical concentration (c^+) from the semidilute domain, approximated as $c^+ \approx 8c^*$ [46,47], ρ remained constant. Thus, the density recorded at $c > c^+$ corresponded to the density in the unperturbed state. The critical concentrations c^* and c are delimited in Figure 3.4a for different temperatures. Figure 3.4b shows the same dependencies for PSFs and CMPSFs with different DS over a high concentration domain. Polymeric coil density in solution was higher for PSFs than for CMPSFs and decreased with increasing the DS.

Modification of ρ was reflected in the variation of R_g with concentration (Figure 3.5). The R_g values decreased with increasing concentration, whereas, at the critical concentration c (identical values with those from Figure 3.4a), they shrank to their unperturbed dimensions.

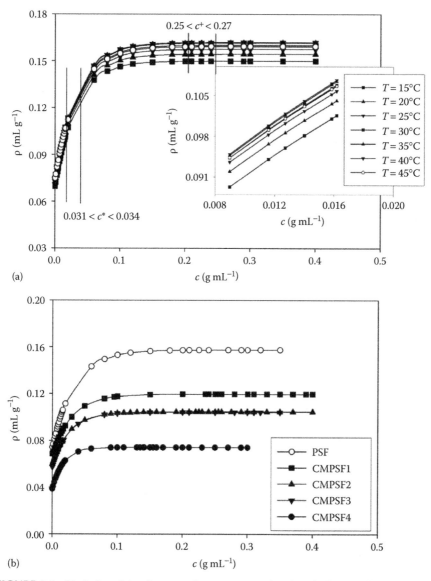

FIGURE 3.4 Variation of density over a large concentration domain for: (a) PSF in DMF at different temperatures. The small plot corresponds to the dilute solution domain; (b) PSF and CMPSFs in DMF at 25°C.

Furthermore, the dimensions in the solution were smaller for PSFs than for CMPSFs and increased with increasing the DS. Nevertheless, the ρ (Figure 3.4) and R_g (Figure 3.5) values of the CMPSF2 and CMPSF3 samples were close. This proximity may have been due to the small differences in DS, together with the possible errors in the analytical determination of the chlorine content.

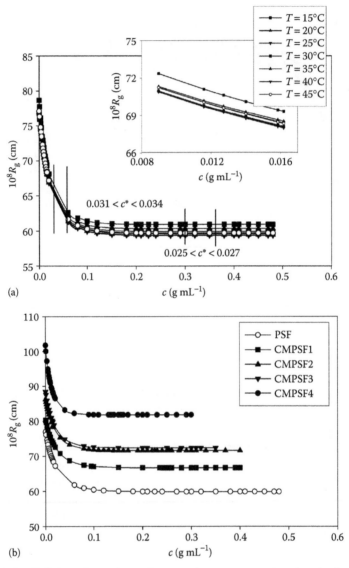

FIGURE 3.5 Variation of gyration radius on a large concentration domain for: (a) PSF in DMF at different temperatures. The small plot corresponds to the dilute solution domain; (b) PSF and CMPSFs in DMF at 25°C.

3.4.3 FLEXIBILITY OF THE UNPERTURBED PSF CHAINS

Generally, in the unperturbed state, the flexibility of macromolecular coils is determined by Flory's characteristic ratio, c_∞, and steric factor, σ. Literature [45] presents for PSFs and modified PSF chains, the effect of the free rotation around a bond, as a result of σ, using different mathematical approximations starting from a tetrahedral structural mode.

$$\sigma = \frac{(<r_0^2>/M)^{1/2}}{(<r_{0f}^2>/M)^{1/2}} \tag{3.56}$$

where:

$<r_0^2>^{1/2}$ is the mean-square end-to-end distance in the unperturbed state

$<r_{0f}^2>^{1/2}$ is the mean-square end-to-end distance in the unperturbed state calculated on the assumption of free rotation

$(<r_0^2>/M)^{1/2}$ was calculated from the Flory–Fox equation (Equation 3.57) considering K_θ from Equation 3.58 (Figure 3.6) and $\phi_0 = 2.87 \cdot 10^{23}$g/mol for $[\eta]$ expressed in mL/g. Figure 3.6 also presents the results obtained for $(<r_0^2>/M)^{1/2}$ at different temperatures.

$$\left(\frac{<r_0^2>}{M}\right)^{1/2} = \left(\frac{K_\theta}{\phi_0}\right)^{1/3} \tag{3.57}$$

$$[\eta]_\theta = K_\theta M^{1/2} \tag{3.58}$$

$(<r_{0f}^2>/M)^{1/2}$ was calculated by considering the different approximations in the tetrahedral model (Scheme 3.2).

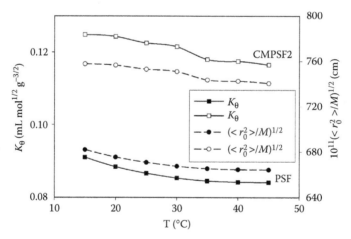

FIGURE 3.6 Variation of unperturbed dimension parameters, K_θ, and $(<r_0^2>/M)^{1/2}$, with temperature, for PSF and CMPSF2 in DMF.

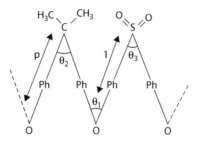

SCHEME 3.2 Structural (tetrahedral) model of the polysulfone chain.

The approximation of Schulz and Horbach [48] on polycarbonates with kindred structure to PSF, assumed that $l = 5.77$Å, corresponding to the bond through the phenylene moiety, $p = 1.43$Å corresponding to the C—O bond and $\theta_1 = \theta_2 = \theta_3 = 109.5$Å.

Thus, $(< r_{0f}^2 > /N) = 35.403 \cdot 10^{-16}$ cm^2 for PSF was obtained from the following relation:

$$\left(\frac{< r_{0f}^2 >}{N} \right) = \left(\frac{l^2 + p^2}{2} \right) \left(\frac{1 + \cos\theta}{1 - \cos\theta} \right) \qquad (3.59)$$

where:

   N is the total number of links or the number of rotating chain elements ($N = M/m_n$, with $m_n = 111$ for PSF)

Berry et al. [49] considered the same values for l, p, and θ angles, but calculated $(< r_{0f}^2 >/N)^{1/2}$ with the following relation:

$$\left(\frac{< r_{0f}^2 >}{N} \right) = \frac{l^2 + p^2}{2} \left[\frac{1 + \cos(\pi - \theta)}{1 - \cos(\pi - \theta)} \right] \left[1 - \frac{(l - p)^2}{(l^2 + p^2)} \right] \cos(\pi - \theta) \qquad (3.60)$$

Applied to PSF, this model gave $(< r_{0f}^2 > /N) = 29.70 \cdot 10^{-16}$ cm^2.

According to Allen et al. [50], the PSF chain consists of three valence angles, $\theta_1 = 123°$, $\theta_2 = 109.5°$ and $\theta_3 = 104°$, and two bond lengths, denoted as $l = 5.87$ Å and $p = 5.64$ Å. Because θ_2 and θ_3 are very close to the tetrahedral angle 109.5°, the first approximation of Allen et al. considered $\theta_1 = \theta_2 = \theta_3 = 109.5$ Å.

Thus, $(< r_{0f}^2 > /N) = 66.31 \cdot 10^{-16}$ cm^2 for PSF, as calculated with Equation 3.61:

$$\left(\frac{< r_{0f}^2 >}{N} \right)^{1/2} = \frac{l^2 + p^2}{2} \left[\frac{1 + \cos(\pi - \theta)}{1 - \cos(\pi - \theta)} \right] \left[1 - \frac{(l - p)^2}{(l^2 + p^2)} \right] \left[\frac{\cos(\pi - \theta)}{1 + \cos(\pi - \theta)} \right] \qquad (3.61)$$

In the second approximation of Allen et al., $\theta_1 = 123°$ and $\theta_2 = \theta_3 = 107°$. Thus, the problem becomes one of a molecule consisting of two valence angles and two bond lengths. In this case, $(< r_{0f}^2 >/N) = 78.64 \cdot 10^{-16}$ cm^2 was obtained from the following equation:

$$\left(\frac{< r_{0f}^2 >}{N} \right)^{1/2} = \left\{ \frac{(l^2 + p^2)\left[1 + \cos(\pi - \theta_1)\right]\left[1 + \cos(\pi - \theta_2)\right]}{2\left[1 - \cos(\pi - \theta_1)\right]\left[\cos(\pi - \theta_2)\right]} \right\}$$

$$\left\{ 1 - \frac{(l - p)^2 \cos(\pi - \theta_1)\left[1 - \cos(\pi - \theta_2)\right]}{(l^2 + p^2)\left[1 + \cos(\pi - \theta_1)\cos(\pi - \theta_2)\right]\left[1 + \cos(\pi - \theta_1)\right]} \right\} \qquad (3.62)$$

TABLE 3.1

Values of m_n, K_θ (mL mol$^{1/2}$ g$^{-3/2}$), $(< r_0^2 >/M)^{1/2}$ (cm), $(< r_{0f}^2 >/M)^{1/2}$ (cm), and σ for PSF and CMPSF Samples at 25°C

Sample	PSF	CMPSF1	CMPSF2	CMPSF3	CMPSF4
m_n	111	116	126	129	133
K_θ	0.0866	0.1114	0.1225	0.1209	0.1677
$(< r_0^2 >/M)^{1/2} \cdot 10^{11}$	670.7	729.4	752.9	749.6	836.0
$(< r_{0f}^2 >/M)^{1/2} \cdot 10^{11}$	565.0[a]	552.7[a]	530.3[a]	524.1[a]	516.1[a]
	517.3[b]	506.0[b]	485.5[b]	479.9[b]	472.6[b]
	772.9[c]	756.1[c]	725.4[c]	717.0[c]	706.1[c]
	841.7[d]	823.4[d]	790.0[d]	780.8[d]	769.0[d]
σ	1.2	1.3	1.4	1.4	1.6
	1.3	1.4	1.6	1.6	1.8
	0.8	0.9	1.0	1.0	1.2
	0.7	0.8	0.9	0.9	1.1

Sources: [a] Schulz, G. V. and Horbach, A., *Die Makromol. Chem.*, 29(1/2), 93–116, 1959.
[b] Berry, G. C. et al., *J. Polym. Sci. A-2 Polym. Phys.*, 5(1), 1–21, 1967.
[c,d] Allen, G. et al., *Eur. Polym. J.*, 5(1), 319–334, 1959.

Table 3.1 presents the $(< r_0^2 >/M)^{1/2}$ values comparable with the existing literature data for PSF [50], and the steric hindrances determined by different approximations. The very small values recorded for steric hindrance show that these polymers possessed very flexible coils and that most of the chain conformations available to the chains with free rotation were accessible to the real chains. These data do not, however, yield information on the height of the rotation barrier, which may be important in other contexts for defining a polymer coil as flexible [51]. However, comparative observations of the results from Table 3.1 revealed that the rigidity of CMPSFs increased with increasing the DS. Also, the approximately similar values obtained for steric hindrance at different temperatures confirm the stability of the molecular chains.

Allen et al. [50] mentioned that it was the phenylene ring system that caused the low value of steric hindrance, and not the nature of X in the polymers containing $-X-Ph-X-$ links. A significant consequence would appear to be the length of the rigid link and the apparently low energy difference between the various rotational isomers, because noticeable characteristic for these polymers was not only the very low value of σ but also the temperature dependence on chain dimensions. This conclusion was supported by the literature results that, for aliphatic PSFs with normal main chain linkages consisting of single σ-bonds, establish a steric hindrance of 1.71 (corresponding to poly(hexane-1 sulfone) [52,53]) or of 2.05, corresponding to poly(2-methyl-1-pentene-1 sulfone) [52].

3.5 THEORETICAL MODELS AND SIMULATIONS OF SPECIFIC INTERACTIONS IN MULTICOMPONENT POLYMER–SOLVENT–SOLVENT SYSTEMS

Investigation of the physicochemical properties of macromolecules in mixed solvents is of a major importance for a number of reasons:

1. Some macromolecules do not dissolve molecularly in single solvents, but molecular solutions can be obtained in mixed solvents.
2. A certain property of the solvent, a definite value of the second virial coefficient, or a particular value of the refractive index, for instance, is more often found in mixed than in single solvents.
3. Such an investigation leads to a better knowledge of the respective affinity of each solvent with regard to the macromolecule and its influence on the molecular dimensions of the polymer.

A dilute polymer solution can be considered as a two-phase system, the microphase being the polymer coil highly swollen with the solvent, and the other phase, the surrounding polymer-free solvent. The introduction of two solvents increases the number of possible interactions in solution; consequently, interactions between each of the two solvents and the polymer, solvent–solvent interactions, interactions between parts of the macromolecular chains, as well as polymer–solvent–solvent ternary interactions occur. The presence of interactions in ternary systems can be expressed by different parameters: preferential (λ_1) and total adsorption (Y), second virial coefficient (A_2), intrinsic viscosity ($[\eta]$), and interaction.

In a mixed solvent, the ratio of the two solvent components, solvent (1) and solvent (2), is different in each phase, due to the fact that generally, the polymer has a higher affinity for one of the solvents. Therefore, the concentration of this component is higher within the polymer molecules than in the surrounding polymer-free solvent. This phenomenon, first observed by Ewart et al. [54], is called *preferential adsorption*. In addition, the preferential adsorption behavior is markedly influenced by various factors [55–57]. One of them is the chemical structure of the polymer, which, apparently, is very important for the number of preferentially adsorbed solvent molecules. Particular interactions are of fundamental importance in the interpretation of preferential adsorption from a thermodynamic viewpoint.

Another characteristic feature of the polymer plus mixed solvent ternary system can be observed if one of the solvents is a good solvent [solvent (1)] and the other a nonsolvent [solvent (2)] of the polymer. In some cases, a mixture of two precipitants is, thermodynamically, a very good solvent for the polymer. These so-called cosolvent mixtures are characterized by an interesting preferential adsorption behavior [58]. In a cosolvent mixture, one component or the other is selectively adsorbed on the polymer, according to the composition of the mixture.

The conclusion to be drawn is that, at a given composition of the cosolvent mixture, the particular component sorbed on the polymer is the one that changes the composition of the mixture in the domain of polymer molecules for obtaining a thermodynamically most effective mixture. In the other cases, the polymer molecules exhibit the tendency of being surrounded by a thermodynamically most efficient solvent.

In the ternary phase, polymer segments are not uniformly distributed, and the magnitude of preferential adsorption in the coil varies from one volume element to another. An integral over the volume of the domain gives the total difference in the content of the component (1) between the coil domain and the same volume of the bulk solvent:

$$\lambda_1 = \frac{N_A}{M} \int (1 - \varphi_3) \varepsilon (\varphi_3) dV \qquad (3.63)$$

where:

λ_1 is the preferential adsorption related to the mass unit of the polymer

N_A is the Avogadro number

M is the molar mass of the polymer

The local preferential adsorption, ε, is defined by $\varepsilon = u_i - \varphi_{10}$, in which $\varphi_i (i = 1,2,3)$ is the volume fraction of component i in the coil domain $(\varphi_1 + \varphi_2 + \varphi_3 = 1)$, $u_i (i = 1,2)$ is the volume fraction of the solvent mixture in ternary phase, $u_i = \phi_i / (1 - \varphi_3)$, and $\varphi_{i0} (i = 1,2)$ is the volume fraction of component i in the bulk solvent, assumed to be equal to the composition of the solvent mixture prior to mixing with the polymer $(\varphi_{10} + \varphi_{20} = 1)$.

For very dilute solutions (very low values of φ_3), local preferential adsorption is proportional to the volume fraction of the polymer, and the proportionality constant A is the coefficient of preferential adsorption.

$$A = \lim_{\varphi_3 \to 0} \frac{\varepsilon}{\varphi_3} = \lim_{\varphi_3 \to 0} \frac{\lambda_1}{v_3} \qquad (3.64)$$

where:

v_3 is the partial specific volume of the polymer

For the given system, A depends only on the composition of the bulk solvent and on temperature.

Total adsorption can be related to the Schultz–Flory potential [59], Y, defined by equation:

$$Y = \lim_{\varphi_3 \to 0} \left(\frac{\Pi}{RT \varphi_3^2} \right) \qquad (3.65)$$

where:

Π is the osmotic pressure of a polymer solution with infinite molar mass

The statistic thermodynamic theory of equilibrium expansion of the coil led to several different equations, in which Y is calculated from the expansion coefficient,

α_s [60,61], and from the values of B (the long-range interaction parameter), according to the following equation:

$$Y = \frac{BV_0 N_A}{2v_3^2} \tag{3.66}$$

where:
V_0 is the molar volume of the solvent mixture, or from the second virial coefficient A_2, according to the following equation:

$$Y = \frac{V_1 A_2}{v_3^2} \frac{1}{F(x)} \tag{3.67}$$

$F(x)$ has given the excluded volume dependence; usually, $F(x) = 1$ [62,63]. It clearly appears that Y is not directly accessible from experiments, but it can be related to experimental parameters (α_s, B, A_2). Thus, the experimental and theoretical values of Y may be compared.

From a phenomenological viewpoint, λ_1 is a parameter directly accessible from experiments, by the dialysis equilibrium method (Equation 3.68), or by light scattering measurements (Equation 3.69).

$$\lambda_1 = \frac{(dn/dc_3)_\mu - (dn/dc_3)\varphi_{10}}{dn/d\varphi_{10}} \tag{3.68}$$

$$\lambda_1 = \frac{(dn/dc_3)_{\varphi_{10}} \left[(M_w^*/M_w)^{1/2} - 1 \right]}{dn/d\varphi_{10}} \tag{3.69}$$

where:
$(dn/dc_3)_{\varphi_{10}}$ is the refractive index increments of a polymer in a mixed solvent at fixed concentration of the low-molecular-weight components in both the solution and the solvent
$(dn/dc_3)_\mu$ is the refractive index increment when all the low-molecular-weight components have the same chemical potentials in both the solution and the solvent
$dn/d\varphi_{10}$ is the refractive index increment of the solvent [component (1)] with respect to the binary solvent of a given composition
M_w is the real molecular weight of the polymer
M_w^* is the apparent molecular weight, obtained by measuring light scattering in a solution of a mixed solvent

3.5.1 THEORY OF MULTICOMPONENT SYSTEMS: PREDICTIVE MOLECULAR THERMODYNAMIC APPROACHES

The theoretical treatment of the excluded volume parameters and preferential adsorption of one solvent components in multicomponent polymer–solvent–solvent systems is usually performed according to the thermodynamic theory—first with the FH model [59], as generalized by Pouchly et al. [64] (FHP) and improved by Campos [64–67] (FHPC), and later on with the equation of state theory [68–70] (Flory, Prigogine, Patterson formalism) (FPP). Generally, the theoretical values of the preferential adsorption coefficient in systems with specific interactions, such as the hydrogen bonding ones, differ from the experimental data. Horta et al. [71] and, recently, Soria et al. [72] and Garcia-Lopera et al. [73] underlined the importance of association phenomena in binary interaction parameters and elaborated the mathematical correction of preferential adsorption, by means of a theory based on multiple association equilibria.

3.5.1.1 FH Model

The theoretical treatment of λ_1 and Y is based on the general conditions of osmotic equilibrium between the volume element of the coil domain and the external solvent. Within the limits of infinite dilution of the polymer, $\varphi_3 \to 0$, one obtains [74–76].

$$\lambda_1 = -\bar{v}_3 \frac{M_{13}}{M_{11}} \tag{3.70}$$

$$Y = \frac{V_1}{2RT}\left(M_{33} - \frac{M_{13}^2}{M_{11}} \right) \tag{3.71}$$

Here, the symbol M_{ij} denotes the limiting values of partial derivatives.

$$M_{ij} = \lim_{u_3 \to 0}\left(\frac{\partial^2 G_u}{\partial u_i \partial u_j} \right) \tag{3.72}$$

where:
  G_u is the Gibbs energy of mixing the polymer with a unit volume of the mixed
    solvent, when molecular weight tends to infinity

Theoretical calculation of preferential and total adsorption with the relations suggested by Flory and Schultz [59] starting from the FH model ignores the existence of the ternary interaction parameter, g_T, but considers the differences in volume and molecular surface between the macromolecules and the solvents. Thus, the preferential adsorption coefficient, λ_1, can be evaluated by the following equation:

$$\lambda_1 = -\bar{v}_3 \varphi_{10}\varphi_{20} \frac{\left(\varphi_{10} - \varphi_{20}\right)g_{12} + g_{13}^o - rg_{23}^o + (r-1)}{r\varphi_{10} + \varphi_{20} - 2g_{12}\varphi_{10}\varphi_{20}} \tag{3.73}$$

where:
  g_{13}^o and g_{23}^o are the polymer–solvent interaction parameters at infinite dilution of
    polymer
  g_{12} is the interaction parameter between the two solvents in the ternary phase
  r is the molar volume ratio of solvents

3.5.1.2 Read Model

Starting again from the FH model, the Read equation [77] for λ_1 introduces a ternary interaction parameter, $g_T \equiv g_{123}$, and includes the concentration dependence of each of the binary interaction parameters.

$$\lambda_1 = -\bar{v}_3 \varphi_{10} \varphi_{20} \frac{\left(\varphi_{10} - \varphi_{20}\right)\left(g_{12} - g_T\right) + g_{13}^{\circ} - r g_{23}^{\circ} + (r-1)}{r\varphi_{10} + \varphi_{20} - 2g_{12}\varphi_{10}\varphi_{20}} \tag{3.74}$$

3.5.1.3 FHP Model

Pouchly, Zivny, and Solc [78] developed a theory of λ_1 and Y based on an extended FH model, including explicitly a ternary interaction parameter, g_T, and considering the concentration dependence of all interaction parameters. This formalism includes the binary polymer–solvent interaction parameters at infinite dilution, g_{13}°, g_{23}°, χ_{13}°, and χ_{23}°, and also the interaction parameter between solvents, g_{12}, which can be evaluated from independent experiments. According to Pouchly model, ternary interaction parameters at polymer infinite dilution, $g_T^{\circ}(u_1)$ and its derivatives, $(\partial g_T/\partial u_1)_{\varphi_3 \to 0}$ and $(\partial g_T/\partial \varphi_3)_{\varphi_3 \to 0}$, can be substituted by constants a_g and a_χ [78,79] (Equations 3.76 through 3.79), but they remain as adjustable constants for experimental data.

$$\chi_{i3}^{\circ} = g_{i3}^{\circ} - \left(\frac{\partial g_{i3}}{\partial \varphi_3}\right)_{\varphi_3 \to 0} , \quad i = 1,2 \tag{3.75}$$

$$g_T^{\circ}(u_1) = a_g g_{12}(u_1) \tag{3.76}$$

$$\left[\frac{\partial g_T(u_1, \varphi_3)}{\partial \varphi_3}\right]_{\varphi_3 \to 0} = a' g_{12}(u_1) \tag{3.77}$$

$$\chi_T^{\circ} = g_T^{\circ} - \frac{1}{2}\left(\frac{\partial g_T}{\partial \varphi_3}\right)_{\varphi_3 \to 0} \tag{3.78}$$

$$a_\chi = a_g - \frac{a'}{2} \tag{3.79}$$

In this way, the model is applied for the determination of preferential and total adsorption coefficients, with the following equations:

$$N_{11} = \frac{M_{11}V_1}{RT} = \frac{1}{\varphi_{10}} + \frac{r}{\varphi_{20}} + \frac{\partial^2\left(\varphi_{10}\varphi_{20}g_{12}\right)}{\partial\varphi_{10}^2} \tag{3.80}$$

$$N_{13} = \frac{M_{13}V_1}{RT} = r - 1 + g_{13}^{\circ} - r g_{23}^{\circ} - \frac{\partial\left[\varphi_{10}\varphi_{20}\left(g_{12}^{\circ} - g_T^{\circ}\right)\right]}{\partial\varphi_{10}} \tag{3.81}$$

$$N_{33} = \frac{M_{33}V_1}{RT} = \frac{1}{2}\left(\varphi_{10} + r\varphi_{20}\right) - \chi_{13}^{\circ}\varphi_{10} - r\chi_{23}^{\circ}\varphi_{20} + \varphi_{10}\varphi_{20}\left(g_{12}^{\circ} - g_T^{\circ} - \chi_T^{\circ}\right) \tag{3.82}$$

where:

$r = V_1 / V_2$

3.5.1.4 FHPC I Model

Figueruelo et al. [80,81] established new equations for g_T^o and $\left(\partial g_T / \partial \varphi_3\right)_{\varphi_3 \to 0}$ [obtained from expressions of $g_T(u_1, \varphi_3)$], proposed as a functions of the binary interaction parameters.

$$g_T^o(u_1) = g_{13}^o g_{23}^o \left\{ g_{12}(u_1) + \left[\frac{\partial g_{12}'(u_1, \varphi_3)}{\partial \varphi_3} \right]_{\varphi_3 \to 0} \right\} \tag{3.83}$$

$$\left[\frac{\partial g_{12}'(u_1, \varphi_3)}{\partial \varphi_3} \right]_{\varphi_3 \to 0} = \left[\frac{\partial g_T(u_1, \varphi_3)}{\partial \varphi_3} \right]_{\varphi_3 \to 0} \tag{3.84}$$

Starting from Equations 3.83 and 3.84, Figueruelo et al. obtained Equations 3.85 and 3.86:

$$\left(\frac{\partial g_T}{\partial \varphi_3} \right)_{\varphi_3 \to 0} = g_{12}(u_1) \frac{D}{1 - D} \tag{3.85}$$

$$g_T^o(u_1) = g_{12}(u_1) \left(\frac{g_{13}^o g_{23}^o}{1 - D} \right) \tag{3.86}$$

where, according to Equations 3.79 and 3.83, constants a_χ and a_g take the form:

$$a_\chi = \frac{2 g_{13}^o g_{23}^o - D}{2(1 - D)} \tag{3.87}$$

$$a_g = \frac{g_{13}^o g_{23}^o}{1 - D} \tag{3.88}$$

and

$$D = g_{13}^o \left(\frac{dg_{23}}{d\varphi_3} \right)_{\varphi_3 \to 0} + g_{23}^o \left(\frac{dg_{13}}{d\varphi_3} \right)_{\varphi_3 \to 0} \tag{3.89}$$

$$\left(\frac{dg_{i3}}{d\varphi_3} \right)_{\varphi_3 \to 0} = g_{i3}^o - \chi_{i3} \tag{3.90}$$

Also, by substituting Equations 3.85 and 3.86 in Equation 3.78, the following equation is obtained:

$$\chi_T^o(u_1) = g_{12}(u_1) \left[\frac{2 g_{13}^o g_{23}^o - D}{2(1 - D)} \right] \tag{3.91}$$

Based on these considerations, N_{13} (Equation 3.81) and N_{33} (Equation 3.82) are expressed as:

$$N_{13} = r - 1 + g_{13}^o - r g_{23}^o - \left(1 - \frac{g_{13}^o g_{23}^o}{1-D}\right) \frac{\partial\left(\varphi_{10}\varphi_{20}g_{12}\right)}{\partial\varphi_{10}} \tag{3.92}$$

$$N_{33} = \frac{1}{2}\left(\varphi_{10} + r\varphi_{20}\right) - \chi_{13}^o\varphi_{10} - r\chi_{23}^o\varphi_{20} + \left[1 - \frac{\left(2g_{13}^o g_{23}^o - D\right)}{1-D}\right]g_{12}\varphi_{10}\varphi_{20} \tag{3.93}$$

3.5.1.5 FHPC II Model

Later on, Campos et al. [65,67] proposed new equations for g_T^o, $\left(\partial g_T / \partial\varphi_3\right)_{\varphi_3\to 0}$, and $\chi_T^o(u_1)$:

$$g_T^o(u_1) = g_{12}(u_1)\frac{g_{13}^o g_{23}^o}{1-D'} \tag{3.94}$$

$$\left(\frac{\partial g_T}{\partial\varphi_3}\right)_{\varphi_3\to 0} = g_{12}(u_1)\frac{g_{13}^o g_{23}^o D'}{1-D'} \tag{3.95}$$

$$\chi_T^o(u_1) = g_{12}(u_1)g_{13}^o g_{23}^o \frac{\left(1 - D'/2\right)}{1-D'} \tag{3.96}$$

so that constants a_χ and a_g from Equations 3.76 and 3.77 take the following form:

$$a_\chi = \frac{g_{13}^o g_{23}^o (1 - D'/2)}{1-D'} \tag{3.97}$$

$$a_g = \frac{g_{13}^o g_{23}^o}{1-D'} \tag{3.98}$$

where:

$$D' = \frac{D}{2g_{13}^o g_{23}^o} \tag{3.99}$$

Finally, in the FHPC II model, N_{13} and N_{33} are expressed as follows.

$$N_{13} = r - 1 + g_{13}^o - r g_{23}^o - \left(1 - \frac{g_{13}^o g_{23}^o}{1-D'}\right) \frac{\partial\left(\varphi_{10}\varphi_{20}g_{12}\right)}{\partial\varphi_{10}} \tag{3.100}$$

$$N_{33} = \frac{1}{2}\left(\varphi_{10} + l\varphi_{20}\right) - \chi_{13}^o\varphi_{10} - r\chi_{23}^o\varphi_{20} + \left[1 - \frac{\left(2g_{13}^o g_{23}^o - D'\right)}{1-D'}\right]g_{12}\varphi_{10}\varphi_{20} \tag{3.101}$$

3.5.1.6   FPP Model

Based on the principles of Prigogine, Flory [4] developed a new approach more adequate to describe the thermodynamics of polymers in solution. Such a theory has been used to predict the variation of the interaction parameters, χ_{i3}, with polymer concentration, which, theoretically, is obtained as a consequence of the dissimilarities in free volume and molecular surface-to-volume ratio or in the contact sites between the polymer and solvents.

The theory of Flory was derived by Horta [69,70] (FPP formalism), who—starting from molecular parameters—considered the dissimilarities in free volume, α, and surface-to-volume ratio, S, between the polymer and solvents, whereas the differences between solvents are neglected, as in the FHP theory.

According to this model, the ternary interaction parameters can be calculated with Equations 3.102 and 3.103:

$$g_T^0(u_1) = g_{12}(u_1)\left[1 - \frac{V_1}{V_3}(S - \alpha)\right] \tag{3.102}$$

$$\left(\frac{\partial g_T}{\partial \varphi_3}\right)_{\varphi_3 \to 0} = \left[1 - 2\frac{V_1}{V_3}(S - \alpha) + \left(\frac{V_1}{V_3}\right)^2 S^2 - \alpha' - S\alpha\right] g_{12}(u_1) \tag{3.103}$$

and with the following expressions for the constants present in the previous equations:

$$a_\chi = \frac{1}{2}\left[1 - \left(\frac{V_1}{V_3}\right)^2 (S^2 - \alpha' - S\alpha)\right] \tag{3.104}$$

$$a_g = 1 - \frac{V_1}{V_3}(S - \alpha) \tag{3.105}$$

$$\alpha = \frac{\partial \ln V_1}{\partial \ln T}\frac{p_3^*}{p_1^*}\left(1 - \frac{T_3^*}{T_{12}^*}\right) \tag{3.106}$$

$$\alpha' = \alpha \frac{p_3^*}{p_{12}^*} \tag{3.107}$$

where:
  $V_i = V_i / V_i^*$ is the reduced volume of component i
  $S = S_i / S_{12}$ with S_i—the molecular surface-to-volume ratio
  p_i^* and T_i^* are characteristic reduced values for pressure and temperature, respectively, and subscript "12" stands for a liquid mixture considered as a single solvent having average properties

Campos et al. [65,67] showed that an empirical relationship exists between $g_T^0(u_1)$, $(\partial g_T / \partial \varphi_3)_{\varphi_3 \to 0}$, and $g_{12}(u_1)$:

$$k = \frac{g_T^0(u_1)}{g_{12}(u_1) + (\partial g_T / \partial \varphi_3)_{\varphi_3 \to 0}} \tag{3.108}$$

According to Horta [71],

$$k = \frac{1}{2}\left\{1 + \frac{1}{2}\left[\frac{(\bar{V}_1 / \bar{V}_3)^2 (S^2 - \alpha' - S\alpha)}{1 - (\bar{V}_1 / \bar{V}_3)(S - \alpha)}\right]\right\}^{-1} \tag{3.109}$$

and the results obtained for k, from Equation 3.108, for a few systems consisting of polymer-mixed solvents, agree with the results of Campos et al. [65,67]. Equation 3.80 for N_{11} is the same both in the FHP and FPP theories when the empirical values of g_{12} and its derivatives, with respect to solvent-mixture composition, are used.

3.5.1.7   FHPC III or FHPC-AE Model

In some cases, the description of ternary systems was not in agreement with the prediction of classical thermodynamic theories (FH formalism, as generalized by Pouchly, and of FPP theory), especially for strongly associating systems when nonrandom effects or specific interactions among the components of the polymer–solvent–solvent system are present. The difficulty of incorporating the effect of specific interactions in the free energy of mixing lies in how to quantify the local ordering effects associated with the formation of such interactions. In this framework, much works have been done to improve the mathematical solution of the lattice problem including chain connectivity and nonrandom mixing [82–84]. Although the established relationships between ternary and their corresponding binary parameters have been ascertained both phenomenologically and semiempirically for polymer-mixed solvents [65,80,81,85] and polymer blends in solution [86–88], the physical origin of the deviations described earlier could be explained by more advanced theories, such as the quasi-chemical model of Barker [3,89] or the association equilibria (AE) theory [72,73].

A thermodynamic treatment of polymer associations in aqueous media has been developed, allowing a quantitative prediction of the association behavior of polymers, starting from their molecular structures and solution conditions. The treatment combines the general thermodynamic principles with detailed molecular models with various contributions to the free energy of mixture. In this context, the AE theory assumes that thermodynamic equilibrium is reached among the complexes, formed from single molecules by hydrogen bonding (or any other strong specific interaction) and the nonassociated species. Therefore, the AE theory has been successfully applied to two main types of ternary polymeric systems:

1. Those in which one of the liquids from the solvent mixture is an active solvent, a self-associating species with proton-donor character, that also interacts specifically with the polymer (a proton-acceptor) [90].
2. A more usual picture consists of a solvent being self-associating and proton-donor, with the other liquid and the polymer being both proton-acceptor species [72,73].

In the AE theory, the existence of association complexes is assumed and the thermo-dynamic functions of mixture, such as the Gibbs free energy, are deduced from the AE constants. Thus, according to this theory, the Gibbs free energy function for a ternary polymeric system with specific interactions is written as follows [73]:

$$
\left(\frac{\Delta G}{RT}\right)_{\text{Ter}} = v_1 \ln\frac{P_1}{P_1^0} + v_2 \ln\frac{P_2}{P_2^0} + v_3 \ln\frac{P_3}{P_3^0} - \sum_q v_q + \varphi_1\left(\sum_q v_q\right)_1^0 + \varphi_2\left(\sum_q v_q\right)_2^0
$$

$$
+ \varphi_3\left(\sum_q v_q\right)_3^0 + v_1\varphi_2 g_{12}' + v_1\varphi_3 g_{13}' + v_2 r_2 \varphi_3 g_{23}'
$$
(3.110)

where:
P_i is the molar fraction of the free component i ($i = 1$, 2, or 3) per mole of total lattice sites ($P_i = n_i/n_T$)
superscript "0" refers to the value of component i when it is alone in the lattice (the pure component)
parameter g_{ij}' expresses all specific binary interactions. Therefore, the three last terms containing g_{ij}' represent the enthalpic term of Gibbs function

Application of Equation 3.110 to ternary polymeric systems requires the statement of all potential specific interactions between the components of the system, which can lead to the formation of multicomponent complexes according to different equilibrium processes. Consequently, the possible thermodynamic equilibria occurring in ternary polymeric system are as follows:

1. Self-association of solvent "1" molecules, according to equilibrium: $S1_{\alpha-1} + S1 \xleftrightarrow{\sigma_{11}} S1_\alpha$. This process may be defined by a single equilibrium constant, σ_{11}, assuming that the equal reactivity principle is valid.
2. Interassociation of solvent "1" and solvent "2" molecules to form a 1–2 complex: $S1 + S2 \xleftrightarrow{\eta_{12}} S1S2$, followed by association of the free molecules of solvent "1" to the above complex: $S1_{\alpha-1}S2 + S1 \xleftrightarrow{\sigma_{12}} S1_\alpha S2$. Both processes are governed by the equilibrium constants, η_{12} and σ_{12}, respectively.
3. Interassociation of solvent "1" and a segment of polymer chain "3" to form a 1–3 complex: $S1 + P3 \xleftrightarrow{\eta_{13}} S1P3$, followed by the association of the free molecules of solvent "1" to the above complex, according to: $S1_{\alpha-1}P3 + S1 \xleftrightarrow{\sigma_{13}} S1_\alpha P3$. In this case, both equilibria are represented by the η_{13} and σ_{13} constants, respectively.

The complete and detailed mathematical derivation of the terms in Equation 3.110 as a function of the association constants necessary to calculate the thermodynamic magnitudes is as follows:

$$
P_1 = \frac{Y + X - \left(X^2 + 2XY\right)^{1/2}}{\sigma_{11}Y}
$$
(3.111)

where:
$$Y = 2\sigma_{11}\varphi_1$$
$$X = 1 + s\eta_{12}\varphi_2 + mr\eta_{13}\varphi_3$$

$$P_2 = s\varphi_2 \left[\frac{1 - \sigma_{12}P_1}{1 - (\sigma_{12} - \eta_{12})P_1} \right] \tag{3.112}$$

$$P_3 = r\phi_3 \left[\frac{1 - \sigma_{13}P_1}{1 - (\sigma_{13} - \eta_{13})P_1} \right]^m \tag{3.113}$$

where:
$$r = V_3/V_1$$
$$s = V_1/V_2$$

Superscript m is derived from component "3," when the polymer with m independent interaction sites manifests a specific polymer–solvent interaction

The corresponding P_1^0 values are deduced from Equations 3.111 through 3.113, reminding that, when $\varphi_i = 1$ (pure component), the rest of the volume fractions are equal to zero, so that

$$P_1^0 = \frac{2\sigma_{11} + 1 - (1 + 4\sigma_{11})^{1/2}}{2\sigma_{11}^2} \tag{3.114}$$

$$P_2^0 = s \tag{3.115}$$

$$P_3^0 = r \tag{3.116}$$

The $\left(P_i/P_i^0 \right)$ ratios for the three components, also present in Equation 3.110, in terms of specific interaction constants, are as follows:

$$\frac{P_1}{P_1^0} = \frac{Y + X - \left(X^2 + 2XY\right)^{1/2}}{\varphi_1 \left[2\sigma_{11} + 1 - (1 + 4\sigma_{11})^{1/2} \right]} \tag{3.117}$$

$$\frac{P_2}{P_2^0} = \varphi_2 \left[\frac{1 - \sigma_{12}P_1}{1(\sigma_{12} - \eta_{12})P_1} \right] \tag{3.118}$$

$$\frac{P_3}{P_3^0} = \varphi_3 \left[\frac{1 - \sigma_{13}P_1}{1 - (\sigma_{13} - \eta_{13})P_1} \right]^m \tag{3.119}$$

Finally, the substitution of these terms into Equation 3.110 allows to obtain the complete expression for the Gibbs free energy of the total process as a function of the association constants (σ_{11}, σ_{12}, η_{12}, σ_{13}, and η_{13}) given by Equation 3.120.

$$\left(\frac{\Delta G}{RT}\right)_{\text{Ter}} = \varphi_1 \ln \left\{ \frac{Y + X - \left(X^2 + 2XY\right)^{1/2}}{\varphi_1 \left[2\sigma_{11} + 1 - \left(1 + 4\sigma_{11}\right)^{1/2}\right]} \right\} + s\varphi_2 \ln \left[\varphi_2 \frac{1 - \sigma_{12}P_1}{1 - \left(\sigma_{12} - \eta_{12}\right)P_1}\right]$$

$$+ r\varphi_3 \ln \left[\varphi_3 \frac{1 - \sigma_{13}P_1}{1 - \left(\sigma_{13} - \eta_{13}\right)P_1}\right]^m - \frac{P_1}{1 - \sigma_{11}P_1} \tag{3.120}$$

$$+ \varphi_1 \left[\frac{2\sigma_{11} + 1 - \left(1 + 4\sigma_{11}\right)^{1/2}}{\sigma_{11}\left(1 + 4\sigma_{11}\right)^{1/2} - \sigma_{11}}\right] + \varphi_1\varphi_2 g_{12}' + \varphi_1\varphi_3 g_{13}' + \varphi_2\varphi_3 g_{23}'$$

Undoubtedly, it is easy to demonstrate that, when the association constants are canceled, Equation 3.120 is transformed into an equation corresponding to the classical FH theory (Equation 3.121).

$$\frac{\Delta G^M}{n_1 + n_2 r_2 + n_3 r_3} = \frac{\Delta G^M}{n_T} = RT \left(\begin{array}{c} \varphi_1 \ln \varphi_1 + \dfrac{V_1}{V_2} \varphi_2 \ln \varphi_2 + \dfrac{V_1}{V_3} \varphi_3 \ln \varphi_3 \\ + \varphi_1\varphi_2 g_{12} + \varphi_1\varphi_3 g_{13} + \varphi_2\varphi_3 g_{23} \end{array} \right) \tag{3.121}$$

Consequently, both theories can be combined to adequately describe ternary systems with specific proton-donor/proton-acceptor interactions. Therefore, the combination of both FH and AE models allows the assessment of a new parameter, named *excess function*, Δg_{ij}, that serves at correcting the contribution of all possible binary specific interactions established among the three components of the system (Equation 3.122):

$$\Delta g_{ij} = g_{ij}' - g_{ij} \tag{3.122}$$

where:
g_{ij}' includes all types of interactions in the system
g_{ij} represents the nonspecific interaction parameter

Literature [72,73] distinguishes the following systems with specific interactions:

- *Proton-donor solvent (1)/proton-acceptor solvent (2) binary system*
  The absence of component "3" ($\varphi_3 = 0$) simplifies Equations 3.120 and 3.121, derived from the FH and AE theories, to the following equation:

$$\left(\frac{\Delta G}{RT}\right)_{12} = \varphi_1 \ln \varphi_1 + s\varphi_2 \ln \varphi_2 + \varphi_1\varphi_2 g_{12} \tag{3.123}$$

$$\left(\frac{\Delta G}{RT}\right)_{12} = \varphi_1 \ln \frac{P_1}{P_1^0} + s\varphi_2 \ln \frac{P_2}{P_2^0} - \frac{P_1}{1 - \sigma_{11}P_1} + \varphi_1 \frac{P_1^0}{1 - \sigma_{11}P_1^0} + \varphi_1\varphi_2 g_{12}' \tag{3.124}$$

Therefore, for the same system composition, by equating Equations 3.123 and 3.124, the excess function, Δg_{12}, is defined as follows:

$$\Delta g_{12} = g'_{12} - g_{12} = \frac{1}{\varphi_2} \ln \frac{P_1}{P_1^0} + \frac{s}{\varphi_1} \ln \frac{P_2}{P_2^0} - \frac{1}{\varphi_1 \varphi_2} \left(\frac{P_1}{1 - \sigma_{11} P_1} \right)$$

$$+ \frac{1}{\varphi_2} \left(\frac{P_1^0}{1 - \sigma_{11} P_1^0} \right) - \frac{\ln \varphi_1}{\varphi_2} - \frac{s \ln \varphi_2}{\varphi_1}$$

(3.125)

This composition-dependent parameter quantifies the specific 1–2 interactions. It is easy to prove from Equation 3.125 that, in the absence of specific interactions, the new parameter should be equal to zero ($\Delta g_{12} = 0$), since, in these circumstances, $\sigma_{11} = \sigma_{12} = \eta_{12} = 0$, $P_1 = \varphi_1$, $P_1^0 = 1$, $P_2 = s \varphi_2$, and $P_2^0 = s$.

- *Proton-donor solvent (1)/proton-acceptor polymer (3) binary system*
  Following the same procedure, the absence of component "2" ($\varphi_2 = 0$) simplifies Equations 3.120 and 3.121:

$$\left(\frac{\Delta G}{RT} \right)_{13} = \varphi_1 \ln \varphi_1 + r \varphi_3 \ln \varphi_3 + \varphi_1 \varphi_3 g_{13}$$

(3.126)

$$\left(\frac{\Delta G}{RT} \right)_{13} = \varphi_1 \ln \frac{P_1}{P_1^0} + r \varphi_3 \ln \frac{P_3}{P_3^0} - \frac{P_1}{1 - \sigma_{11} P_1} + \varphi_1 \frac{P_1^0}{1 - \sigma_{11} P_1^0} + \varphi_1 \varphi_3 g'_{13}$$

(3.127)

Now, Equations 3.126 and 3.127 can be equated for a given system composition, whereas, by the subtraction of $\left(g'_{13} - g_{13} \right)$, another new excess function which quantifies the specific 1–3 interactions, Δg_{13}, is defined by Equation 3.128.

$$\Delta g_{13} = g'_{13} - g_{13} = \frac{1}{\varphi_3} \ln \frac{P_1}{P_1^0} + \frac{r}{\varphi_1} \ln \frac{P_3}{P_3^0} - \frac{1}{\varphi_1 \varphi_3} \left(\frac{P_1}{1 - \sigma_{11} P_1} \right)$$

$$+ \frac{1}{\varphi_3} \left(\frac{P_1^0}{1 - \sigma_{11} P_1^0} \right) - \frac{\ln \varphi_1}{\varphi_3} - \frac{r \ln \varphi_3}{\varphi_1}$$

(3.128)

In the absence of specific interactions, $\Delta g_{13} = 0$; in this case, $\sigma_{11} = \sigma_{13} = \eta_{13} = 0$, $P_1 = \varphi_1$, $P_1^0 = 1$, $P_3 = r \varphi_3$, and $P_3^0 = r$.

According to Equations 3.125 and 3.128, it can be argued that the lower values of the excess function and free energy and, therefore, the more stabilized system are a consequence of the specific *i–j* interactions. Concomitantly, the values of $\Delta g_{13} < \Delta g_{12}$ demonstrate that the specific 1–3 interactions are stronger than the 1–2 ones and are dominant to a higher extent.

- *Proton-donor solvent (2)/proton-acceptor polymer (3) binary system*
  Finally, following the same methodology, the absence of component "1" ($\varphi_1 = 0$) leads to the following expressions for the Gibbs free energy, according to the FH and EA theories:

$$\left(\frac{\Delta G}{RT}\right)_{23} = s\varphi_2 \ln\varphi_2 + r\varphi_3 \ln\varphi_3 + \varphi_2\varphi_3 g_{23} \tag{3.129}$$

$$\left(\frac{\Delta G}{RT}\right)_{23} = s\varphi_2 \ln\frac{P_2}{P_2^0} + r\varphi_3 \ln\frac{P_3}{P_3^0} + \varphi_2\varphi_3 g_{23}' \tag{3.130}$$

$$= s\varphi_2 \ln\varphi_2 + r\varphi_3 \ln\varphi_3 + \varphi_2\varphi_3 g_{23}'$$

For this system, at a given composition, the Δg_{23} excess function is defined by the following equation:

$$\Delta g_{23} = g_{23}' - g_{23} = \frac{1}{\varphi_3}\ln\frac{P_2}{P_2^0} + \frac{r}{\varphi_2}\ln\frac{P_3}{P_3^0} - \frac{1}{\varphi_2\varphi_3}\left(\frac{P_2}{1-\sigma_{11}P_2}\right)$$

$$+ \frac{1}{\varphi_3}\left(\frac{P_2}{1-\sigma_{11}P_2^0}\right) - \frac{\ln\varphi_2}{\varphi_3} - \frac{r\ln\varphi_3}{\varphi_2} \tag{3.131}$$

It is assumed that, if the two equations (3.129 and 3.130) are equated, the subtraction of $\left(g_{23}' - g_{23}\right)$ is equal to zero. This suggests that nonspecific interactions are established between components "2" and "3," because both are proton-acceptor species.

3.5.2 THEORETICAL CONTRIBUTIONS TO SPECIFIC INTERACTIONS IN TERNARY SYSTEM FUNCTIONALIZED PSF-MIXED SOLVENTS

Preferential adsorption, expressed in terms of thermodynamic functions, can be theoretically evaluated and discussed *versus* experimental data obtained on the basis of various approximations, in order to establish the experiment-theory correspondence. In this context, the literature [91–93] shows that theoretical and experimental results on the preferential adsorption coefficients, λ_1, of quaternized polysulfones (PSFQ) *versus* solvent's composition can be discussed in correlation with the interaction parameters of polymer-mixed solvents. The solvent systems were selected according to the ionic chlorine content of quaternized PSFs, which dictated the solubility in *N*,*N*-dimethylformamide (DMF)/methanol (MeOH), DMF/water, or MeOH/water solvent mixtures. Thus, DMF solvates quaternized PSF with an ionic chlorine content of 2.15% (PSFQ1), while increasing the quaternization degree augments the solubility in MeOH; thus, MeOH solvates quaternized PSF with content in ionic chlorine of 5.71% (PSFQ2).

In order to determine the theoretical preferential adsorption coefficients, the knowledge of the solvent–solvent interaction parameter, g_{12}, of the polymer–solvent interaction parameters, g_{i3} and χ_{i3} (subscript $i = 1$ refers to DMF or MeOH, whereas subscript $i = 2$ refers to water, and subscript "3" refers to quaternized PSFs), and of the ternary interaction parameters, g_T and χ_T, is necessary.

The solvent–solvent interaction parameter, g_{12}, is determined by FH equation [71]:

$$g_{12} = \left[\frac{G^E}{RT} + x_1\ln\left(\frac{x_1}{\varphi_1}\right) + x_2\ln\left(\frac{x_2}{\varphi_2}\right)\right]\frac{1}{x_1\varphi_2} \tag{3.132}$$

where:

x_{1,2} and $\varphi_{1,2}$ are the mole and volume fractions of the mixture solvents, respectively
G^E is the Gibbs free energy of the mixture solvents, calculated from the following
equation [94]:

$$\frac{G^E}{V_m \varphi_1 \varphi_2} = (\delta_1 - \delta_2)^2 \tag{3.133}$$

where:

V_m is the molar volume of the mixed solvents
$\delta_1 = 24.7 \sqrt{J/cm^3}$ or $\delta_1 = 29.7 \sqrt{J/cm^3}$ is the solubility parameter of DMF
or MeOH, respectively
$\delta_2 = 47.9 \sqrt{J/cm^3}$ is the solubility parameter of water [95]

Excess free energy, $G^E > 0$, for DMF/MeOH (Figure 3.7a), and DMF/water or
MeOH/water solvent mixtures (Figure 3.7b) is depicted as a function of the volume
fraction of DMF and water, respectively.

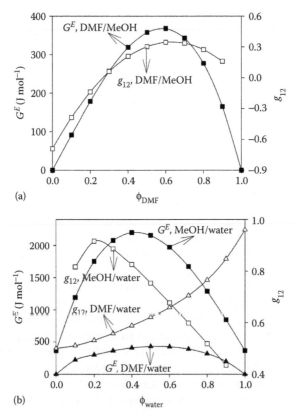

(a)

(b)

FIGURE 3.7 Excess free energy and solvent–solvent interaction parameters as a function of
the DMF volume fraction for DMF/MeOH binary mixtures (a), and as a function of the water
volume fraction for DMF/water and MeOH/water binary mixtures (b).

A decrease of G^E from the maximum value, corresponding to $\lambda_1 = 0$, to zero, leads to a thermodynamically more stable system. Thus, the preferential adsorption coefficient is related to this variation and to the magnitude of G^E. The g_{12} functions obtained at $T = 298K$, presented in Figure 3.7, are as follows:

$$g_{12} = -0.69 + 3.29\varphi_1 - 2.61\varphi_1^2, \text{ for DMF (1)/MeOH (2) system} \tag{3.134}$$

$$g_{12} = 0.95 - 1.12\varphi_1 + 1.10\varphi_1^2 - 0.44\varphi_1^3, \text{ for DMF(1)/water (2) system} \tag{3.135}$$

$$g_{12} = 2.45 + 0.09\varphi_1 + 6.36\varphi_1^2 - 5.67\varphi_1^3, \text{ for MeOH (1)/water (2) system} \tag{3.136}$$

The polymer–solvent interaction parameters, χ_{i3}, are calculated considering the entropic and enthalpic contributions [95]:

$$\chi_{i3} = \frac{V_1}{RT}\left(\delta_{1,2} - \delta_3\right)^2 + 0.34 \tag{3.137}$$

where:
R is the gas constant
T is Kelvin temperature
V_1 is the molar volume of solvent "1"

Also, the quaternized PSF–solvent interaction parameter, g_{i3}, is calculated from Equation 3.138 with the lattice coordination number $z = 8$:

$$\chi_{i3} = \left(1 - \frac{2}{z}\right)g_{i3} \tag{3.138}$$

The solubility parameter for quaternized PSFs, δ_3, is calculated by applying the group contributions of Fedors and van Krevelen–Hoftyzer [92,96], which involves the following steps:

- Calculation of the zero-order connectivity indices ${}^0\chi$ and ${}^0\chi^v$ and the first-order connectivity indices ${}^1\chi$ and ${}^1\chi^v$.

$$ {}^0\chi \equiv \sum\left(\frac{1}{\sqrt{\delta}}\right) \tag{3.139}$$

$$ {}^0\chi^v \equiv \sum\left(\frac{1}{\sqrt{\delta^v}}\right) \tag{3.140}$$

$$ \beta_{ij} \equiv \delta_i\delta_j \tag{3.141}$$

$$ \beta_{ij}^v = \delta_i^v\delta_j^v \tag{3.142}$$

$$^1\chi \equiv \sum \left(\frac{1}{\sqrt{\beta}} \right) \tag{3.143}$$

$$^1\chi^v \equiv \sum \left(\frac{1}{\sqrt{\beta^v}} \right) \tag{3.144}$$

The values of simple connectivity atomic indices, δ, and the valence connectivity indices, δ^v, used in the calculations, are listed in Table 3.2.

- Calculation of cohesive energy by two methods: (a) Equations 3.145 through 3.147 and (b) Equations 3.148 and 3.149, as follows:
  - Calculation of cohesive energy by applying the group contributions of Fedors (Equations 3.145 through 3.147):

$$E_{coh}(1) \approx 9882.5 \ ^1\chi + 358.7(6N_{atomic} + 5N_{group}) \tag{3.145}$$

$$N_{atomic} \equiv 4N_{(-S-)} + 12N_{sulfone} - N_F + 3N_{Cl} + 5N_{Br} + 7N_{cyanide} \tag{3.146}$$

where:

$N_{(-S-)}$ is the number of sulfur atoms in the lowest (divalent) oxidation state

$N_{sulfone}$ is the number of sulfur atoms in the highest oxidation state (commonly in $-SO_2$)

N_F is the number of fluorine atoms

N_{Cl} is the number of chlorine atoms

N_{Br} is the number of bromine atoms

$N_{cyanide}$ is the number of $-C\equiv N$ groups

TABLE 3.2

Values of δ and δ^v Used for the Calculation of Zero- and First-Order Connectivity Indices

Atom	Hy[a]	N_H[b]	δ	δ^v	Atom	Hyb	N_H	δ	δ^v
C	sp^3	3	1	1	N	sp^3	0	3	5
		2	2	2	O	sp^3	1	1	5
		0	4	4			0	2	6
	sp^2	1	2	3	S	sp^{3c}	0	4	8/3
		0	3	4	Cl	–	0	1	7/9

Sources: Bicerano, J., *J. Macromol. Sci. Part C Polym. Rev.*, 36(1), 161–196, 1996.

[a] Hybridization state

[b] The number of hydrogen atoms

[c] These numbers refer to sulfur in its highest oxidation state, as typically encountered in the bonding configuration $R-SO_2-R'$.

$$N_{group} \equiv 4N_{hydroxyl} + 12N_{amide} + 2N_{(nonamide\text{-}(NH)\text{-}unit)}$$

$$+ 4N_{(nonamide\text{-}(C=O)\text{-}next\ to\ nitrogen)}$$

$$+ 7N_{(\text{-}(C=O)\text{-}in\ carboxylic\ acid,\ ketone,\ or\ aldehyde)} \qquad (3.147)$$

$$+ 2N_{(other\text{-}(C=O)\text{-})} - N_{(alkyl\ ether\text{-}O\text{-})}$$

$$- N_{C=C} + 4N_{(nitrogen\ atoms\ in\ six\text{-}membered\ aromatic\ rings)}$$

where:

$N_{hydroxyl}$ is the number of $-OH$

N_{amide} is the number of amide groups

$N_{(nonamide\text{-}(NH)\text{-}unit)}$ is the number of NH units from the nonamide structure

$N_{(nonamide\text{-}(C=O)\text{-}next\ to\ nitrogen)}$ is the number of C=O units from the nonamide structure next to nitrogen

$N_{(\text{-}(C=O)\text{-}in\ carboxylic\ acid,\ ketone\ or\ aldehyde)}$ is the number of C=O groups in carboxylic acid, ketone, or aldehyde structures

$N_{(other\text{-}(C=O)\text{-})}$ is the number of other C=O groups

$N_{(alkyl\ ether\text{-}O\text{-})}$ is the number of alkyl ether $-O-$ groups

$N_{C=C}$ is the number of carbon–carbon double bonds, excluding any such bonds found along the edges of the rings

$N_{(nitrogen\ atoms\ in\ six\text{-}membered\ aromatic\ rings)}$ is the number of nitrogen atoms in six-membered aromatic rings

- Calculation of cohesive energy applying the group contributions of van Krevelen and Hoftyzer (Equations 3.148 and 3.149):

$$E_{coh}(2) \approx 10570.9(^{0}\chi^{v} - {}^{0}\chi) + 9072.8(2{}^{1}\chi - {}^{1}\chi^{v}) + 1018.2N_{VKH} \qquad (3.148)$$

$$N_{VKH} \equiv N_{Si} + 3N_{(\text{-}S\text{-})} + 36N_{sulfone} + 4N_{Cl} + 2N_{Br}$$

$$+ 12N_{cyanide} + 16N_{(nonamide\text{-}(C=O)\text{-}next\ to\ nitrogen)}$$

$$+ 7N_{(nitrogen\ atoms\ in\ six\text{-}membered\ aromatic\ rings)}$$

$$+ 12N_{cyanide} + 2N_{(nitrogen\ with\ \delta\ =\ 2,\ but\ not\ adjacent\ to\ C=O,\ and\ not\ in\ a\ six\text{-}membered\ aromatic\ rings)} \qquad (3.149)$$

$$+ 20N_{(carboxylic\ acid)} + 33N_{HB} - 4N_{cyc}$$

$$+ 19N_{anhydride} + \sum (4 - N_{row})_{(substituents\ with\ \delta=1\ attached\ to\ aromatic\ rings\ in\ the\ backbone)}$$

where:

N_{Si} is the number of silicon atoms

$N_{(carboxylic\ acid)}$ is the number of carboxylic acids

N_{HB} is the total number of strongly hydrogen-bonded structural units, such as alcohol or phenol-type hydroxyl (—OH) groups and amide groups (the —OH groups in carboxylic acid and sulfonic acid moieties are not counted in N_{HB})

N_{cyc}—number of nonaromatic rings (i.e., *cyclic* structures) with no double bonds along any of the ring edges. When more than one such ring shares the edges, N_{cyc} is determined by using simple counting rules, which avoids double counting of any of the shared edges, and may result in a noninteger value of N_{cyc}

$N_{anhydride}$ is the number of anhydride groups

N_{row} is the row of an atom in the periodic table. The methyl (—CH$_3$) groups and halogen atoms are substituents with $\delta = 1$, bonded to only one nonhydrogen atom, commonly encountered in polymers

$N_{(nitrogen\ with\ \delta\ =\ 2,\ but\ not\ adjacent\ to\ C=O,\ and\ not\ in\ a\ six-membered\ aromatic\ rings)}$ is the number of nitrogen atoms with specification from subscript.

- Calculation of the molar volume, V_3, at room temperature (298K), according to the following equations:

$$V_3(298K) \approx 3.642770\ ^0\chi + 9.798697\ ^0\chi^v - 8.542819\ ^1\chi$$
$$+ 21.693912\ ^1\chi^v + 0.978655\,N_{MV} \tag{3.150}$$

$$N_{MV} \equiv 24N_{Si} - 18N_{(-S-)} - 5N_{sulfone} - 7N_{Cl} - 16N_{Br} + 2N_{(backbone\ ester)}$$
$$+ 3N_{ether} + 5N_{carbonate} + 5N_{C=C} - 11N_{cyc} - 7(N_{fused} - 1) \tag{3.151}$$

(last term only to be used if $N_{fused} \geq 2$)

where:
  $N_{(backbone\ ester)}$ is the number of ester (—COO—) groups in the backbone of the repeating units

  N_{ether} is the total number of ether (—O—) linkages in the polymeric repeating unit. Note that only the (—O—) linkages between two carbon atoms will be counted as ether linkages in N_{ether}

  $N_{carbonate}$ is the number of carbonate (—O—COO—) groups

  N_{fused} is the number of rings in fused-ring structures. A *fused-ring* structure is defined in the present context as any ring structure containing at least one aromatic ring that shares at least one edge with another ring and with all the other rings with which it shares an edge.

- Calculation of solubility parameter, δ_3, at room temperature [2,97]:

$$\delta_3(298K) \equiv \left[\frac{E_{coh}}{V_3(298K)}\right]^{1/2} \tag{3.152}$$

The resulting values obtained for the polymer–solvent interaction parameters (Equations 3.137 and 3.138) are presented in Table 3.3.

The values of the ternary interaction parameters, g_T and χ_T, (Table 3.4) are calculated according to the FHPC II model [91,92], with coefficients a_g and a_χ from Equations 3.97 through 3.99.

Figures 3.8 and 3.9 plot graphically the theoretical values of the preferential adsorption coefficients calculated according to the FHPC II model. For both studied ternary systems, PSFQ1/DMF/MeOH (Figure 3.8a) and PSFQ2/DMF/MeOH (Figure 3.8b), the experimental results for λ_1, determined from refractive index increments, both before and after attaining dialysis equilibrium (Equation 3.68), are better fitted by the FHPC II model. However, the most important deviations between

TABLE 3.3

Binary Polymer–Solvent Interaction Parameters

Ternary System	PSFQ1(3)/ DMF(1)/MeOH(2)	PSFQ2(3)/ DMF(1)/MeOH(2)	PSFQ1(3)/ DMF(1)/Water(2)	PSFQ2(3)/ MeOH(1)/Water(2)
χ_{13}	0.347	0.370	0.347	0.895
χ_{23}	0.804	0.895	0.586	0.517
g_{13}	0.463	0.493	0.463	1.193
g_{23}	1.072	1.193	0.781	0.689

TABLE 3.4

Theoretical Values of Ternary Interaction Parameters g_T and χ_T

Sample	ϕ_1 (DMF)	g_T	χ_T	ϕ_2 (water)	g_T	χ_T
	0.2	−0.0958	−0.0838	0.1	0.246	0.215
	0.3	0.0499	0.0436	0.2	0.256	0.224
	0.4	0.1312	0.1148	0.3	0.269	0.235
	0.5	0.1843	0.1612	0.4	0.284	0.248
PSFQ1	0.6	0.2197	0.1922	0.5	0.299	0.262
	0.7	0.2361	0.2066	0.6	0.318	0.278
	0.8	0.2177	0.1905	0.7	0.340	0.297
	0.9	0.0078	0.0681	0.8	0.369	0.323
	1	Indefinite	Indefinite			
	0	Indefinite	Indefinite	0.2	4.142	3.624
	0.1	−0.2978	−0.2606	0.3	4.055	3.548
	0.2	−0.1134	−0.0992	0.4	3.877	3.393
	0.3	0.0590	0.0517	0.5	3.667	3.209
PSFQ2	0.4	0.1553	0.1359	0.6	3.443	3.013
	0.5	0.2182	0.1910	0.7	3.213	2.811
	0.6	0.2601	0.2276	0.8	2.979	2.606
	0.7	0.2796	0.2447			
	0.8	0.2578	0.2256			

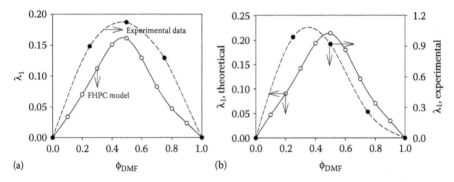

FIGURE 3.8 Theoretical (FHPC II model) and experimental values of the preferential adsorption coefficients as a function of the volume fraction of DMF for: (a) PSFQ1/DMF/MeOH and (b) PSFQ2/DMF/MeOH ternary systems.

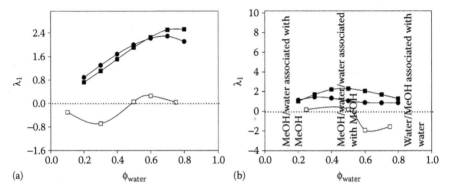

FIGURE 3.9 Theoretical [(■)—FHPC I and (●)—FHPC II] and experimental (□) values of the preferential adsorption coefficients as a function of the volume fraction of water for: (a) PSFQ1/DMF/water and (b) PSFQ2/MeOH/water ternary systems.

theoretical and experimental data appear for quaternized PSFs with a higher content of charged groups (PSFQ2), due to the electrostatic interactions (negligible in the calculation of the polymer–solvent interaction parameters).

Unlike these systems, in the case of ternary systems containing polar components (e.g., PSFQ1/DMF/water and PSFQ2/MeOH/water), the specific interactions between polar groups are important, and the formation of hydrogen bonds should be taken into account. In addition, three distinct ranges of water composition, in which the solvent mixture will show highly different interactive properties, may be clearly evidenced in Figure 3.9b.

Theoretical calculation of the preferential adsorption coefficient starting from the FHP model ignores the existence of electrostatic interactions. Therefore, the experimental results for λ_1 (Figure 3.9) do not fit with the FHP model for both studied systems. Important deviations appear in the theoretical data, due to the electrostatic interactions that are neglected in the calculation of the interaction parameters, g_{i3} and χ_{i3}, and also due to some association phenomena, when alcohol is a component of the system, which influences the g_{12} interaction parameters.

3.5.3   MOLECULAR DYNAMICS SIMULATIONS OF ASSOCIATION PHENOMENA IN FUNCTIONALIZED PSF SOLUTIONS

Theoretical studies of polyelectrolytes through molecular dynamics are important for their use in high-performance fields. Realistic models on the charge density of polyelectrolytes suggest that the ions in the conductive process situated along a polymer chain determine breaking bonds between ions and polymer segments and the renewal of these bonds with other segments of the same or another polymer [98–100]. Models that depict particle motion as hopping between neighboring sites or ion sites on a two-dimensional lattice have been reported. Chain motions are simulated by periodical redistribution at different times, so that the model reproduces the dependence of ion transport on polymer motion [101]. Accordingly, there is a strong coupling between ion motion and segmental relaxation in such a way that the understanding of ionic behavior in polyelectrolytes requires a detailed knowledge of all specific interactions from these systems.

In addition, in water-organic solvent binary mixtures, molecular associations are easily formed as a result of the balance of intermolecular interactions, depending on the water-organic solvent mixing ratio [102,103]. These structural formations influence the solvation and preferential adsorption of solvents. Generally, the theoretical values of the preferential adsorption coefficient in systems with specific interactions, such as hydrogen bonding, differ from the experimental ones.

From this reason, recent researches [72,73,104,105] stated the importance of association phenomena in theoretical evaluation of interaction parameters, and elaborated the mathematical correction of preferential adsorption by means of a theory based on multiple association equilibria (FHPC-AE), developed for neutral polymers. This investigation represents a new method for understanding the behavior of quaternized PSFs compound. In this context, the investigations can be correlated with the computerized chemical structure of quaternized PSFs, which provides a generalized view on the chemical conformations of the repeating units (Scheme 3.3). These molecular

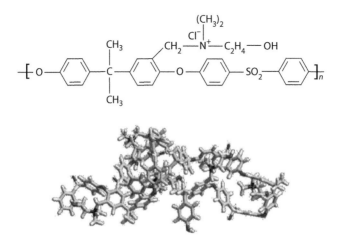

SCHEME 3.3   Chemical structure of the monomer unit of polysulfones with quaternary groups (PSFQ) and conformational structure with minimized energies, considering four repeating units.

simulations were performed with the HyperChem 8.0.7 professional program (demo version) (a graphic professional program that allows for rapid structure building, geometry optimization, and molecular display), with Amber 99 force field approximation and Polak-Ribiere conjugate gradient, in vacuum, at 0K [106]. This representation helps to identify the aspects of molecular structure that may be relevant to the interactions problem here under consideration.

Differences observed between the experimental and theoretical data obtained by the FHPC I and II models (Figure 3.9) for quaternized PSFs (3) (proton-acceptor)/ DMF (1) or MeOH (1) (proton-donor)/water (2) (proton-acceptor) ternary systems can be interpreted by this new approach. Therefore, the possible specific interactions, such as hydrogen bonding and dispersive interactions from ternary systems, and also the electrostatic interactions induced by the ionic groups from the polymeric structure, which generate association phenomena, are established. Consequently, different association constants are considered for the correction of binary and ternary interaction parameters, g_{12}, g_{13}, g_{23} and g_T, as follows:

- σ_{11}, obtained by the self-association of solvent (1) molecules (Scheme 3.4a).
- η_{12}, obtained by the interassociation of solvent (1) molecules with solvent (2) molecules, leading to the 1–2 complex (Scheme 3.4b).
- σ_{12}, obtained by the association of the free molecules of solvent (1) to the 1–2 aforementioned complex (Scheme 3.4b).
- η_{13}, obtained by the interassociation of solvent (1) molecules with segments of the polymer chain (3), leading to the 1–3 complex (Scheme 3.4c).
- σ_{13}, obtained by the association of the free molecules of solvent (1) to the 1–3 aforementioned complex (Scheme 3.4c).

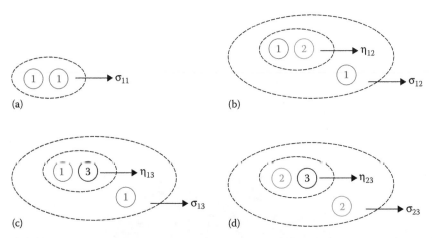

SCHEME 3.4 Graphical representation of molecular associations: (a) the self-association of solvent (1) molecules; (b) the interassociation of solvent (1) molecules with solvent (2) molecules; (c) the interassociation of solvent (1) molecules with segments of the polymer chain (3); (d) the interassociation of solvent (2) molecules with polymer chain segment (3). "1" is solvent (1) (DMF or MeOH), "2" is solvent (2) (MeOH or water), and "3" is polymer (PSFQ1 or PSFQ2).

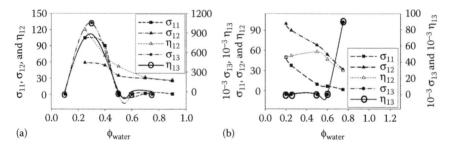

FIGURE 3.10 Association constants determined by mathematical simulations, as adjusted parameters, to fit the theoretical values of preferential adsorption to the experimental data, for: PSFQ1/DMF/water (a) and PSFQ2/MeOH/water (b) ternary systems.

- η_{23}, obtained by the interassociation of solvent (2) molecules with polymer chain segment (3), leading to the 2–3 complex (Scheme 3.4d).
- σ_{23}, obtained by the association of the free molecules of solvent (2) to the 2–3 aforementioned complex (Scheme 3.4d).

The hydrogen bonding, dispersive interactions, and electrostatic interactions are reciprocally influenced, depending on the mixed solvents composition and on PSFQ charge density. Figure 3.10 presents association constants determined by mathematical simulations, as parameters adjusted to fit the theoretical values of preferential adsorption to the experimental data.

As known, the mixing of DMF or MeOH with water will induce changes in the formation of hydrogen bonding and dipolar interactions [107]. Figure 3.10a illustrates the association phenomena generated by hydrogen bonding, dispersive interactions, and electrostatic interactions, for PSFQ1/DMF/water ternary system, by the σ_{11}, η_{12}, σ_{12}, η_{13}, and σ_{13} constants, as a function of the composition of solvent mixtures. In the absence of polymer, the DMF molecules may exhibit hydrogen bonding interactions with the coexistent water associations. At a low DMF content, isolated associations, represented by DMF–water associations and the self-association of water [102], appear, whereas at a higher DMF content, the association structure is obviously reorganized, and DMF self-association is remarkably promoted.

On the other hand, the preferential adsorption of PSFQ1 (with low charge density) will be controlled by the hydrogen bonding and weak electrostatic interactions, which occur especially at high water content. Thus, Figure 3.10a, depicting the different association constants reorganized by the presence of PSFQ1, evidences the following:

1. $\eta_{23} = 0$ and $\sigma_{23} = 0$, as no specific interactions are established between components "2" and "3"; both are proton-acceptor species, and the electrostatic interactions are negligible, due to the low charge density of PSFQ1.
2. Instead, influenced by the presence of the polymer, η_{12} and σ_{12} decrease with increasing the DMF content.
3. σ_{11}, η_{13}, and σ_{13} can be correlated with preferential adsorption; an inflexion point is observed for these association constants at $\varphi_2 = 0.48$, as in the case of the preferential adsorption coefficient (Figure 3.9a).

Second, water provides strong polar interactions but very weak dispersive interactions, whereas methanol, besides providing polar interactions, evidences dispersive interactions; by increasing the methanol content of the mixture, the dispersive character increases. However, the interactive character of the methanol/water mixtures is complicated by strong associations between methanol and water [104]. Thus, at high water contents, mixed solvents are formed from water and methanol associated with water. Reversely, at high methanol compositions, the mixture consists largely of methanol and water associated with methanol. Only at intermediate compositions (40%–80% v/v methanol), the system can be considered as a ternary mixture of methanol, water, and, predominantly, water associated with methanol (Figure 3.9b).

PSFQ2, with a 5.71% ionic chlorine content, could be studied over the MeOH/water composition range of 25%–80% v/v, where:

1. The methanol–water associations are predominant and the unassociated methanol and water may generate less electrostatic interactions with PSFQ2.
2. The hydrogen bondings contribute to η_{13}, σ_{13}, being nonsignificant for η_{23} and σ_{23}.
3. The reduced electrostatic interactions and the absence of hydrogen bonding between components "2" and "3" explain why $\eta_{23} = 0$ and $\sigma_{23} = 0$.

Figure 3.10b reflects the hydrogen bonding and the possible electrostatic interactions on the basis of the σ_{11}, η_{12}, σ_{12}, η_{13}, and σ_{13} association constants. The preferential adsorption illustrated in Figure 3.9b, influenced by these estimations, can be explained in terms of the specific interactions balance.

Finally, the excess functions, Δg_{12}, Δg_{13}, and Δg_{23}, and implicitly the new binary interaction parameters, g'_{12}, g'_{13}, and g'_{23}, are corrected on the basis of these association constants (Equations 3.125, 3.128, and 3.131) for the PSFQ1 (3)/DMF (1)/water (2) (Figure 3.11a) and PSFQ2 (3)/MeOH (1)/water (2) (Figure 3.11b) ternary systems. In addition, one should mention that, for the aforementioned ternary systems, $\Delta g_{23} = g'_{23} - g_{23} = 0$, as both component "2" (water) and "3" (PSFQ1 and PSFQ2) are proton-acceptor species.

The Gibbs free energy of the total process and, implicitly, the preferential adsorption coefficients are corrected on the basis of these association constants. Thus, Figure 3.12 shows the theoretical adsorption coefficients calculated with the new interaction parameters, g'_{12}, g'_{13}, and g'_{23}, introduced in Equations 3.125, 3.128, and 3.131—FHPC-AE, as well as those based on the FHPC theory.

An optimum agreement is observed between the predicted values obtained with the association constants and the experimental data. As a result, mathematical simulations allow a good theoretical description of the preferential adsorption coefficients, in agreement with experimental data. Therefore, for attaining a thorough agreement between the experimental and the theoretical data, the AE theory has been successfully applied to systems, in which one of the liquids of the solvent mixture is an active solvent- a self-associating species with proton-donor character (i.e., DMF or MeOH)-, which also interacts specifically with the polymer (a proton acceptor). On the contrary [91], when both solvents have a proton-donor character and the polymer has a proton-acceptor character, that is, in PSFQ1/DMF/MeOH and PSFQ2/DMF/MeOH systems, the experimental results for λ_1 are better fitted to the original FHPC model (Equations 3.70, 3.100, and 3.101).

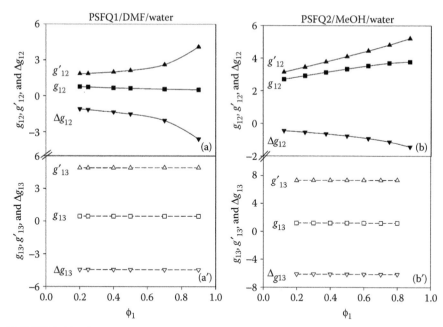

FIGURE 3.11 Interaction parameters for: (a), (a') PSFQ1 (3) in DMF (1)/water (2) mixed solvents: (a) g_{12}—noncorrected DMF–water interaction parameters (FHPC), g'_{12}—DMF–water interaction parameters corrected according to FHPC-AE, Δg_{12}—excess functions; (a') g_{13}—noncorrected DMF–PSFQ1 interaction parameters (FHPC), g'_{13}—DMF–PSFQ1 interaction parameters corrected according to FHPC-AE, Δg_{13}—excess functions; (b), (b') PSFQ2 (3) in MeOH/water mixed solvents: (b) g_{12}—noncorrected MeOH–water interaction parameters, g'_{12}—MeOH–water interaction parameters corrected according to FHPC-AE, Δg_{12}—excess functions; (b') g_{13}—noncorrected MeOH-PSFQ2 interaction parameters, g'_{13}—MeOH–PSFQ2 interaction parameters corrected according to FHPC-AE, Δg_{13}—excess functions.

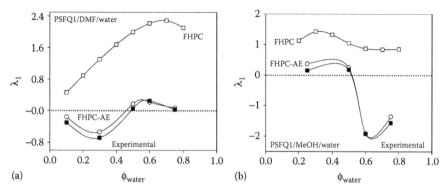

FIGURE 3.12 Theoretical [FHPC II (□) and FHPC-AE (o) models] and experimental (■) values of the preferential adsorption coefficients as a function of the volume fraction of water for: (a) PSFQ1/DMF/water and (b) PSFQ2/MeOH/water ternary systems.

Unlike aforementioned systems, which contain functionalized PSFs with different ionic chlorine content, other AE were identified in the literature [105], with different implications of the association constants on the specific interactions for systems of PSFs with different alkyl side groups.

The inductive effect of the alkyl groups with eight carbon atoms from the quaternized polysulfone PSF-DMOA, is higher than that of the alkyl group with two carbon atoms from the quaternized polysulfone PSF-DMEA. This effect determines the proton-acceptor character of both samples, in which the electronegativity of PSF-DMOA is higher than that of PSF-DMEA. As a result, ternary systems are formed by proton-acceptor (PSF-DMEA or PSF-DMOA) in proton-donor (DMF)/proton-donor (MeOH) or in proton-donor (DMF)/proton-acceptor (water) solvent mixtures. Scheme 3.5 presents the general chemical and conformational structures of PSF-DMEA and PSF-DMOA, obtained by a computerized method [106].

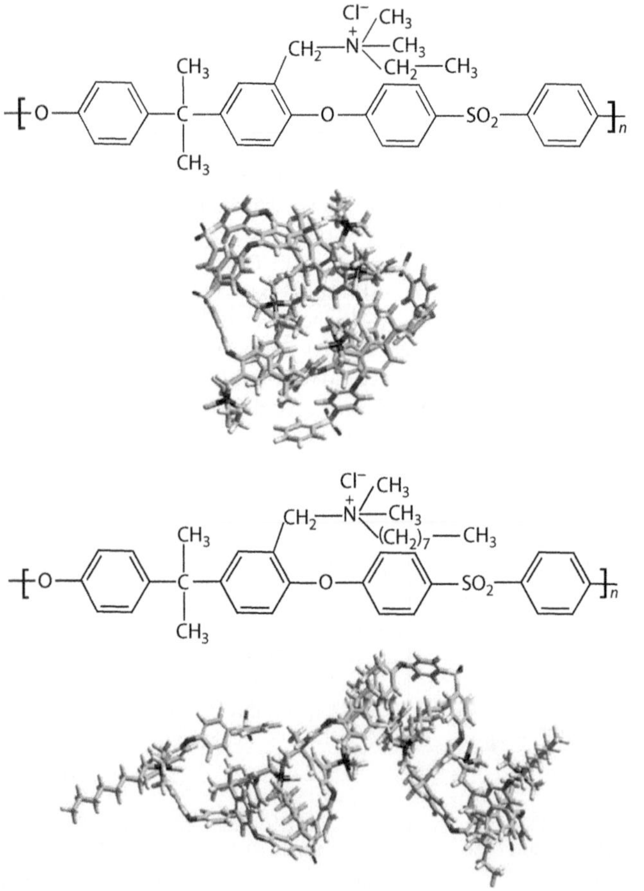

SCHEME 3.5 Chemical structures of the monomer unit of polysulfones with quaternary groups (PSF–DMEA and PSF–DMOA) and conformational structures with minimized energies, considering four repeating units.

In the mentioned research [105], the theoretical and experimental aspects of the association phenomena generated by hydrogen bonding, dispersive, and electrostatic interactions in ternary systems consisting of a proton-donor solvent (DMF or MeOH), a proton-acceptor solvent (water), and a proton-acceptor polymer (PSFs with different alkyl side groups, PSF-DMEA or PSF-DMOA) were investigated. In this context, binary and ternary thermodynamic interaction parameters are corrected on the basis of the different association constants (defined by the graphical representation of molecular associations—Scheme 3.4), and the numerical values of these constants are evaluated as a function of system composition, by mathematical simulations.

Figure 3.13a, a′, b, and b′ illustrates the association phenomena generated by hydrogen bonding, dispersive interactions, and electrostatic interactions, for PSF-DMEA/DMF/MeOH and PSF-DMOA/DMF/MeOH ternary systems by means of the σ_{11}, σ_{13}, η_{13}, σ_{23}, and η_{23} constants, as a function of solvent mixtures composition. Examination of Figure 3.13a and b reveals the following:

- $\sigma_{12} = 0$ and $\eta_{12} = 0$, because both solvents are proton–donor species.
- Self-association of DMF molecules by hydrogen bonding is defined by the σ_{11} association constant, which decreases in the presence of MeOH; moreover, increasing the MeOH content in the mixture favored the occurrence of dispersive interactions.
- For the PSF-DMEA/DMF/MeOH system, the electrostatic interactions significantly influenced the σ_{13}, σ_{23}, and η_{23} association constants and insignificantly the η_{13} association constant (Figure 3.13a).
- For the PSF-DMOA/DMF/MeOH system, the influence was significant for the σ_{13} and σ_{23} association constants and insignificant for the η_{13} and η_{23} association constants (Figure 3.13b).

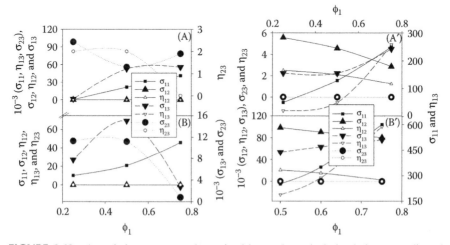

FIGURE 3.13 Association constants determined by mathematical simulations, as adjusted parameters, to fit the theoretical values of preferential adsorption to the experimental data, for: (A) PSF-DMEA/DMF/MeOH, (A′) PSF-DMEA/DMF/water, (B) PSF-DMOA/DMF/MeOH, and (B′) PSF-DMOA/DMF/water ternary systems.

Water provides strong polar interactions. Therefore, the interactivity between DMF and water is complicated due to the phenomenon of mutual associations. Figure 3.13a' and b' depicts the association constants from PSF-DMEA/DMF/water and PSF-DMOA/DMF/water ternary systems, where:

- The different composition domains of DMF/water solvent mixtures were imposed by the nature of the alkyl radicals and content of nonsolvent from the systems.
- In the absence of polymer, the DMF molecules may exhibit hydrogen bonding interactions with the coexistent water associations, and also dispersive interactions, expressed by association constant η_{12}. Also, the association of free molecules of DMF to the above 1–2 complex, characterized by η_{12}, is defined by the association constant σ_{12}. Variation of the η_{12} and σ_{12} association constants is influenced by the self-association of water and DMF molecules and also by the association between DMF and water, which appear as prevalent phenomena over different composition domains of the binary mixture.
- For a low DMF content, isolated associations, represented by DMF–water association, and self-association of water, appear [102,104] while, for a higher DMF content, the association structure is obviously reorganized, and DMF self-association is predominant.
- σ_{13} and η_{13} increase with increasing the DMF content (Figure 3.13a' and b'), being influenced by the presence of the polymer.
- $\eta_{23} = 0$ and $\sigma_{23} = 0$, as due to the weak dispersive and electrostatic interactions, without hydrogen bonding between components "2" and "3."

Based on these association constants, the excess functions Δg_{12}, Δg_{13}, and Δg_{23}, and also the corrected binary interaction parameters g'_{12}, g'_{13}, and g'_{23} were evaluated by Equations 3.125, 3.128, and 3.131, respectively (FHPC-AE) for the PSF-DMEA (3)/DMF (1)/MeOH (2) and PSF-DMOA (3)/DMF (1)/MeOH (2) (Figure 3.14), and PSF-DMEA (3)/DMF (1)/water (2) and PSF-DMOA (3)/DMF (1)/water (2) (Figure 3.15) ternary systems.

Figure 3.16 shows the theoretical adsorption coefficients calculated with the newly corrected interaction parameters, g'_{12}, g'_{13}, and g'_{23}, as well as with those based on the FHPC theory.

Excellent agreement is observed between the predicted values obtained with the association constants and the experimental data. The electrostatic interactions depended on the charge density and the number of carbon atoms present in the alkyl groups of PSF-DMEA or PSF-DMOA, as well as on the association–dissociation capacity of both solvents.

A comparative analysis with the corresponding experiments shows that simulations shed light on the thermodynamic behavior of the charged polymeric systems with specific interactions and helped to understand the properties of cationic PSFs in solution and/or solvent mixtures, for their numerous applications in different fields.

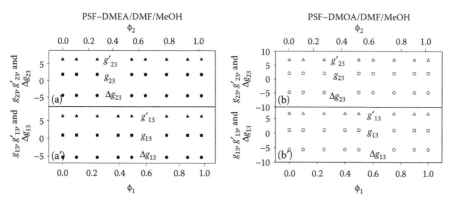

FIGURE 3.14 Interaction parameters for: (a), (a′) PSF–DMEA (3) in DMF (1)/MeOH (2) mixed solvents: (a) g_{23}—noncorrected MeOH–PSF–DMEA interaction parameters (FHPC), g'_{23}—MeOH–PSF–DMEA interaction parameters corrected according to FHPC-AE, Δg_{23}—excess functions, and (a′) g_{13}—noncorrected DMF–PSF–DMEA interaction parameters (FHPC), g'_{13}—DMF–PSF–DMEA interaction parameters corrected according to FHPC-AE, Δg_{13}—excess functions; (b), (b′) PSF–DMOA (3) in DMF (1)/MeOH (2) mixed solvents: (b) g_{23}—noncorrected MeOH–PSF–DMOA interaction parameters (FHPC), g'_{23}—MeOH–PSF–DMOA interaction parameters corrected according to FHPC-AE, Δg_{23}—excess functions, and (b′) g_{13}—noncorrected DMF–PSF–DMOA interaction parameters (FHPC), g'_{13}—DMF–PSF–DMOA interaction parameters corrected according to FHPC-AE, Δg_{13}—excess functions.

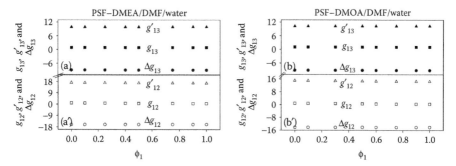

FIGURE 3.15 Interaction parameters for: (a), (a′) PSF–DMEA (3) in DMF (1)/water (2) mixed solvents: (a) g_{13}—noncorrected DMF–PSF–DMEA interaction parameters (FHPC), g'_{13}—DMF–PSF–DMEA interaction parameters corrected according to FHPC-AE, Δg_{13}—excess functions, and (a′) g_{12}—noncorrected DMF–water interaction parameters (FHPC), g'_{12}—DMF–water interaction parameters corrected according to FHPC-AE, Δg_{12}—excess functions; (b), (b′) PSF–DMOA (3) in DMF (1)/water (2) mixed solvents: (b) g_{13}—noncorrected DMF–PSF–DMOA interaction parameters (FHPC), g'_{13}—DMF–PSF–DMOA interaction parameters corrected according to FHPC-AE, Δg_{13}—excess functions, and (b′) g_{12}—noncorrected DMF–water interaction parameters (FHPC), g'_{12}—DMF–water interaction parameters corrected according to FHPC-AE, Δg_{12}—excess functions.

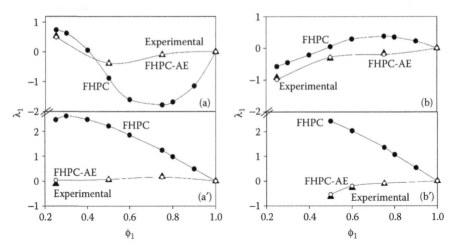

FIGURE 3.16 Theoretical [FHPC (●) and FHPC-AE (○) models] and experimental (▲) values of the preferential adsorption coefficients as a function of the volume fraction of DMF for: (a) PSF–DMEA/DMF/MeOH, (a′) PSF–DMEA/DMF/water, (b) PSF–DMOA/DMF/MeOH, and (b′) PSF–DMOA/DMF/water ternary systems.

3.6   GENERAL REMARKS

This chapter reflects the current state of knowledge and the development of different theories and models applicable to multicomponent systems of neutral and charged PSFs. Using an evolutionary strategy as an alternative optimization procedure, it has been shown that it is possible to improve the classical theories by applying molecular modeling and numeric simulations. In other words, this approach can better characterize materials, providing a detailed knowledge on the specific interactions, which modify the different thermodynamic, equilibrium, and transport properties of solutions polymers. Therefore, molecular dynamic simulations, combined with mathematical methods, have proven to be an effective way to provide global solutions for multicomponent polymers systems.

Finally, it can be pointed out that this chapter is part of my PhD thesis [108]. Also, the content is useful for studies in both academic and industry fields, because it contributes to a better understanding and knowledge of the specific interactions, developed via hydrogen bonding, dispersive, and electrostatic interactions, which generate and modify the properties of PSF and functionalized PSFs, required by applications in different domains.

ACKNOWLEDGMENT

This work was supported by a grant of the Romanian National Authority for Scientific Research, CNCS—UEFISCDI (project number PN-II-RU-TE-2012-3-143).

REFERENCES

1. Guo, W. W. Multiscale, multiphysics and multidomain models I: Basic theory. *J. Theor. Comput. Chem.*, 12(8), 1341006-1–1341006-34, 2013.
2. Vebber, G. C., Pranke, P., and Pereira, C. N. Calculating Hansen solubility parameters of polymers with genetic algorithms. *J. Appl. Polym. Sci.*, 131(1), 39696–39707, 2014.
3. Milczewska, K., Voelkel, A., and Piedzia, K. Interactions in PEG/aerosil and PLA/aerosil composites described by IGC-determined Flory-Huggins χ_{23} parameter. *J. Polym. Res.*, 21(3), 394–400, 2014.
4. Flory, P. J. *Principles of Polymer Chemistry.* Cornell University Press, Ithaca, NY,1953.
5. Yamakawa, H. *Modern Theory of Polymer Solutions.* Harper and Row, New York, 1971.
6. Bohdanecky, M. and Kovar, J., *Viscosity of Polymer Solutions.* Elsevier, Amsterdam, the Netherlands, 1982.
7. Wolf, B. A. and Adam, H. J. Second osmotic virial coefficient revisited: Variation with molecular weight and temperature from endothermal to exothermal conditions. *J. Chem. Phys.*, 75(8), 4121–4129, 1981.
8. Wolf, B. A. Second osmotic virial coefficient revisited. 2. Buildup from contributions of inter- and intramolecular contacts between polymer segments. *Macromolecules*, 18(12), 2474–2478, 1985.
9. Gundert, F. and Wolf, B. A. Second virial coefficient revisited 3. Viscosity of dilute polymer solutions: Molecular weight dependence of the Huggins coefficient. *Macromol. Chem. Phys.*, 187(12), 2969–2990, 1986.
10. Gundert, F. and Wolf, B. A. On the molecular weight dependence of the thermodynamic and of the hydrodynamic pair interaction between chain molecules. IV. Second virial coefficients revisited. *J. Chem. Phys.*, 87(10), 6156–6165, 1987.
11. Ahmadloo, E. and Sobhanifar, N. Thermodynamic modeling of vapor–liquid equilibrium for binary polyethylene glycol/solvent solutions using cubic equations of state: Optimization and comparison of CEoS models. *Polym. Bull.*, 71(4), 887–905, 2014.
12. Tsivintzelis, I. and Kontogeorgis, G. M. Modeling the vapor–liquid equilibria of polymer–solvent mixtures: Systems with complex hydrogen bonding behavior. *Fluid Phase Equil.*, 280(1), 100–109, 2009.
13. Gupta, R. B. and Prausnitz, J. M. Vapor–liquid equilibria of copolymer + solvent and homopolymer + solvent binaries: New experimental data and their correlation. *J. Chem. Eng. Data*, 40(4), 784–791, 1995.
14. Se, R. A. G. and Aznar, M. Vapor-liquid equilibrium of polymer + solvent systems: Experimental data and thermodynamic modeling. *Polymer*, 48(18), 5646–5652, 2007.
15. Hirano, T., Kamikubo, T., Fujioka, Y., and Sato, T. Hydrogen-bond-assisted of N-isopropylacrylamide: The solvent effect on the stereospecificity. *Eur. Polym. J.*, 44(5), 1053–1059, 2008.
16. Romero, R. B., Leite, C. A. P., and Goncalves, M. D. C. The effect of the solvent on the morphology of cellulose acetate/montmorillonite nanocomposites. *Polymer*, 50(1), 161–170, 2009.
17. Tsivintzelis, I., Marras, S. I., Zuburtikudis, I., and Panayiotou, C. Porous poly(L-lactic acid) nanocomposite scaffolds prepared by phase inversion using supercritical CO_2 as anti-solvent. *Polymer*, 48(21), 6311–6318, 2007.
18. Ho Chang, B. and Chan Bae, Y. Vapor–liquid equilibria and liquid–liquid equilibria calculations of binary polymer solutions. *Polymer*, 43(24), 6627–6634, 2002.
19. Wolf, B. A. Unified thermodynamic modeling of polymer solutions: Polyelectrolytes, proteins, and chain molecules. *Ind. Eng. Chem. Res.*, 52(9), 3530–3536, 2013.

20. Bereau, T., Kramer, C., Monnard, F. W., Nogueira, E. S., Ward, T. R., and Meuwly, M. Scoring multipole electrostatics in condensed-phase atomistic simulations. *J. Phys. Chem. B*, 117(18), 5460–5471, 2013.

21. Antonov, Y., Eckelt, J., Sugaya, R., and Wolf, B. A. Liquid/gas and liquid/liquid phase equilibria of the system water/bovine serum albumin. *J. Phys. Chem. B*, 117(18), 5497–5502, 2013.

22. Teraoka, I. *Polymer Solutions: An Introduction to Physical Properties.* Wiley, Brooklyn, NY, 2002.

23. Striolo, A. and Prausnitz, J. M. Vapor–liquid equilibria for some concentrated aqueous polymer solutions. *Polymer*, 41(3), 1109–1117, 2000.

24. Lieu, J. G., Prausnitz, J. M., and Gauthier, M. Vapor–liquid equilibria for binary solutions of arborescent and linear polystyrenes. *Polymer*, 41(1), 219–224, 2000.

25. Fornasiero, F., Halim, M., and Prausnitz, J. M. Vapor–sorption equilibria for 4-vinylpyridine-based copolymer and cross-linked polymer/alcohol systems. Effect of intramolecular repulsion. *Macromolecules*, 33(22), 8435–8442, 2000.

26. Kruger, K. M., Pfohl, O., Dohrn, R., and Sadowski, G. Phase equilibria and diffusion coefficients in the poly(dimethylsiloxane) plus n-pentane system. *Fluid Phase Equil.*, 241(1), 138–146, 2006.

27. Champetier, G. and Monnerie, L., *Introduction a la Chimie Macromoleculaire.* Masson Ed., Partea a II-a, Cap. I, Paris, France, p. 95, 1968.

28. Flory, P. J. Thermodynamics of dilute solutions of high polymers. *J. Chem. Phys.*, 13(11), 453–465, 1945.

29. Huggins, M. L. Comparison of the structures of stretched linear polymers. *J. Chem. Phys.*, 13(11), 37–42, 1945.

30. Barrat, J.-L. and Joanny, J.-F. Theory of polyelectrolyte solutions. *Adv. Chem. Phys.*, 94(1), 1–66, 1996.

31. Forster, S. and Schmidt, M. Polyelectrolytes in solution. *Adv. Chem. Phys.*, 120(1), 51–133, 1995.

32. Freed, K. *Renormalization Group Theory of Macromolecules.* Wiley, New York, 1987.

33. Flory, P. J. *Statistical Mechanics of Chain Molecules*, Interscience, New York, 1969.

34. Flory, P. J. Theory of elasticity of polymer networks. The effect of local constraints on junctions. *J. Chem. Phys.*, 66(3), 5720–5729, 1977.

35. Yamakawa, H. Excluded volume effects and binary cluster integrals in dilute polymer solutions. *Pure Appl. Chem.*, 31(1), 179–199, 1972.

36. Barrett, A. J. and Domb, C. Statistical properties of a polymer chain in the two-parameter approximation. *Proc. Roy. Soc. Lond.*, 376(2), 361–375, 1981.

37. Domb, C. and Barrett, A. J. Universality approach to the expansion factor of a polymer chain. *Polymer*, 17(3), 179–184, 1976.

38. Douglas, J. F. and Freed, K. F. Renormalization and the two-parameter theory. *Macromolecules*, 17(11), 2344–2354, 1984.

39. Wang, S. Q., Douglas, J. F., and Freed, K. F. Influence of draining and excluded volume on the intrinsic viscosity of flexible polymers. *Macromolecules*, 18(12), 2464–2474, 1985.

40. Wang, S. Q., Douglas, J. F., and Freed, K. F. Influence of variable draining and excluded volume on the hydrodynamic radius within Kirkwood-Riseman model: Dynamical renormalization group description to order ε^2. *J. Chem. Phys.*, 87(2), 1346–1354, 1987.

41. Stapper, M. and Liverpool, T. B. Renormalized field theory of polyelectrolyte solutions, Max-Planck-Institut fur Polymerforschung, Postfach 3148, D-55021 Mainz, 2006.

42. Liverpool, T. B. and Stapper, M. The scaling behaviour of screened polyelectrolytes. *Europhys. Lett.*, 40(5), 485–490, 1997.

43. Simionescu, B. C., Ioan, C., Ioan, S., and Simionescu, C. I. Specific interactions in dilute polymer solutions. *Macromol. Symp.*, 98(1), 1045–1068, 1995.

44. Qian, J. W., Wang, M., Han, D. L., and Cheng, R. S. A novel method for estimating unperturbed dimension $[\eta]_\theta$ of polymer from the measurement of its $[\eta]$ in a non-theta solvent. *Eur. Polym. J.*, 37(7), 1403–1407, 2001.

45. Ioan, S., Filimon, A., and Avram, E. Influence of the degree of substitution on the solution properties of chloromethylated polysulfone. *J. Appl. Polym. Sci.*, 101(1), 524–531, 2006.

46. Qian, J. W. and Rudin, A. Prediction of hydrodynamic properties of polymer solutions. *Eur. Polym. J.*, 28(7), 733–738, 1992.

47. Qian, J. W. and Rudin, A. Prediction of thermodynamic properties of polymer solutions. *Eur. Polym. J.*, 28(7), 725–732, 1992.

48. Schulz, G. V. and Horbach, A. Die molekularen Konstanten von Polycarbonaten in Lösung. *Die Makromol. Chem.*, 29(1/2), 93–116, 1959.

49. Berry, G. C., Nomura, H., and Mayhan, K. G. Dilute solution studies on a polycarbonate in good and poor solvents. *J. Polym. Sci. A-2 Polym. Phys.*, 5(1), 1–21, 1967.

50. Allen, G., McAinsh, J., and Strazielle, C. Dilute solution properties of the polyether from bisphenol A and 4,4′-dichlorodiphenyl sulphone. *Eur. Polym. J.*, 5(1), 319–334, 1959.

51. Ioan, S., Bercea, M., Simionescu, B. C., and Simionescu, C. I. In *The Polymeric Materials Encyclopedia: Synthesis, Properties and Applications*, Salamone, J. C., Ed., CRC Press, Boca Raton, FL, Vol. 11, p. 8417, 1996.

52. Bates, T. W., Biggins, J., and Ivin, K. J. The coil dimensions of poly(olefin sulphones) in theta-solvents. II. Poly(hexene-1 sulphone) and poly(2-methylpentene-1 sulphone). *Macromol. Chem. Phys.*, 87(1), 180–189, 1965.

53. Ende, H. A., Ivin, K. J., and Meyerhoff, G. The solution properties of olefin polysulphones I—hexene-1 polysulphone. *Polymer*, 3(1), 129–141, 1962.

54. Ewart, R. H., Roe, C. P., Debye D., and McCartney, J. R. The determination of polymeric molecular weights by light scattering in solvent-precipitant systems. *J. Chem. Phys.*, 14(5), 687–694, 1946.

55. Dondos, A. and Benoit, H. Linear representation of viscosity data as a function of molecular weight. *Polymer*, 19(5), 523–525, 1978.

56. Gargallo, L. and Radic, D. Preferential adsorption of vinyl polymers in binary solvents. *Adv. Colloid Interface Sci.*, 21(1), 1–53, 1984.

57. Katime, I., Gargallo, L., Radic, D., and Horta, A. Preferential adsorption behaviour of poly(alkyl methacrylate)s in 1,4-dioxane/methanol. *Macromol. Chem. Phys.*, 186(10), 2125–2131, 1985.

58. Tuzar, Z. and Kratochvil, P. Determination of the composition of copolymers by differential refractometry in mixed solvents. *J. Polym. Sci. Part B: Polym. Lett.*, 7(12), 825–828, 1969.

59. Schultz, A. R. and Flory, P. J. Polymer chain dimensions in mixed-solvent media. *J. Polym. Sci.*, 15(1), 231–242, 1955.

60. Tanford, C. H. *Physical Chemistry of Macromolecules*, Wiley, New York, p. 343, 1961.

61. Tanaka, G., Imai, S., and Yamakawa, H. Experimental test of the two-parameter theory of dilute polymer solutions: Poly-p-methylstyrene. *J. Chem. Phys.*, 52(5), 2639–2650, 1970.

62. Cowie, J. M. G. and McCridle, J. T. Polymer cosolvent systems—I. Selective adsorption in methyl cyclohexane (1), acetone (2), polystyrene (3) *Eur. Polym. J.*, 8(10), 1185–1191, 1972.

63. Cowie, J. M. G. and McCridle, J. T. Polymer co-solvent systems—II: An asymmetric solubility parameter system: Acetone (1), cyclohexanol (2), polystyrene (3). *Eur. Polym. J.*, 8(12), 1325–1331, 1972.

64. Pouchly, L., Zivny, A., and Solc, K. Thermodynamic equilibrium in the system macromolecular coil–binary solvent. *J. Polym. Sci. Part C: Polym. Symp.*, 23(1), 245–256, 1968.

65. Campos, A., Gavara, R., Tejero, R., Gomez, C., and Celda, B. A Flory–Huggins thermodynamic approach for predicting sorption equilibrium in ternary polymer systems. *J. Polym. Sci. Part B Polym. Phys.*, 27(8), 1559–1597, 1989.

66. Celda, B., Gavara, R., Gomez, C., Tejero, R., and Campos, A. Comparative study of the formalism of Flory-Huggins as generalized by Pouchly and the formalism of Flory-Prigogine-Patterson in ternary polymer systems, n-alkane-butanone-poly(dimethylsiloxane). *Polymer*, 30(5), 897–904, 1989.
67. Campos, A., Gavara, R., Tejero, R., Gomez, C., and Celda, B. A procedure for predicting sorption equilibrium in ternary polymer systems from Flory–Huggins binary interaction parameters and the inversion point of preferential salvation. *J. Polym. Sci. Part B Polym. Phys.*, 27(8), 1599–1610, 1989.
68. Pouchly, J. and Patterson, D. Effect of long-range interactions in the determination of unperturbed dimensions. *Macromolecules*, 6(3), 465–467, 1973.
69. Horta, A. Statistical thermodynamics of preferential sorption. *Macromolecules*, 12(4), 785–789, 1979.
70. Horta, A. Statistical thermodynamics of preferential sorption. 2. *Macromolecules*, 18(12), 2498–2504, 1985.
71. Horta, A., Radic, D., and Gargallo, L. Association equilibria theory of preferential adsorption in systems with solvent–solvent and solvent–polymer interactions. *Macromolecules*, 22(11), 4267–4272, 1989.
72. Soria, V., Figueruelo, J. E., Abad, C., and Campos, A. Association equilibria theory for polymers in mixed solvents with specific interactions. *Macromol. Theory Simul.*, 13(5), 441–452, 2004.
73. Garcia-Lopera, R., Monzo, I. S., Abad, C., and Campos, A. A thermodynamic approach to study hydrogen-bonding interactions in solvent/solvent/polymer ternary systems. *Eur. Polym. J.*, 43(1), 231–242, 2007.
74. Pouchly, J. Sorption equilibria in ternary systems: Polymer/mixed solvent. *Pure Appl. Chem.*, 61(6), 1085–1095, 1989.
75. Pouchly, J. and Zivny, A. Theoretical analysis of sorption of a binary solvent in a polymer phase. I. Occurrence and character of inversion in preferential sorption. *J. Polym. Sci. Part A Polym. Chem.*, 10(8), 1467–1480, 1972.
76. Pouchly, J. and Zivny, A. Theoretical analysis of sorption of a binary solvent in a polymer phase. II. Occurrence of maxima and minima in the curve of total sorption. *J. Polym. Sci. A-2 Polym. Phys.*, 10(8), 1481–1495, 1972.
77. Read, B. E. A light-scattering study of preferential adsorption in the system benzene+cyclohexane+polystyrene. *Trans. Faraday Soc.*, 56(1), 382–390, 1960.
78. Pouchly, J. and Zivny, A. Correlation of data on preferential sorption using the modified Flory-Huggins equation. *Die Makromol. Chem.*, 183(12), 3019–3040, 1982.
79. Pouchly, J. and Zivny, A. Correlation of data on intrinsic viscosities in mixed solvents by means of the modified Flory-Huggins equation. *Die Makromol. Chem.*, 184(10), 2081–2096, 1983.
80. Figueruelo, J., Celda, B., and Campos, A. Predictability of properties in ternary solvent (1)/solvent (2)/polymer (3) systems from interaction parameters of the binary systems. 1. General considerations and evaluation of preferential solvation coefficients *Macromolecules*, 18(12), 2504–2511, 1985.
81. Figueruelo, J., Campos, A., and Celda, B. Predictability of properties in ternary solvent (1)/solvent (2)/polymer (3) systems from interaction parameters of the binary systems. 2. Evaluation of total sorption parameters and related magnitudes *Macromolecules*, 18(12), 2511–2515, 1985.
82. Brinke, T. G. and Karasz, F. E. Lower critical solution temperature behavior in polymer blends: Compressibility and directional-specific interactions. *Macromolecules*, 17(4), 815–820, 1984.
83. Goldstein, R. E. On the theory of lower critical solution points in hydrogen-bonded mixtures. *J. Chem. Phys.*, 80(10), 5340–5341, 1984.

84. Sanchez, I. C. and Balazs, A. C. Generalization of the lattice-fluid model for specific interactions. *Macromolecules*, 22(5), 2325–2331, 1989.

85. Barth, C. and Wolf, B. A. Evidence of ternary interaction parameters for polymer solutions in mixed solvents from headspace-gas chromatography. *Polymer*, 41(24), 8587–8596, 2000.

86. Gomez, C. M., Verdejo, E., Figueruelo, J. E., Campos, A., and Soria, V. On the thermodynamic treatment of poly(vinylidene fluoride)/polystyrene blend under liquid—liquid phase separation conditions. *Polymer*, 36(7), 1487–1498, 1995.

87. Campos, A., Gomez, C. M., Garcia, R., Figueruelo, J. E., and Soria, V. Extension of the Flory-Huggins theory to study incompatible polymer blends in solution from phase separation data. *Polymer*, 37(15), 3361–3372, 1996.

88. Gomez, C. M., Figueruelo, J. E., and Campos, A. Evaluation of thermodynamic parameters for blends of polyethersulfone and poly(methyl methacrylate) or polystyrene in dimethylformamide. *Polymer*, 39(17), 4023–4032, 1998.

89. Barker, J. A. Cooperative orientation effects in solutions. *J. Chem. Phys.*, 20(10), 1526–1531, 1952.

90. Pouchly, J. and Zivny, A. The effect of specific interactions on the sorption equilibrium in the polymer/mixed solvent system. *Die Makromol. Chem.*, 186(1), 37–52, 1985.

91. Ioan, S., Filimon, A., and Avram, E. Conformational and viscometric behavior of quaternized polysulfone in dilute solution. *Polym. Eng. Sci.*, 46(7), 827–836, 2006.

92. Filimon, A., Avram, E., and Ioan, S. Influence of mixed solvents and temperature on the solution properties of quaternized polysulfones. *J. Macromol. Sci. Part B Phys.*, 46(3), 503–520, 2007.

93. Filimon, A., Albu, R. M., Avram, E., and Ioan, S. Effect of alkyl side chain on the conformational properties of polysulfones with quaternary groups. *J. Macromol. Sci. Part B Phys.*, 49(1), 207–217, 2010.

94. Katime, I., Ochoa, J. R., Cesteros, L. C., and Penafiel, J. Polymer cosolvent systems 3. PMMA(3)/CCl4(1)/n-butyl chloride(2). *Polym. Bull.*, 6(1), 429–436, 1982.

95. Grulke, E. A. Solubility parameter values. In *Polymer Handbook*, Brandrup, J., Immergut, E. H. (Eds.), Wiley, New York, Chapter VII, p. 675, 1999.

96. Bicerano, J. Prediction of the properties of polymers from their structures. *J. Macromol. Sci. Part C Polym. Rev.*, 36(1), 161–196, 1996.

97. Hansen, C. M. *Hansen Solubility Parameters-A User's Handbook*, 2nd ed., CRC Press, Boca Raton, FL, 2007.

98. Pozuelo, J., Riande, E., Saiz, E., and Compan, V. Molecular dynamics simulations of proton conduction in sulfonated poly(phenyl sulfone)s. *Macromolecules*, 39(26), 8862–8866, 2006.

99. Kryven, I. and Iedema P. D. Topology evolution in polymer modification. *Macromol. Theory and Simul.*, 23(1), 7–14, 2014.

100. Leeuw, S. W., van Zon, A., and Bel, G. J. Structural relaxation in poly(ethyleneoxide) and poly(ethyleneoxide)–sodium iodide systems: A molecular dynamics study. *Electrochim. Acta*, 46(10/11), 1419–1426, 2001.

101. Synder, J. F., Ratner, M. A., and Shriver, D. F. Polymer electrolytes and polyelectrolytes: Monte Carlo simulations of thermal effects on conduction. *Solid State Ionics*, 147(3/4), 249–257, 2002.

102. Kobara, H., Wakisaka, A., Takeuchi, K., and Ibusuki, T. Preferential solvation of Na$^+$ in *N,N*-Dimethylformamide–water binary mixture. *J. Phys. Chem. B*, 107(43), 11827–11829, 2003.

103. Durlak, P., Mierzwicki, K., and Latajka, Z. Investigations of the very short hydrogen bond in the crystal of nitromalonamide via Car–Parrinello and path integral molecular dynamics. *J. Phys. Chem. B*, 117(20), 5430–5440, 2013.

104. Filimon, A., Avram, E., and Ioan, S. Specific interactions in ternary system quaternized polysulfones/mixed solvent. *Polym. Eng. Sci.*, 49(1), 17–25, 2009.
105. Filimon, A., Albu, R. M., Avram, E., and Ioan, S. Impact of association phenomena on the thermodynamic properties of modified polysulfones in solutions. *J. Macromol. Sci. Part B Phys.*, 52(4), 545–560, 2013.
106. HyperChem. *HyperChem Professional Program*, Hypercube, Gainesville, FL, 2001.
107. Bhuiyan, M. M. H. and Uddin, M. H. Excess molar volumes and excess viscosities for mixtures of *N,N*-dimethylformamide with methanol, ethanol and 2-propanol at different temperatures. *J. Molec. Liq.*, 138(1/3), 139–146, 2008.
108. Filimon, A. *Polymer's Conformation in Solution Under the Influence of the Solvent, Concentration and Temperature*. PhD Thesis, "Petru Poni" Institute of Macromolecular Chemistry, Romanian Academy, Iasi, Romania, Supervisor Ioan., S, 2009.

4 Structure–Property Relationships of Functionalized Polysulfones

Anca Filimon, Raluca Marinica Albu, and Silvia Ioan

CONTENTS

4.1 IMPACT OF CHEMICAL FUNCTIONALIZATION OF POLYSULFONES: FROM NEUTRAL TO POLYELECTROLYTE STRUCTURES

The literature has shown that each time a major new architecture is discovered the event has been accompanied by the emergence of a plethora of new properties, concepts, applications, products, and activities, all of which have led to new technologies and enhanced quality of life. Over time, macromolecular architectures have evolved, leading to well-known classes of thermoplastic or thermoset polymers, beginning with linear, cross-linked, branched, and now dendritic topologies, as illustrated in Figure 4.1 [1].

Consequently, in recent years, there has been a spurt in the demand for polymers with unique physicochemical properties and high potential, to be used in obtaining valuable end products, that is, biocompatible and biodegradable plastics, and so on

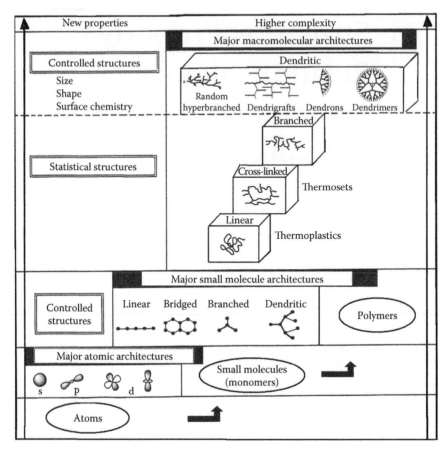

FIGURE 4.1 Development stages of major architecture for atoms, small molecules, and macromolecules (polymers) as a function of their new properties and complexity.

with applications in quite different areas, such as the food and the pharmaceutical and biomedical fields [2]. In most applications, a polymer, once designed as a product, has to be stable and has to maintain its structure and morphology under various temperatures and other environmental conditions during the lifetime of the product. However, the recent interest is also manifested in changing the shape or morphology of the molecule, instantaneously and reversibly, without any memory or hysteresis effects, with electrical, optical, or mechanical stimuli. These *smart* materials are aimed at applications such as information processing, storage and retrieval, and molecular recognition similar to the biological systems.

In this context, aromatic polysulfones (PSFs) [polysulfones, poly(ethersulfone)s, or poly(phenyl sulfone)s] appear as high-performance polymers with excellent chemical and thermal stability, increased strength and flexibility, transparency, as well as high glass transition temperature and good film-forming properties [3–5]. Owing to these properties, PSFs are used in materials science, biology, and polymer science, constituting the basis of numerous applications, such as filtration membranes [6–10], coatings [11,12], composites [13–15], microelectronic devices [16], thin-film technology [17], biomaterials [18,19], and fuel cells [20–22].

Polysulfonic membranes have been developed for a wide variety of applications in separation technology, biological processes, medical devices, and blood purification. Systems generally composed of a polymer, a solvent, and a nonsolvent are usually used to obtain asymmetrical membranes, the process being governed by the diffusion of the various low-molecular-weight components. Introduction of nonsolvents plays an important role in membrane formation through the occurrence of specific interactions in the three-component system [23].

Despite tremendous progress in their synthesis and applications, PSFs have some limitations related to their intrinsic hydrophobic nature, which precludes their use in membrane applications (requiring a hydrophilic character). Therefore, the applicability of these polymers in the aqueous phase—restricted by their hydrophobicity—may be improved by either modifying them through different processes or blending with an additional polymer [24,25].

Synthetic effort in designing polymers with functional groups in the main or side chain, for providing superior properties, has been an active area in recent years [26]. Thus, the introduction of functional groups into PSFs not only solves these limitations but also extends the range of potential applications of these high-performance materials through the specific properties gained, and provides a wider scope [27–30]. Therefore, chemical modifications can be easily achieved *via* reacting simple chemicals with a reactive pendant group, such as vinyl, carbonyl, and halomethyl, present on the polymer. Among these reactive groups, the chloromethyl one is especially useful, because it can be readily modified by a substitution reaction with various nucleophilic reactants. Therefore, polymers with chloromethyl pendant groups are often used as starting materials for synthesizing new functional polymers bearing amino, azomethyne, siloxane, or carboxylic groups [31–34]. Additionally, the chloromethylation reaction is a subject of considerable interest from both theoretical and practical points of view; there is an interest in obtaining precursors for functional membranes, coatings, ion-exchange resins, ion-exchange fibers, and selectively permeable membranes [4,35,36]. By grafting poly(ethylene glycol) on chloromethylated polysulfone (CMPSF), a hydrophilic yet water-insoluble membrane with enhanced porosity and resistance to protein absorption can be obtained [37].

Chemical modification of CMPSFs through quaternization with ammonium groups is an efficient method for increasing their hydrophilicity. Several studies [38,39] reported that quaternary ammonium functionalized PSFs are useful as anion exchange membranes. This approach not only enables the control of the amount of quaternary ammonium groups and their location along the polymer backbone, but it also provides environmentally friendly conditions, as it avoids the use of chloromethyl methyl ethers, which are hazardous.

On the other hand, quaternary ammonium cations may improve the thermal stability of polymers, being preferred for use in long-term applications [40] or as an aid in matrix reinforcement of ionomers [41]. Due to the enhanced thermal stability of ammonium cations, quaternary ammonium-containing polymers have a significant technological importance as phase-transfer catalysts, antistatic agents, biocides, humidity sensors, and water filtration membranes [42]. Moreover, functionalized compounds have been recently shown to possess an attractive combination of properties, which motivates the investigation of quaternized polymers as proton conductors [43]. Also, the different components of a block or graft copolymer may segregate in bulk to yield nanometer-sized patterns or mesophasic structures. Numerous applications involve nanodomained solids [28]. By matching the periodicity of the patterns with the wavelength of visible light, literature studies have demonstrated that block copolymers, including PSFs, act as photonic crystals. Segregated block copolymers, PSFs included, have also been used as precursors for the preparation of various nanostructures, including nanospheres, nanofibers, annotates, and thin membrane-containing nanochannels. Nanochannels have been used as membranes, pH sensors, and templates for the preparation of metallic nanorods.

Consequently, polymers carrying functional groups have quite different properties than those with PSFs and, from a practical viewpoint, some distinct features, such as high flexibility, hydrophilicity, and lack of crystallinity, permitting to functionalized PSFs the capacity to form thin layers, electrospun nanofibers, nanoparticles, flexible coatings, stand-alone films, and three-dimensional objects [2] (Figure 4.2).

The polymer blend concept has been extended in recent years in order to improve the properties of membranes by developing advanced membrane materials for the products of our everyday life. Therefore, polymer blending is a proven tool to obtain new types of materials with a large range of properties, intermediate among those

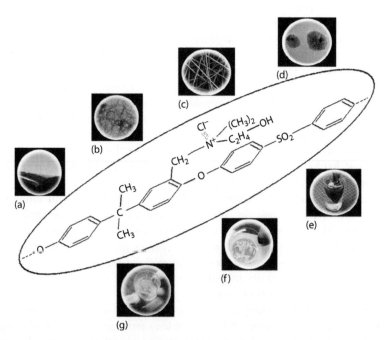

FIGURE 4.2 Representative illustrations of different forms of organization of quaternized polysulfones [thin layers (a), bundles (b), electrospun nanofibers (c), and micro-, nanoparticles doped with active compounds (d)] with potential application in industrial fields [coating on food (e), generation of stand-alone films (f), and fabrication of three-dimensional objects (g)].

of the pure components. Polymer blending is designed to generate materials with optimized structural, mechanical, morphological, and biological properties [44,45]. As a consequence, the blending of functionalized PSFs with other synthetic polymers has wide applications, as a versatile method to tailor materials for specific uses [46,47] and for further developments in biomedical applications. Accordingly, for example, poly(4-vinylpyridine) (P4VP) has a wide range of applications—from electronics to medicine—as a homopolymer, a copolymer, or blended with other polymers. P4VP is considered as a common hydrophobic additive for enhancing the properties of polysulfonic materials, which recommends it for different applications, for example, as a coating or an additive to coatings [48]. On the other hand, polystyrene (PS) is a rigid, transparent thermoplastic material, possessing hydrophobic characteristics, good electrical properties, low dielectric loss, and excellent resistance to gamma radiations [49]. Therefore, it is of interest to find out whether functionalized PSFs can be designed for specific applications, in blends with synthetic polymers (e.g., PS and P4VP), and to establish their impact on different properties.

From these reasons, this chapter will present the properties of some new functionalized PSFs and biomaterial composites (functionalized PSFs/synthetic polymers) used for obtaining performant membranes with applications in biomedical fields. Results would provide an insight into the development of high-performance membranes with enhanced biocompatibility and bacterial resistance assured by antibacterial agents.

4.2 EFFECT OF SIDE CHAINS ON THE CONFORMATIONAL PROPERTIES OF PSFs WITH QUATERNARY GROUPS IN MIXED SOLVENTS

As known, the physical properties of a polymer depend not only on the type of monomer(s) forming it but also on the secondary and tertiary structures, that is, the stereochemistry of the linkage, chain length and its distribution, its ability to crystallize or remain amorphous under various conditions, and the conformation or distribution of the chain conformations in solution [50]. Through the progress recorded in polymer chemistry in the last two decades, polymers with specific properties can be designed, and the control of their physicochemical properties in solution allows anticipation of their conformational properties. [50].

Charged polymers display complex conformations, due to electrostatic interactions and rearrangement of counterions in solution. Studies performed in solutions of polyelectrolytes are of particular importance, considering their complex behavior, influenced by the chemical structure of the polycation, size, and charge density, as well as the complex interpretation of the obtained parameters [51]. In this context, the literature [52–55] has pointed out intense interest in investigating new functionalized PSFs, in particular PSFs synthesized by quaternization of CMPSFs with *N,N*-dimethylethanolamine, *N,N*-dimethylethylamine, and *N,N*-dimethyloctylamine [56,57].

The viscometric behavior is related to the structural characteristics of the polycation, but also to environmental properties, such as ionic strength, pH, and addition of other solvents or salts [51]. One should emphasize that viscometry probably represents the most widely used experimental methods to assess the conformational modification of charged polymers in the solution.

In the aforementioned researches [52–55], the hydrodynamic volume of macromolecules in dilute solution, and the size and conformation of PSFs and quaternized PSFs chains in the solutions of solvent/nonsolvent mixtures, are evaluated from the modification of viscometric parameters, that is, specific viscosity, η_{sp}; intrinsic viscosity, $[\eta]$; and the Huggins constant, k_H. In this context, Figure 4.3 gives indications on the electrolyte effect of quaternized PSFs by application of the Huggins equation [58] (Equation 4.1).

$$\frac{\eta_{sp}}{c} = [\eta]_{\text{Huggins}} + k_H [\eta]^2_{\text{Huggins}} c \qquad (4.1)$$

where:
   η_{sp} is the specific viscosity
   k_H is the Huggins constant
   c is the concentration of polymer solution

An examination of Huggins plots for solutions of polyelectrolytes revealed the balance between the forces acting in polymeric complex systems over a concentration domain. Thus, Figure 4.3a and b exemplifies the linear dependencies with positive

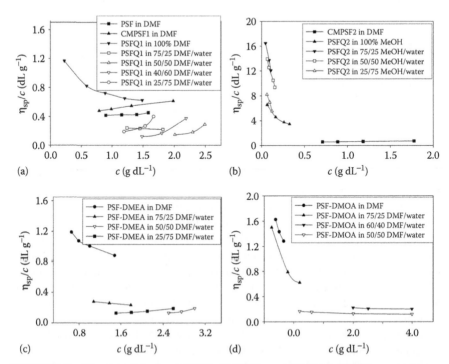

FIGURE 4.3 Huggins plots for: (a) PSF, CMPSF1, and PSFQ1 in DMF/water mixture; (b) CMPSF2 and PSFQ2 in DMF and MeOH/water mixture; (c) PSF-DMEA in DMF/water mixture; and (d) PSF-DMOA in DMF/water mixture at 25°C.

slopes from Huggins plots for polysulfone (PSF) and chloromethylated polysulfones (CMPSF1 and CMPSF2) in N,N-dimethylformamide (DMF), as expected for neutral polymers [52,54]. The specific behavior of the polyelectrolyte is also illustrated in Figure 4.3a and b for quaternized polysulfones (PSFQ1 and PSFQ2) with different ionic chlorine content in DMF/water and methanol (MeOH)/water solvent mixtures, where a decrease of η_{sp}/c with increasing polymer concentration appears [53]. In addition, this specific behavior of the polyelectrolyte is presented, too, in Figure 4.3c and d for PSF-DMEA and PSF-DMOA in DMF and DMF/water mixtures [55].

The solvent/nonsolvent systems are selected as a function of the ionic chlorine content of quaternized polysulfones (PSFQ1—Cl_i = 2.15% and PSFQ2—Cl_i = 5.71%), the alkyl chain length being attached to the PSF backbone (PSF-DMEA—with two carbon atoms in the alkyl side chain, and PSF-DMOA—with eight carbon atoms in the alkyl side chain), although the composition domains of these mixtures were imposed by polymer solubility. Moreover, the different domains of concentrations plotted in Figure 4.3 are imposed under the condition: $1.25 < \eta_{rel} < 1.9$.

The polyelectrolyte effect is generated by an expansion of the polyionic chain, caused by the progressively enhanced dissociation of the ionizable groups, as concentration decreases, and, therefore, by the intensification of the intramolecular repulsive interactions between the ionized groups; that is, the ammonium groups spread all along the chain [59].

On the other hand, solvents or solvent/nonsolvent mixtures contribute essentially to the modification of solution behavior (association, complex, micelle, and core-shell structure of the polymer chains). Thus, Figure 4.3a–d shows the influence of solvent mixture composition on η_{sp}/c. Therefore, the affinity of the DMF, MeOH or DMF/MeOH, DMF/water, and MeOH/water mixtures for the quaternized samples depends both on the neutral segment and on the charged groups.

Deviations from linearity, shown in Figure 4.3 for quaternized PSFs in the dilute concentration domain, can be eliminated by the Rao approximation [60] (Equation 4.2)— slightly sensitive to the possible errors occurring in relative viscosity data, η_{rel}—for the determination of intrinsic viscosity.

$$\frac{1}{2\left(\eta_{rel}^{1/2}-1\right)} = \frac{1}{[\eta]_{Rao}c} - \frac{(a-1)}{2.5} \qquad (4.2)$$

where:
   $a = 1/\Phi_m$ and Φ_m the maximum volume fraction to which the particles can pack, expressed as $\Phi_m = ([\eta]/2.5)c_m$

The values of intrinsic viscosity are affected by the charged groups from the studied quaternized samples and by the composition of the solvent mixtures (Figure 4.4). Moreover, Figure 4.4a and b reflects the modification of intrinsic viscosity with increasing the bulky alkyl side chain for the studied quaternized PSFs. Thus, precipitation is caused by the nature of the alkyl radicals and by the higher content of nonsolvent in the system.

Intrinsic viscosities and their dependence on temperature are interpreted in terms of a conformational change of the polymer chain. The results seem to indicate that the prevailing factor is the polarity of solvent in solvation power. Therefore, for a given

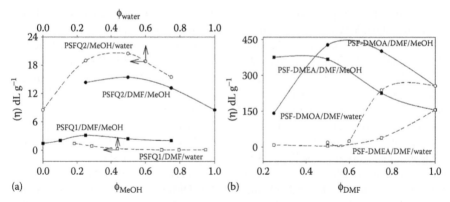

FIGURE 4.4 Influence of composition of solvent/nonsolvent mixtures on intrinsic viscosity for: (a) PSFQ1 and PSFQ2 in DMF/MeOH, DMF/water, and MeOH/water; (b) PSF-DMEA and PSF-DMOA in DMF/MeOH and DMF/water at 25°C.

composition of the solvent/nonsolvent mixtures (e.g., DMF/MeOH, DMF/water, or MeOH/water), one of the components is preferentially adsorbed to the quaternized PSF molecules, in the direction of a thermodynamically most effective mixture.

4.3 CONFORMATIONAL RESTRUCTURATIONS OF CATIONIC POLYELECTROLYTES/MIXED SOLVENTS SYSTEMS

Molecular structure and the conformation of polymers are important parameters in the flow behavior of polymer solutions. Chain stiffness, expansion of macromolecular coils, and the space occupied by them determine the hydrodynamic volume of individual molecules, which affect the flow behavior of polymer solutions compared to the pure solvent. The dependence between the structure of individual molecules in solution and molecular parameters is described using structure–property relationships. In this respect, in relation with the molecular structure of PSFs, all intra- and intermolecular-specific interactions, influencing various properties, should be mentioned [61,62]. Accordingly, the conformational restructurations generated by hydrogen bonding, electrostatic interactions, and association phenomena occurring in polyelectrolytes/solvent/nonsolvent ternary systems are evidenced by rheological properties. In addition, some studies [63,64] indicated that the cumulative effect of the specific interactions and the chemical structure of quaternized PSFs with N,N-dimethylethanolamine (PSFQ1 and PSFQ2), N,N-dimethylethylamine (PSF-DMEA), and N,N-dimethyloctylamine (PSF-DMOA) pendant groups are optimized for establishing processing-property relationships to be used in future research in biomedical fields. Knowledge concerning the conformational properties of quaternized PSFs in solution is essential in the understanding of surface morphology of the corresponding films with important role in various applications, such as membranes in medicine [5,10,16].

Consequently, the flow behavior of quaternized PSFs with different compositions of the solvent/nonsolvent mixtures was observed from the dynamic viscosity-shear rate dependence. Generally, according to Figure 4.5a, PSFQ1 and PSFQ2 exhibit a Newtonian behavior in DMF, MeOH, and DMF/MeOH solvent mixtures, with a constant viscosity region over the entire shear rate range, at 25°C [63].

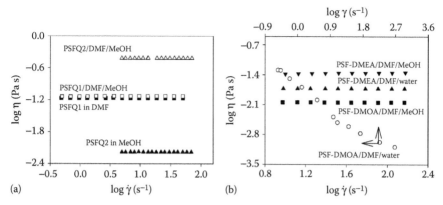

FIGURE 4.5 Double logarithmic plot of dynamic viscosity *versus* shear rate for: (a) PSFQ1 in DMF and 35/65 DMF/MeOH, and PSFQ2 in MeOH and 75/25 DMF/MeOH; (b) PSF-DMEA in 25/75 DMF/MeOH and 40/60 DMF/water, and PSF-DMOA in 45/55 DMF/MeOH and 50/50 DMF/water for different concentration values, at 25°C.

On the contrary, the lower flexibility of PSF-DMOA, compared with that of PSF-DMEA, as well as of the different compositions of solvent mixtures (DMF/MeOH and DMF/water), influences dynamic viscosity (Figure 4.5b) [64]. In this context, all solutions exhibit a constant viscosity region for the studied shear rates and different concentrations, revealing a Newtonian behavior, except for the sample PSF-DMOA in DMF/water. In this last case, for all compositions of the solvent mixture, shear thinning is observed at low shear rates. According to the studies of Witten and Cohen [47] on the mechanism of shear thinning, shear flow could decrease the probability of interchain association at the expense of intrachain association reduction, thus leading to the lowering of viscosity. At the same time, it is observed that, as shear rate increases, the slope of curves decreases and a Newtonian plateau appears. This plateau shrinks and moves toward higher shear rates as water composition increases.

Recent studies [64,65] show that the investigation of the rheological properties of pure components is essential for a better understanding of the viscoelastic properties developed by quaternized PSFs/synthetic polymer blends (i.e., PSF-DMEA or PSF-DMOA blends with PS and/or P4VP). These combined studies contribute to the knowledge on the nature of the interactions manifested in the system. Thus, the flow behavior, in DMF, of quaternized PSF blends with PS or P4VP obtained at the same concentration values is presented in Figure 4.6a and b [64]. For different compositions of the PSF-DMEA/PS, PSF-DMOA/PS, PSF-DMEA/P4VP, and PSF-DMOA/P4VP blends, a Newtonian behavior appears, whereas increasing the amount of PS or P4VP decreases the viscosity.

Flow behavior is reflected in the values obtained for the flow behavior (n) and consistency (k) indices obtained from the dependence of shear stress, σ, on shear rate, $\dot{\gamma}$, according to the Ostwald-de Waele model (Equation 4.3).

$$\sigma = k\dot{\gamma}^n \tag{4.3}$$

It is estimated that $n = 1$ for a Newtonian behavior of fluids, $n < 1$ for a thinning behavior, and $n > 1$ for a thickening behavior [65]. In this context, the results

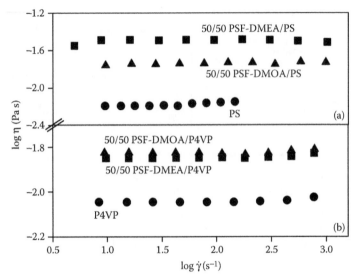

FIGURE 4.6 Log–log plot of viscosity as a function of shear rate, of the PSF-DMEA/PS and PSF-DMOA/PS blends in DMF (a), PSF-DMEA/P4VP and PSF-DMOA/P4VP blends in DMF (b) at equal concentrations and 25°C.

TABLE 4.1

Flow Behavior Index, Consistency Index, and Activation Energy of Quaternized PSFs for the Same Concentrations, at 25°C

Ternary System	Mixed Solvent Ratios	n	k	E_a (kJ mol^{-1})
PSFQ1/DMF/MeOH	100/0	0.99	0.21	−34.78
	36/65	0.97	0.33	−76.27
PSFQ2/DMF/MeOH	0/100	1.08	0.13	−103.76
	75/25	1.04	0.15	−26.67
PSF-DMEA/DMF/MeOH	25/75	–	–	9.30
PSF-DMEA/DMF/water	40/60	–	–	69.88
PSF-DMOA/DMF/MeOH	45/55	–	–	11.67
PSF-DMOA/DMF/water	50/50	0.71	0.03	−0.40

Source: Filimon, A. et al. *Polym. Bull.*, 70(10), 1835–1851, 2013; Albu, R. M. et al. *Polym. Compos.*, 32(10), 1661–1670, 2011.

presented in Table 4.1 confirm that the flow behavior indices are close to unity, as expected for a Newtonian fluid, and decrease, indicating a shear thinning behavior (which agrees with the rheological behavior evidenced in Figures 4.5 and 4.6).

These results, influenced by both composition and solution concentrations of the polymer, are a consequence of the modification of polymer interactions in the system, such as hydrogen-bonding interactions.

The interactions between chain segments, which involve the size of the energy barrier for the movement of an element of the fluid, can be described by the apparent activation energy, E_a, using the Arrhenius equation [66,67].

$$\ln \eta = \ln \eta_0 + \frac{E_a}{RT} \tag{4.4}$$

where:

$\eta_0 \propto e^{\Delta S/R}$ represents a preexponential constant

ΔS is the flow activation entropy

R is the universal gas constant

T is absolute temperature

This barrier is related to the interactions between chain segments and polymer entanglements or specific interactions, such as hydrogen bonding. Accordingly, the overall activation energy involves two processes:

$$E_a = E_{dis} + E_{ass} \tag{4.5}$$

where:

E_{dis} is the positive contribution from disengagement

E_{ass} is a negative contribution from the associated formations

Analysis of polymer entanglements provides an interesting perspective on the effects generated by the interactions from systems. Thus, in PSFQ1/DMF/MeOH and PSFQ2/DMF/MeOH ternary systems, different types of interactions appear, generating specific molecular associations, that is, interactions between DMF and MeOH, interactions between these solvents and PSFQ1 or PSFQ2, and electrostatic interactions due to the charged groups attached to the main polymer chain. As a consequence, in the case of these ternary systems, association phenomena were manifested among the components of the complex polymeric system; moreover, the presence of electrostatic interactions induced by the ionic groups leads to negative values of the activation energy (Table 4.1). In this situation, a negative contribution of the associated formations, E_{ass}, becomes preponderant, compared to the positive contribution of disengagement, E_{dis}.

Similar to dynamic viscosity, activation energy gets modified, being affected by the nature and size groups from quaternized PSFs, and by the composition of solvent/nonsolvent mixtures. In this context, for PSF-DMEA and PSF-DMOA in DMF/MeOH and DMF/water solvent mixtures, the slopes of Arrhenius plots take positive values, which lead to different values of the activation energy, depending on the type of pendant groups from quaternized PSFs, alkyl radical size, solution concentrations, and the composition of solvent mixtures (Table 4.1). Thus, water contributes to the specific molecular rearrangement of the system with the modification of temperature, favoring the formation of associated molecules at high concentration and high water content.

The pendant groups from quaternized PSFs (different radical alkyl) influence the solubility process in DMF/water mixtures, generating molecular restructurations in solution, under the influence of hydrogen bonding, electrostatic interactions, and association phenomena. In addition, one can mention that the rheological properties are influenced by the hydrophobic characteristics of the modified PSFs, which decrease in the following order: PSF-DMOA > PSF-DMEA > PSFQ. Thus, for a more hydrophobic character of polymers, association phenomena become predominant.

Physical chain entanglements behave in a similar manner to chemical cross-links, although the chains can also slide one over another, affecting the viscoelastic behavior. This aspect can be evaluated using oscillatory rheometric measurements, which allow the characterization of polymers as a function of frequency. In this context, viscoelastic measurements can significantly contribute to the knowledge and differentiation of polymer systems, completing the rheological studies developed in the shear regime. The effect of polymer structural characteristics and the composition of solvent/nonsolvent mixtures on the mobility of the segments from the shear field are reflected in the storage, G', and loss, G'', moduli. Thus, the literature [63] exemplifies the variation of storage and loss moduli *versus* frequency for quaternized PSFs (PSFQ1 and PSFQ2) with different ionic chlorine content, at different compositions of mixed solvents (Figure 4.7a and b). Typically, at lower frequencies, the values of G'' exceed those of G'; moreover, the storage, G', and the loss moduli, G'', are proportional to f^2 and f^1, respectively (Figure 4.7a). Consequently, for these systems,

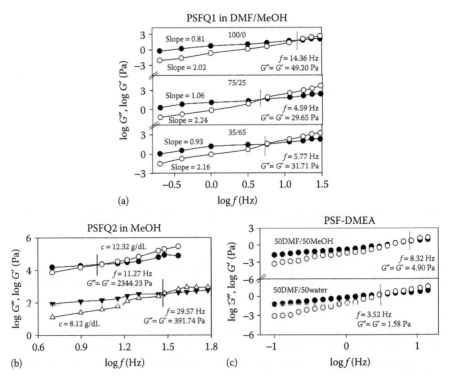

FIGURE 4.7 Log–log plot of the storage (G'—o) and loss (G''—•) moduli as a function of frequency, at 25°C, for: (a) PSFQ1 in 100/0, 75/25, 35/65 (v/v) DMF/MeOH solvent mixture at about 15 g/dL concentration; (b) PSFQ2 in 0/100 DMF/MeOH mixed solvent; and (c) PSF-DMEA sample in 50 DMF/50 MeOH and 50 DMF/50 water solvent mixtures at 13.05 g/dL concentration.

moduli variation with frequency is typical for viscoelastic Maxwellian fluids [67]. At higher values of frequency, G' becomes higher than G'', and the frequency corresponding to their overlapping increases with decreasing concentration (Figure 4.7b).

According to previous assertions, when concentration increases, expansion of the polyionic chain decreases, concomitantly with the dissociation of the ionizable groups from the modified PSFs, generating a higher $G' = G''$ value. In addition, these figures show the influence of the chemical structures of quaternized PSFs and the solvent/nonsolvent mixtures. For example, Figure 4.7c shows that, for the PSF-DMEA in DMF/MeOH and DMF/water solvent mixtures, at the same concentrations (e.g., 13.05 g/dL), the frequencies corresponding to the crossover point, which delimit the viscous flow from the elastic one, and for which $G' = G''$, exhibit lower values in DMF/water than in DMF/MeOH; moreover, these frequencies take lower values at higher concentrations, in both solvent mixtures [64]. Thereby, the aspect of the curves for both moduli could be related to polymer topological entanglements [68]. Moreover, the electronegativity of the pendant groups, generated by their electron-donor character, influences the dissolution of quaternized PSFs in DMF. Addition of water modifies solubility. Once known that water provides strong polar interactions, the DMF molecules may exhibit hydrogen bonding interactions with water and also mutual association phenomena, which affect dissolution. These interactions modify the flow properties, especially through enhancing the water content and concentration.

All these aspects reflect the specific molecular rearrangements in the system, through the modification of the mixing ratio of solvents, under the influence of hydrogen bonding interactions between the polymer components and the solvent. Knowledge of the structural peculiarities of quaternized PSFs becomes important for establishing the correlation between rheological characteristics, surface hydrophobicity, and specific surface topography. In this context, knowledge of the rheological properties of these solutions, in correlation with morphological aspects, represents the basis of their future applications, such as obtaining semipermeable membranes designed for biomedical fields.

4.4 TOPOGRAPHIC REORGANIZATIONS OF POLYSULFONIC MEMBRANES INDUCED BY THE PRESENCE OF DIFFERENT FUNCTIONAL GROUPS

The design of novel structures with specific macroscopic properties, such as texture, appearance, chemical and microbiological stabilities, and their pharmacological or physiological effectiveness, continues to be a major challenge for modern technologists. Depending on the structure created, a unique set of properties arises, which may or may not fully fulfill the requirements set by the intended user [69]. In particular, the design of novel structures has gained an enormous interest because it allows for the creation of structures at various scales, including the nano-, colloidal-, and microscopic levels [69,70].

In addition, there are reports indicating that the chain shape of a polymer in solution could affect the morphology of polymer in bulk [71,72]. Consequently, the investigation of the rheological properties of quaternized PSFs in both mixed solvents and polymer blends is essential for a better understanding of the morphology developed by

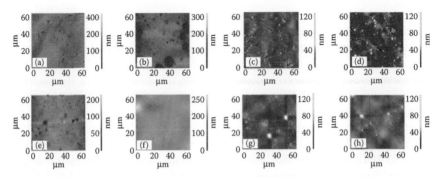

FIGURE 4.8 2D AFM images for PSFQ membranes obtained from different solvent mixtures at various compositions: (a) PSFQ1 in 60/40 DMF/MeOH; (b) PSFQ1 in 20/80 DMF/MeOH; (c) PSFQ2 in 40/60 DMF/MeOH; (d) PSFQ2 in 80/20 DMF/MeOH; (e) PSFQ1 in 60/40 DMF/water; (f) PSFQ1 in 40/60 DMF/water; (g) PSFQ2 in 60/40 MeOH/water; and (h) PSFQ2 in 20/80 MeOH/water.

quaternized PSF films. These combined studies extend the knowledge on the nature of the interactions manifested in the system and on the relation between shear deformation and texture. Therefore, atomic force microscopy (AFM) investigations of the PSFQ films prepared from solutions in solvent/nonsolvent mixtures can reflect the influence of these interactions on the morphological properties. Thus, the 2D AFM images (Figure 4.8) reveal the morphology of films modifications, caused by the charge density of PSFQ and the nature and composition of solvent/nonsolvent mixtures [19].

Each micrograph shows that the film surface is not smooth, appearing as an ordered domain, within which pores and nodules with different size and intensity are distributed. Mention has been made in the beginning of the work that MeOH is a weak solvent for PSFQ1 (with an ionic chlorine content of 2.15%), becoming a better solvent with increasing ionic chlorine content for PSFQ2 (with an ionic chlorine content of 5.71%). In addition, the increase of the nonsolvent content in DMF/MeOH or DMF/water solvent mixtures (MeOH, water for PSFQ1 or DMF, water for PSFQ2) increases the solvation power, as observed from viscometric studies in dilute solutions [43,54]. In particular, it was found that increasing the nonsolvent content in the casting solutions favored the modification of the ordered domains; increasing the MeOH content favored the increase of pore number and their characteristics—area, volume, and diameter—whereas their depth decreased (Table 4.2; Figure 4.8b). This changing trend in morphology is due to the modification of chain conformation of PSFQs in solution, influenced by the quality of the mixed solvents and by the specific interactions, including hydrogen bonding [71]. In addition, it allowed the establishment of optimal composition of solvent/nonsolvent mixtures for obtaining surfaces with controlled dimensions, according to the applied field.

As known, mixing of DMF with MeOH will induce changes in the formation of hydrogen bonding and dipolar interactions [73]. Methanol, besides providing polar interactions, evidences dispersive interactions; by increasing the methanol content of the mixture, the dispersive character increases. Moreover, in the presence of the polymer, addition of DMF to MeOH leads to self-association and increased hydrogen bonding between the two components. Moreover, the strong electrostatic

TABLE 4.2

Surface Roughness Parameters[a] and Pore Characteristics[b] of Membranes Prepared from Quaternized PSFs with Different Solvent Mixtures

Membrane-Forming Solution	Surface Roughness			Pore Characteristics			
	S_q	nhp	nhh	Area	Volume	Depth	Diameter
PSFQ1/60DMF/40MeOH	12.36	279	253	0.50	74.72	237.62	0.79
PSFQ1/20DMF/80MeOH	18.36	205	180	1.44	83.47	88.54	1.35
PSFQ1/60DMF/40water	8.83	170	135	0.34	8.85	46.21	0.67
PSFQ1/40DMF/60water	6.53	200	190	0.16	4.60	45.74	0.46
PSFQ2/40DMF/60MeOH	5.45	66	50	0.19	1.00	6.82	0.49
PSFQ2/80DMF/20MeOH	5.62	64	42	0.22	0.88	6.99	0.53
PSFQ2/60MeOH/40water	9.72	104	50	0.48	5.84	20.07	0.78
PSFQ2/20MeOH/80water	2.72	45	30	0.15	0.25	3.01	0.43

Source: Filimon, A. et al. *J. Appl. Polym. Sci.*, 112(3), 1808–1816, 2009.

[a] Includes root-mean-square roughness (S_q, nm), nodules height from the height profile (nhp, nm), and nodules average height from the histogram (nhh, nm).

[b] Includes area (μm × μm), volume (μm × μm × μm), depth (nm), and diameter (μm).

interactions from the PSFQ2/DMF/MeOH system are generated by the pronounced electron-donor character of PSFQ2, comparatively with PSFQ1.

On the other hand, a higher charge density in PSFQ2 determines the occurrence of nodules, as illustrated in Figure 4.8c and d.

The presence of water as a nonsolvent in the solutions used for casting membranes influenced the AFM images; increasing the water content led to the formation of pores with lower area for both polymer membranes under study (Figure 4.8f for the PSFQ1 membranes and Figure 4.8h for the PSFQ2 membranes), and also to fewer nodules in the PSFQ2 membranes (Figure 4.8g and h). Also, it may be assumed that the association of MeOH with water over different composition domains of their mixtures might have been one of the factors affecting the morphology of the PSFQ2 membrane surface. Thus, mixed solvents were formed from water and MeOH associated with water at high water contents; in contrast, at high MeOH compositions, the mixtures consisted largely of MeOH and water associated with MeOH. Therefore, these phenomena changed the PSFQ2 solubility, determining the modification of solution properties (Figure 4.4a), as well as of surface morphology.

Figure 4.9 exemplifies the bi-dimensional structures evidenced by AFM investigations for the following:

- PSF-DMEA films prepared in 75/25 and 25/75 DMF/MeOH solvent mixtures and in 75/25 and 40/60 DMF/water solvent mixtures (Figure 4.9a, b, e, and f)
- PSF-DMOA films prepared in 75/25 and 45/25 DMF/MeOH solvent mixtures and in 75/25 and 50/50 of DMF/water solvent mixtures (Figure 4.9c, d, g, and h)

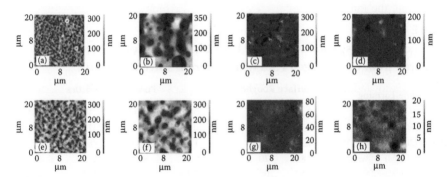

FIGURE 4.9 2D AFM images for quaternized polysulfone membranes obtained from different solvent mixtures at various compositions: (a) PSF-DMEA in 75/25 DMF/MeOH; (b) PSF-DMEA in 25/75 DMF/MeOH; (c) PSF-DMOA in 75/25 DMF/MeOH; (d) PSF-DMOA in 45/55 DMF/MeOH; (e) PSF-DMEA in 75/25 DMF/water; (f) PSF-DMEA in 40/60 DMF/water; (g) PSF-DMOA in 75/25 DMF/water; and (h) PSF-DMOA in 50/50 DMF/water.

According to these images, increasing the nonsolvent content in the casting solutions favors the modification of surface morphology. Thus, the average surface roughness decreases with increasing MeOH content, favoring the increase of pore number and their characteristics—area, depth, diameter, and mean width, as shown in Table 4.3. It should also be noted that the quality of the solvent mixtures over the studied domain increases with the addition of a nonsolvent (Figure 4.4b). Moreover, the presence of water as a nonsolvent in the solutions used for casting films influenced the AFM images presented in Figure 4.9; a higher water content decreases the thermodynamic quality of the DMF/water solvent mixtures (Figure 4.4b), so that, for PSF-DMEA in 40/60 DMF/water, the average surface roughness, the number of pores, and their depths take maximum values with minimum area (Table 4.3). It may be assumed that the specific interactions with the mixed solvents employed in the study modify the PSF-DMOA solubility and determine the modification of the solution properties, as illustrated in Figure 4.4b [55].

Recently, the influence of synthetic polymers on the morphology of quaternized PSF/synthetic polymer blend films has been studied [64], as well as their ability to improve the film-forming characteristics, necessary for a better understanding and control of their prospective application in plasma separation or biomedicine. In this context, the AFM images (Figure 4.10) of the PSF-DMEA/PS, PSF-DMOA/PS, PSF-DMEA/P4VP, and PSF-DMOA/P4VP films at a 50/50 wt/wt mixing ratio, prepared from DMF solutions, exhibit different structures.

Pure PSF-DMEA film prepared under the same conditions exhibits a larger number of pores and higher surface roughness, compared with PSF-DMOA (Table 4.4). In addition, for all blending systems from Table 4.4, the number of pores is lower than for the pure components, PSF-DMEA and PSF-DMOA, whereas the surface roughness increases, especially in the presence of PS.

The pore characteristics for both polymer blends are different; the presence of PS in polymer blends leads to higher values of the average depths and mean widths, compared with those generated by the presence of P4VP. Moreover, the low hydrophilic characteristics given by the ethyl radical from the N-dimethylethylammonium

TABLE 4.3

Pore Characteristics[a] and Surface Roughness Parameters[b] of PSF-DMEA and PSF-DMOA Films Prepared from Solutions in DMF/MeOH and DMF/Water, with 20 × 20 μm² Scanned Areas, Corresponding to 2D AFM Images

Solvent Mixtures	Number of Pores	Area	Depth	Diameter	Length	Mean Width	S_a	S_q	H_a
		Pore Characteristics					Surface Roughness		
				PSF-DMEA in DMF/MeOH					
75/25	268	0.27	259.59	0.62	0.94	0.32	31.89	41.47	217.26
25/75	37	1.10	242.07	1.18	1.73	0.62	48.36	59.80	193.33
				PSF-DMEA in DMF/Water					
75/25	147	0.51	245.19	0.86	1.25	0.48	37.41	47.76	227.79
40/60	42	2.19	230.10	1.64	2.43	0.86	44.98	57.61	281.80
				PSF-DMOA in DMF/MeOH					
75/25	–	–	–	–	–	–	14.43	19.90	82
45/55	44	0.80	16.02	0.98	1.53	0.49	2.77	4.24	28
				PSF-DMOA in DMF/Water					
75/25	5	3.12	13.65	1.97	3.26	0.96	1.59	2.34	15
50/50	18	2.09	5.55	1.46	2.63	0.64	1.52	2.17	8

Source: Albu, R. M. et al. *Polym. Compos.*, 32(10), 1661–1670, 2011.

[a] Include number of pores, area (μm²), depth (nm), diameter (μm), length (μm), mean width (μm).

[b] Include average roughness (S_a, nm), root-mean-square roughness (S_q, nm), and average height from the height histogram (H_a, nm).

chloride pendant group and by the octyl radical from the *N*-dimethyloctylammonium chloride pendant group, respectively (where the electron-donor interactions are lower than the electron-acceptor ones for PSF-DMEA, and the electron-donor interactions exceed the electron-acceptor interactions for PSF-DMOA), influence films morphology. Thus, the electron-acceptor characteristics of PSF-DMEA or the electron-donor ones of PSF-DMOA and the zero polarity of PS increase the surface roughness in film surface blends, more distinctly in the PSF-DMOA/PS blend. Moreover, the polarization properties of both quaternized PSFs and the low electron-donor properties of P4VP led to a different modification of the blending process; the same characteristics of polarity generates a slightly higher surface roughness, the electron-donor and electron-acceptor characteristics of the blends inducing a much higher growth in roughness. Thus, the molecular interactions of such systems are reflected in the predictable performance of blending materials.

Consequently, surface morphology depends on the history of film preparation, including the characteristics of quaternized PSFs, the type of pendant groups from quaternized PSFs, and thermodynamic quality of solvents.

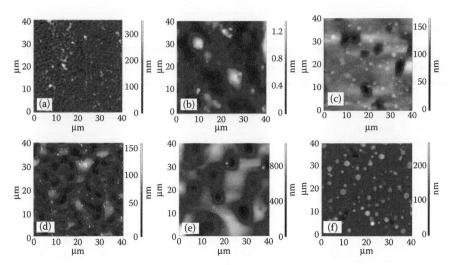

FIGURE 4.10 2D AFM images for: (a) PSF-DMEA film; (b) PSF-DMEA/PS; (c) PSF-DMEA/P4VP; (d) PSF-DMOA film; (e) PSF-DMOA/PS; and (f) PSF-DMOA/P4VP blend films.

TABLE 4.4
Surface Roughness Parameters[a] and Pore Characteristics[b] for PSF-DMEA, PSF-DMOA, and Their Blends with PS and P4VP Films [at a 50/50 (wt/wt) Mixing Ratio] Prepared from Solutions in DMF, Corresponding to 2D AFM Images

Samples	Surface Roughness					Pore Characteristics			
	Gpa	Aars	Ah	S_a	S_q	No. p	Ad	Al	Wm
PSF-DMEA	1600	1640.35	145.85	30.68	38.78	512	114	1.26	1.02
PSF-DMEA/PS	1600	1617.35	467.84	168.58	211.96	7	524	12.11	5.17
PSF-DMEA/P4VP	1600	1600.16	132.60	8.03	13.97	8	84	6.87	3.95
PSF-DMOA	1600	1600.59	54.13	14.08	17.35	36	33	7.36	4.22
PSF-DMOA/PS	1600	1604.61	450.21	103.42	131.65	9	432	13.53	10.05
PSF-DMOA/P4VP	1600	1601.24	110.98	16.93	22.47	4	61	4.74	3.61

Source: Albu, R. M. et al. *Polym. Compos.*, 32(10), 1661–1670, 2011.

[a] Include geometrically projected area (Gpa, μm^2), actual area of roughness surface (Aars, μm^2), average height (Ah, nm), average roughness (S_a, nm), root-mean-square roughness (S_q, nm).

[b] Include number of collected pores (No. p), average depth (Ad, nm), average length (Al, μm), and mean width (Wm, μm).

This type of membranes represents an excellent scaffold for applications in both cellular and tissue engineering. It should be mentioned that fibroblasts and chondrocyte cells have been shown to grow well in porous membranes, which evidences their superior properties (specific molecular microarchitecture and controlled porosity) for tissue regeneration applications [74].

The results reveal that, considering the traditional processes and the recently developed techniques, the improved ability to control the porosity and molecular microarchitecture of functionalized PSFs/synthetic polymers membranes will drive the research closer to proposed goals. With these techniques, it is possible not only to specifically control individual and group pore architecture but also to take the next step to create microvascular features to improve integration within host tissues. Also, structural improvement and increased pore interconnectivity of the porous scaffolds are claimed for the development of artificial blood vessels or peripheral nerve growth.

4.5 SURFACE AND INTERFACIAL PROPERTIES OF FUNCTIONALIZED PSFs

Surface and interfacial tension data for polymers are essential to many aspects of the production and the application of elastomers, plastics, textiles, films and coatings, foams, polymer blends, adhesives, and sealants [75,76]. Additionally, the measurement of surface properties of polymers, correlated with the shear process and the molecular structure of polymers, provide a source of engineering design properties for various applications [75].

It has been shown that, in most cases of practical interest, the rheological and morphological properties are influenced by the hydrophobic/hydrophilic characteristics. In this context, some studies have discussed the wettability of the surfaces of PSFs and functionalized PSFs using a combined approach—contact angle/theoretical analysis [77], permitting quantification of the contribution of each physicochemical phenomenon involved at the solid–liquid interface. Absorption and/or spreading were identified as the major effects occurring upon the deposition of liquid droplets on the surfaces of PSFs. Moreover, the polarization effect, arising from the dipole orientation and charge carriers of quaternized PSFs, generates different electron-donor/electron-acceptor interactions—as shown in Tables 4.5 and 4.6 [64,77]. Therefore, the Lifshitz-van der Waals/acid-base method (LW/AB) (Equations 4.6 through 4.8) [46,78] can be used to calculate the surface tension parameters of functionalized PSFs using the surface tension parameters of test liquids provided in the literature [79] and the measured contact angles between these liquids and the prepared polysulfonic films [77].

$$1 + \cos\theta = \frac{2}{\gamma_{lv}}\left(\sqrt{\gamma_{sv}^{LW}\gamma_{lv}^{LW}} + \sqrt{\gamma_{sv}^{+}\gamma_{lv}^{-}} + \sqrt{\gamma_{sv}^{-}\gamma_{lv}^{+}}\right) \tag{4.6}$$

$$\gamma_{sv}^{AB} = 2\sqrt{\gamma_{sv}^{+}\gamma_{sv}^{-}} \tag{4.7}$$

$$\gamma_{sv}^{LW/AB} = \gamma_{sv}^{LW} + \gamma_{sv}^{AB} \tag{4.8}$$

where:
Superscript LW/AB indicates the total surface tension
Superscripts AB and LW represent the polar component, obtained from the interactions between the electron-donor, γ_{sv}^{-}, and the electron-acceptor, γ_{sv}^{+}, and the disperse component, respectively

TABLE 4.5

Surface Tension Parameters (mN/m)[a], Surface Free Energy (ΔG_w, mJ m^{-2}), and Interfacial Free Energy between Two Particles of PSFs in Water Phase (ΔG_{sls}, mJ m^{-2}) for Polysulfone (PSF), Chloromethylated Polysulfone (CMPSF1, CMPSF2, and CMPSF3) Films Prepared from Solutions in Chloroform, and Quaternized Polysulfone Films (PSFQ1, PSFQ2, and PSFQ3) Prepared from Solutions in Methanol

Samples	γ_{sv}^{LW}	γ_{sv}^{AB}	γ_{sv}^{-}	γ_{sv}^{+}	$\gamma_{sv}^{LW/AB}$	ΔG_w	ΔG_{sls}
PSF	18.77	9.34	8.74	28.10	33.23	−86.28	−25.08
CMPSF1	21.27	7.46	11.43	28.73	25.97	−88.35	−20.38
CMPSF2	16.85	12.38	17.02	29.23	42.35	−91.64	−19.20
CMPSF3	15.79	14.14	17.56	29.93	47.23	−81.67	−21.23
PSFQ1	12.70	19.29	27.24	31.98	60.31	−105.09	−21.02
PSFQ2	8.15	42.56	29.98	43.71	97.38	−105.09	−50.32
PSFQ3	7.82	56.82	49.34	64.74	82.70	−137.28	−60.08

Source: Ioan et al. *e-Polymers*, 031, 1–13, 2007.

[a] Include parameters such as total surface tension, $\gamma_{sv}^{LW/AB}$; disperse component of surface tension, γ_{sv}^{LW}; and polar component of surface tension, γ_{sv}^{AB}, with their electron-donor, γ_{sv}^{-}, electron-acceptor, γ_{sv}^{+}, contributions.

According to the observations made by the authors, the surface tension of PSF evidences the lowest hydrophilicity, induced by the aromatic rings connected by one carbon and two methyl groups, oxygen elements, and sulfonic groups, whereas the chloromethylation of PSF with the $-CH_2Cl$ functional group increases hydrophilicity (see the values of surface tension for PSF and CMPSF given in Table 4.5). Moreover, the results indicate that the PSFQ membranes are the most hydrophilic ones among all studied samples (lowest water contact angle), due to the N,N-dimethylethanolamine hydrophilic side groups. Hence, it is observed that total surface tension, $\gamma_{sv}^{LW/AB}$, and the polar component, γ_{sv}^{AB}, increase with the substitution degree of CMPSF and with the quaternization degree of the ammonium groups for PSFQ samples. The apolar component, γ_{sv}^{LW}, decreases from PSF to CMPSF and PSFQ. The total surface tensions of PSF and CMPSF1, at a substitution degree DS < 1, are dominated by the apolar component, whereas the total surface tensions of CMPSF2, CMPSF3 (DS > 1), and PSFQ are dominated by the polar term, with the electron-donor interactions, γ_{sv}^{-}, lower than the electron-acceptor ones, γ_{sv}^{+}. Thus, the $-CH_2Cl$ functional groups attached through chloromethylation increase the polarity of CMPSFs with a substitution degree DS > 1; moreover, the N,N-dimethylethanolamine side groups introduced by the quaternization process increase polarity. The change is moderate for CMPSFs with DS > 1, at different chloride contents.

The PSF-DMEA films (with two carbon atoms in the alkyl side chain) possess low polar surface-tension parameters, yet slightly higher than those for PSF-DMOA (with eight carbon atoms in the alkyl side chain), as shown in

TABLE 4.6

Surface Tension Parameters (mN/m), Surface Free Energy (ΔG_w, mJ m^{-2}), and Interfacial Free Energy between Two Particles of Quaternized Polysulfones in Water Phase (ΔG_{sls}, mJ m^{-2}) for PSF-DMEA and PSF-DMOA Quaternized Polysulfone Films Prepared from Solutions in DMF/MeOH and DMF/Water

Solvent mixtures	γ_{sv}^{LW}	γ_{sv}^{AB}	γ_{sv}^{-}	γ_{sv}^{+}	$\gamma_{sv}^{LW/AB}$	ΔG_w	ΔG_{sls}
			PSF-DMEA in DMF/MeOH				
100/0	42.5	6.2	2.6	3.6	48.7	−67	−51.90
75/25	41.3	6.9	2.8	4.3	48.1	−68	−48.52
50/50	41.8	9.9	2.5	9.9	51.7	−75	−36.94
25/75	40.6	10.4	4.1	6.5	51.0	−74	−38.30
			PSF-DMEA in DMF/Water				
75/25	41.5	3.18	0.1	21.4	44.68	−77	−32.30
50/50	42.3	3.83	0.2	19.0	46.08	−76	−35.20
40/60	42.7	4.15	0.2	25.4	46.85	−79	−31.14
			PSF-DMOA in DMF/MeOH				
100/0	42.4	1.5	1.4	0.4	43.9	−95.30	−53.84
75/25	42.7	0.8	0.8	0.2	43.5	−87.94	−64.12
50/50	43.1	1.8	2.0	1.5	44.9	−111.38	−74.30
45/55	41.3	1.4	0.5	1.0	42.7	−89.18	−59.82
			PSF-DMOA in DMF/Water				
75/25	41.4	1.5	1.2	0.5	42.9	−102.41	−43.32
60.40	40.2	3.3	3.5	0.8	43.6	−103.57	−40.16
50/50	42.8	1.6	1.3	0.5	44.4	−97.70	−50.60

Source: Albu, R. M. et al. *Polym. Compos.*, 32(10), 1661–1670, 2011.

Table 4.6. The hydrophobic character is given by the ethyl radical from the N-dimethylethylammonium chloride pendant group and by the octyl radical from the N-dimethyloctylammonium chloride pendant group, respectively. Furthermore, the electron-donor interactions, γ_{sv}^{-}, are lower than the electron-acceptor ones, γ_{sv}^{+}, for PSF-DMEA, whereas, for PSF-DMOA, the electron-donor interactions, γ_{sv}^{-}, exceed the electron-acceptor ones, γ_{sv}^{+}, due to the inductive phenomena from the alkyl radical. These results reflect the capacity of the N-dimethylethylammonium or N-dimethyloctylammonium chloride pendant groups to determine the acceptor or donor character of the polar terms, generated by such inductive phenomena [64].

These parameters are influenced by the solvent/nonsolvent composition from which the films had been prepared. Thus, Table 4.6 shows that the polar components of surface tensions slightly increase for films prepared in DMF/MeOH solvents mixtures. On the contrary, for films prepared in DMF/water solvent mixtures, no significant changes were observed in the polar component. These results show that the studied samples evidence high hydrophobicity; a maximum hydrophobicity of the PSFs with pendant groups would be advantageous, for example, for dielectric performance, as a low water absorption causes a significant decrease in the dielectric constant and, implicitly, low adhesion to different interfaces.

The effects of the chemical structure and history of films prepared from solutions on the surface and interfacial properties, evaluated by Equations 4.9 through 4.11, evidence the balance between the hydrophobicity and hydrophilicity of the surface of quaternized PSFs, characterized by a surface free energy (ΔG_w) higher than -113 mJ m^{-2} [79], and negative values of the interfacial free energy (ΔG_{sls}), denoting attraction between the two surfaces of the quaternized PSF, s, immersed in water, l (Tables 4.5 and 4.6).

$$\Delta G_w = -\gamma_{lv}(1 + \cos\theta_{water}) \tag{4.9}$$

$$\Delta G_{sls} = -2\gamma_{sl} \tag{4.10}$$

$$\gamma_{sl} = \left(\sqrt{\gamma_{lv}^p} - \sqrt{\gamma_{sv}^{AB}}\right)^2 + \left(\sqrt{\gamma_{lv}^d} - \sqrt{\gamma_{sv}^{LW}}\right)^2 \tag{4.11}$$

where:
γ_{sl} indicates the solid–liquid interfacial tension.

The surface free energy for PSF and CMPSF samples possesses low wettability. Moreover, all functionalized PSFs (PSFQ) are characterized by scarce wettability. On the other hand, the N,N-dimethyloctylamine group—corresponding to PSF-DMOA—determines a higher wettability than the N,N-dimethylethylamine group—corresponding to PSF-DMEA. This wettability depends on the surface morphology of the samples prepared from different compositions of DMF/MeOH and DMF/water solvent mixtures (Table 4.6).

These results show that functionalized PSFs evidence high hydrophilicity, which increases with increasing substitution degrees. A maximum hydrophilicity of the PSFs with quaternary ammonium pendant groups would be advantageous, for example, for obtaining semipermeable membranes with superior performance suitable in biomedical applications, including the evaluation of bacterial adhesion onto the surface.

4.6 GENERAL REMARKS

The construction of advanced materials is a current challenge in the field of polymers. The approaches to such structures vary widely, depending on the modes of binding the components, which can be generated by changes in the environment, such as temperature, pH, and ionic strength.

This chapter summarizes the recently developed researches devoted to polymer chains consisting of water-soluble PSFs. Knowledge and understanding of the interactions manifested in these complex systems constitute the essential elements for the conception and optimization of new structures. Different characterization techniques have allowed the complete evaluation of the mechanisms involved in multicomponent systems with specific interactions, such as hydrogen bonding, electrostatic interactions, and association phenomena, and the manner in which these interactions affect the properties of final compounds.

This chapter reveals the relationship between molecular–structural parameters (nature and size of the functionalized groups, quaternization degree, and charge density) and the physicochemical properties of functionalized PSFs, which represent an important challenge from both scientific and industrial perspectives. Such responsive systems could be specifically engineered for the particular functions required, which could be tailored more efficiently to suit different requirements in various applications, for example, for high-potential applications in biomedical fields.

The future challenge lies in exploiting this class of chemical compounds for the control of bacterial adhesion, drug delivery, developing biomedical devices, hybrid materials, and so on.

ACKNOWLEDGMENT

This work was supported by a grant of the Romanian National Authority for Scientific Research, CNCS—UEFISCDI (project number PN-II-RU-TE-2012-3-143).

REFERENCES

1. Tomalia, D. A. The emergence of a new macromolecular architecture: "The Dendritic State." In *Properties of Polymers Handbook*, Second Edition; Mark, E. J. Ed., Springer, Cincinnati, OH, Chapter 42, p. 671, 2007.
2. Dizman, C., Tasdelenc, M. A., and Yagcia, Y. Recent advances in the preparation of functionalized polysulfones. *Polym. Int.*, 62 (7), 991–1007, 2014.
3. Barikani, M. and Mehdipour-Ataei, S. Synthesis, characterization and thermal properties of novel arylene sulfone ether polyimides and polyamides. *J. Polym. Sci. Part A Polym. Chem.*, 38 (9), 1487–1492, 2000.
4. Väisänen, P. and Nyström, M. Comparison of polysulfone membranes and polysulfone films. *Acta Polytech. Scand.*, 247 (1), 25–34, 1997.
5. Higuchi, A., Koga, H., and Nakagawa, T. Surface-modified polysulfone hollow fibers. IV. Chloromethylated fibers and their derivatives. *J. Appl. Polym. Sci.*, 46 (3), 449–457, 1992.
6. Du, R. H. and Zhao, J. S. Properties of poly (*N,N*-dimethylaminoethyl methacrylate)/polysulfone positively charged composite nanofiltration membrane. *J. Membr. Sci.*, 239 (2), 183–188, 2004.
7. Du, R. H. and Zhao, J. S. Positively charged composite nanofiltration membrane prepared by poly(*N,N*-dimethylaminoethyl methacrylate)/polysulfone. *J. Appl. Polym. Sci.*, 91 (4), 2721–2728, 2004.
8. Ohya, H., Shiki S., and Kawakami H. Fabrication study of polysulfone hollow-fiber microfiltration membranes: Optimal dope viscosity for nucleation and growth. *J. Membr. Sci.*, 326 (2), 293–302, 2009.
9. Sikder, J., Pereira, C., Palchoudhury, S., Vohra, K., Basumatary, D., and Pal, P. Synthesis and characterization of cellulose acetate-polysulfone blend microfiltration membrane for separation of microbial cells from lactic acid fermentation broth. *Desalination*, 249 (2), 802–808, 2009.

10. Nady, N., Franssen, M. C. R., Zuilhof, H., Eldin, M. S. M., Boom, R., and Schroen, K. Modification methods for poly(arylsulfone) membranes: A mini-review focusing on surface modification. *Desalination*, 275 (1–3), 1–9, 2011.

11. Sivaraman, K. M., Kellenberger, C., Pané, S., Ergeneman, O., Lühmann, T., Luechinger, N. A., Hall, H., Stark, W. J., and Nelson, B. J. Porous polysulfone coatings for enhanced drug delivery. *Biomed. Microdevices*, 14 (3), 603–612, 2012.

12. Tomaszewska, M. and Jarosiewicz, A. Polysulfone coating with starch addition in CRF formulation. *Desalination*, 163 (1–3), 247–252, 2004.

13. Aerts, P., Van Hoof, E., Leysen, R., Vankelecom, I. F. J., and Jacobs, P. A. Polysulfone–aerosil composite membranes: Part 1. The influence of the addition of aerosil on the formation process and membrane morphology. *J. Membr. Sci.*, 176 (1) 63–73, 2000.

14. Sanchez, S., Pumera, M., Cabruja, E., and Fabregas, E. Carbon nano-tube/polysulfone composite screen printed electrochemical enzyme biosensor. *Analyst*, 132 (2), 142–147, 2007.

15. Filimon, A., Avram, E. A., and Stoica, I. Rheological and morphological characteristics of multicomponent polysulfone/poly(vinyl alcohol) systems. *Polym. Int.*, 63 (10), 1856–1868, 2014.

16. von Kraemer, S., Puchner, M., Jannasch, P., Lundblad, A., and Lindbergh, G. Gas diffusion electrodes and membrane electrode assemblies based on a sulfonated polysulfone for high-temperature PEMFC. *J. Electrochem. Soc.*, 153 (11), A2077–A2084, 2006.

17. Kuroiwa, T., Miyagishi, T., Ito, A., Matsuguchi, M., Sadaoka, Y., and Sakai, Y. A thin-film polysulfone-based capacitive-type relative-humidity sensor. *Sens. Actuators, B*, 25 (1–3), 692–695, 1995.

18. Claes, L. Carbonfibre reinforced polysulfone—A new biomaterial. Patent 0013–5585, 1989.

19. Filimon, A., Avram, E., Dunca, S., Stoica, I., and Ioan, S. Surface properties and antibacterial activity of quaternized polysulfones. *J. Appl. Polym. Sci.*, 112 (3), 1808–1816, 2009.

20. Karlsson, L. E. and Jannasch, P. Polysulfone ionomers for proton-conducting fuel cell membranes: Sulfoalkylated polysulfones. *J. Membr. Sci.*, 230 (1–2), 61–70, 2004.

21. Lufrano, F., Gatto, I., Staiti, P., Antonucci, V., and Passalacqua, E. Sulfonated polysulfone ionomer membranes for fuel cells. *Solid State Ionics*, 145 (1–4), 47–51, 2001.

22. Manea, C. and Mulder, M. Characterization of polymer blends of polyethersulfone/sulfonated polysulfone and polyethersulfone/sulfonated polyetheretherketone for direct methanol fuel cell applications. *J. Membr. Sci.*, 206 (1–2), 443–453, 2002.

23. Madaeni, S. S. and Rahimpour, A. Effect of type of solvent and non-solvents on morphology and performance of polysulfone and polyethersulfone ultrafiltration membranes for milk concentration. *Polym. Adv. Technol.*, 16 (10) 717–724, 2005.

24. Malaisamy, R., Mahendran, R., and Mohan, D. J. Cellulose acetate and sulfonated polysulfone blend ultrafiltration membranes. II. Pore statistics, molecular weight cutoff, and morphological studies. *Appl. Polym. Sci.*, 84 (2), 430–444, 2002.

25. Arthanareeswaran, G., Velu, S., and Muruganandam, L. Performance enhancement of polysulfone ultrafiltration membrane by blending with polyurethane hydrophilic polymer. *J. Polym. Eng.*, 31 (2–3), 125–131, 2011.

26. Mark, E. J. *Properties of Polymers Handbook*, Second Edition, Springer, Cincinnati, OH, 2007.

27. Sotiroiu, K., Pispas, S., and Hadjichristidis, N. Effect of the end-positioning of a lithium sulfonate group on the aggregation and micellization behaviour of x-lithium sulfonate polystyrene block polyisoprenes. *Macromol. Chem. Phys.*, 205 (1), 55–62, 2004.

28. Ismail, A. F. and Hafiz, W. A. Effect of polysulfone concentration on the performance of membrane-assisted lead acid battery. *J. Sci. Technol.*, 24 (Suppl), 815–821, 2002.

29. Savariar, S., Underwood, G. S., Dickinson, E. M., Schielke, P. J., and Hay, A. S. Polysulfone with lower levels of cyclic dimer: Use of MALDI-TOF in the study of cyclic. *Desalination*, 144 (1–3), 15–20, 2002.

30. Ydens, I., Moins, S., Degee, P., and Dubois, P. Solution properties of well-defined 2-(dimethylamino)ethyl methacrylate-based (co)polymers: A viscometric approach. *Eur. Polym. J.*, 41 (7), 1502–1509, 2005.

31. Avram, E., Butuc, E., Luca, C., and Druta, I. Polymers with pendant functional group. III. Polysulfones containing viologen group. *J. Macromol. Sci. Part A Pure Appl. Chem.*, 34 (9), 1701–1714, 1997.

32. Cozan, V. and Avram, E. Side chain thermotropic liquid crystalline polysulfone obtained from polysulfone Udel by chemical modification. *Eur. Polym. J.*, 39 (1), 107–114, 2003.

33. Racles, C., Avram, E., Marcu, M., Cozan, V., and Cazacu, M. New siloxane-ester modified polysulfones by phase transfer catalysis. *Polymer*, 41 (23), 8205–8211, 2000.

34. Guiver, M. D., Black, P., Tam, C. M., and Deslandes, Y. Functionalized polysulfone membranes by heterogeneous lithiation. *J. Appl. Polym. Sci.*, 48 (9), 1597–1606, 1993.

35. Higuchi, A., Shirano, K., Harashima, M., Yoon, B. O., Hara, M., Hattori, M., and Imamura, K. Chemically modified polysulfone hollow fibers with vinylpyrrolidone having improved blood compatibility. *Biomaterials*, 23, 2659–2666, 2002.

36. Tomaszewska, M., Jarosiewicz, A., and Karakulski, K. Physical and chemical characteristics of polymer coatings in CRF formulation. *Desalination*, 146 (1–3), 319–323, 2002.

37. Wavhal, D. S., and Fisher, E. R. Hydrophilic modification of polyethersulfone membrane by low temperature plasma-induced graft polymerization. *J. Membr. Sci.*, 209 (1), 255–269, 2002.

38. Zhang, Q., Li, S., and Zhang, S. A novel guanidinium grafted poly(aryl ether sulfone) for high-performance hydroxide exchange membranes. *Chem. Commun.*, 46 (11), 7495–7497, 2010.

39. Zhang, Q. F., Zhang, S. B., Dai, L., and Chen, X. S. Novel zwitterionic poly(arylene ether sulfone)s as antifouling membrane material. *J. Membr. Sci.*, 349 (1–2), 217–224, 2010.

40. Xie, W., Xie, R., Pan, W., Hunter, D., Koene, B., Tan, L., and Vaia, R. Thermal stability of quaternary phosphonium modified montmorillonites. *Chem. Mater.*, 14 (11), 4837–4845, 2002.

41. Eisenberg, A., Hird, B., and Moore, R. B. A new multiple-cluster model for the morphology of random ionomers. *Macromolecules*, 23 (18), 4098–4107, 1990.

42. Cheng, S., Beyer, F. L., Mather, B. D., Moore, R. B., and Long, T. E. Phosphonium-containing ABA triblock copolymers: Controlled free radical polymerization of phosphonium ionic liquids. *Macromolecules*, 44 (16), 6509–6517, 2011.

43. Schuster, M., Rager, T., Noda, A., Kreuer, K. D., and Maier, J. About the choice of the protogenic group in PEM separator materials for intermediate temperature, low humidity operation: A critical comparison of sulfonic acid, phosphonic acid and imidazole functionalized model compounds. *Fuel Cells*, 5 (3), 355–365, 2005.

44. Meredith, J. C., Sormana, B. J., Keselowsky, L. G., Garcia, A. J., Tona, A., Karim, A., and Amis, E. J. Combinatorial characterization of cell interactions with polymer surfaces. *J. Biomed. Mater. Res.*, 66A (3), 483–490, 2003.

45. Averous, L. Blends of thermoplastic starch and polyesteramide: Processing and properties. *J. Appl. Polym. Sci.*, 76 (7), 1117–1128, 2000.

46. van Oss, C. J., Ju, L., Chaudhury, M. K., and Good, R. J. Interfacial Lifshitz-van der Waals and polar interactions in macroscopic systems. *Chem. Rev.*, 88 (6), 927–941, 1988.

47. Witten, T. A. and Cohen, M. H. Crosslinking in shear-thickening ionomers. *Macromolecules*, 18 (10), 1915–1918, 1985.

48. Cox, J. A. and Kulkarni, K. R. Comparison of inorganic films and poly(4-vinylpyridine) coatings as electrode modifiers for flow-injection systems. *Talanta*, 33 (11), 911–913, 1986.

49. Ashley, K. M., Meredith, J. C., Amis, E., Raghavan, D., and Karim, A. Combinatorial investigation of dewetting: Polystyrene thin films on gradient hydrophilic surfaces. *Polymer*, 44 (3), 769–772, 2003.
50. Sundararajan, P. R. Chain structures. In *Properties of Polymers Handbook*, Second Edition; Mark, E. J. Ed., Springer, Cincinnati, OH, Chapter 1, p. 3, 2007.
51. Kotlyarevskaya, O. O., Navrotskii, V. A., Orlyanskii, M. V., Navrotskii, A.V., and Novakov, I. A. Hydrodynamic behavior of *N,N*-dimethylaminoethyl methacrylate polylectrolytes in mixed solvents. *Polym. Sci., Series A*, 47 (3), 313–318, 2005.
52. Ioan, S., Filimon, A., and Avram, E. Influence of the degree of substitution on the solution properties of chloromethylated polysulfone. *J. Appl. Polym. Sci.*, 101 (1), 524–531, 2006.
53. Filimon, A., Avram, E., and Ioan, S. Influence of mixed solvents and of temperature on the solution properties of quaternized polysulfones. *J. Macromol. Sci. Part B*, 46 (3), 503–520, 2007.
54. Ioan, S., Filimon, A., and Avram, E. Conformational and viscometric behavior of quaternized polysulfone in dilute solution. *Polym. Eng. Sci.*, 46 (7), 827–836, 2006.
55. Filimon, A., Albu, R. M., Avram, E., and Ioan, S. Effect of alkyl side chain on the conformational properties of polysulfones with quaternary groups. *J. Macromol. Sci. Part B*, 49 (1), 207–217, 2010.
56. Avram, E. Polymers with pendent functional groups. VI. A comparative study on the chloromethylation of linear polystyrene and polysulfone with paraformaldehyde/Me$_3$SiCl. *Polym. Plast. Technol. Eng.*, 40 (3), 275–281, 2001.
57. Luca, C., Avram, E., and Petrariu, I. Quaternary ammonium polyelectrolytes. V. Amination studies of chloromethylated polystyrene with *N,N*-dimethylalkylamines. *J. Macromol. Sci. Part A Chem.*, 25 (4), 345–361, 1988.
58. Huggins, M. L. The viscosity of dilute solutions of long-chain molecules. IV. Dependence on concentration. *J. Am. Chem. Soc.*, 64 (11), 2716–2718, 1942.
59. Ise, N. On the solution viscosity of ionic polymers and their conformation in solutions. *Proc. Jpn. Acad. B*, 74 (8), 192–200, 1998.
60. Rao, M. V. S. Viscosity of dilute to moderately concentrated polymer solutions. *Polymer*, 34 (3), 592–596, 1993.
61. Filimon, A., Avram, E., and Ioan, S. Specific interactions in ternary system quaternized polysulfones/mixed solvent. *Polym. Eng. Sci.*, 49 (1), 17–25, 2009.
62. Filimon, A., Albu, R. M., Avram, E. and Ioan, S. Impact of association phenomena on the thermodynamic properties of modified polysulfones in solutions. *J. Macromol. Sci. Part B Phys.*, 52 (4), 545–560, 2013.
63. Filimon, A., Avram, E., and Ioan S. Structure-rheology relationship in complex quaternized polysulfones/solvent/nonsolvent systems. *Polym. Bull.*, 70 (10), 1835–1851, 2013.
64. Albu, R. M., Avram, E., Stoica, I., Ioanid, E. G., and Ioan, S. Miscibility and morphological properties of quaternized polysulfone blends with polystyrene and poly(4-vinylpyridine). *Polym. Compos.*, 32 (10), 1661 1670, 2011.
65. Lue, A. and Zhang, L. Rheological behaviors in the regimes from dilute to concentrated in cellulose solutions dissolved at low temperature. *Macromol. Biosci.*, 9 (5), 488–496, 2009.
66. de Vasconcelos, C. L., Martins, R. R., Ferreira, M. O., Pereira, M. R., and Fonseca, J. L. C. Rheology of polyurethane solutions with different solvents. *Polym. Int.*, 51 (1), 69–74, 2002.
67. Gupta, K. and Yaseen, M. Viscosity-temperature relationship of dilute solution of poly(vinyl chloride) in cyclohexanone and in its blends with xylene. *J. Appl. Polym. Sci.*, 65 (13), 2749–2760, 1997.

68. Cassagnau, P. and Melis F. Non-linear viscoelastic behaviour and modulus recovery in silica filled polymers. *Polymer*, 44 (21), 6607–6615, 2003.

69. Aguilera, J. M. Seligman lecture 2005 food product engineering: Building the right structures. *J. Sci. Food Agr.*, 86 (8), 1147–1155, 2006.

70. Mc Clements, D. J., Decker, E. A., Park, Y., and Weiss, J. Structural design principles for delivery of bioactive components in nutraceuticals and functional foods. *Crit. Rev. Food Sci. Nutr.*, 49 (6), 577–606, 2009.

71. Qian, J. W., An, Q. F., Wang, L. N., Zhang, L., and Shen, L. Influence of the dilute-solution properties of cellulose acetate in solvent mixtures on the morphology and per-vaporation performance of their membranes. *J. Appl. Polym. Sci.*, 97 (5), 1891–1898, 2005.

72. Huang, D. H., Ying, Y. M., and Zhuang, G. Q. Influence of intermolecular entanglements on the glass transition and structural relaxation behaviors of macromolecules. 2. Polystyrene and phenolphthalein poly(ether sulfone). *Macromolecules*, 33 (2), 461–464, 2000.

73. Bhuiyan, M. M. H. and Uddin, M. H. Excess molar volumes and excess viscosities for mixtures of *N,N*-dimethylformamide with methanol, ethanol and 2-propanol at different temperatures. *J. Mol. Liquids*, 138 (1–3), 139–146, 2008.

74. Annabi, N., Nichol, J. W., Zhong, X., Ji, C., Koshy, S., Khademhosseini, A., and Dehghani, F. Controlling the porosity and microarchitecture of hydrogels for tissue engineering. *Tissue Eng. Part B*, 16 (4), 371–383, 2010.

75. Couper, A. Physical methods of chemistry. In: *Investigations of Surfaces and Interfaces-Part A*, Rossiter, B. W. and Baetzold, R. C. Eds., Wiley, New York, Vol. IX, p. 1, 1993.

76. Falsafi, A., Mangipudiy, S., and Owenz, M. J. Surface and interfacial properties. In: *Properties of Polymers Handbook*, Second Edition; Mark, E. J. Ed., Springer, Cincinnati, OH, Chapter 59, p. 1011, 2007.

77. Ioan, S., Filimon, A., Avram, E., and Ioanid, G. Effects of chemical structure and plasma treatment on the surface properties of polysulfones. *e-Polymers*, 031, 1–13, 2007.

78. van Oss, C. J., Good, R. J., and Chaudhury, M. K. Additive and nonadditive surface tension components and the interpretation of contact angles. *Langmuir*, 4 (4), 884–891, 1988.

79. Rankl, M., Laib, S., and Seeger, S. Surface tension properties of surface-coatings for application in biodiagnostics determined by contact angle measurements. *Colloids Surf. B*, 30 (3), 177–186, 2003.

5 Phosphorus-Containing Polysulfones for High-Performance Applications in Advanced Technologies

Luminita-Ioana Buruiana

CONTENTS

5.1 PHOSPHORUS-CONTAINING POLYMERS—AN INTRODUCTION

In recent years, phosphorus-containing polymers have aroused increasing interest in different application domains [1]. Certainly, various chemical applications of phosphorus in the environment have led to attractive properties, which makes phosphorus highly interesting. Studies made on phosphorus-containing polymers are steadily in development, which reflect the diversification and characterization of the range of polymers available and their use in various domains. In this context, phosphorus-containing polymers can be employed for a wide range of technological applications: in industry, because of their aptitude to bind metals [2], in flame retardancy—where phosphorus is known to be extremely efficient [3–5], and as proton-conducting fuel cell membranes [6–8]; at the

same time, those functionalized polymers have found applications as phase-transfer catalysts, antistatic agents, biocides, humidity sensors, and water filtration membranes [9].
Moreover, phosphonated compounds have been recently shown to possess an attractive
combination of properties that motivates the investigation of phosphonated polymers for
use as proton conductors under low-humidity conditions [10].

Research interest in phosphorus-based polymers (polyphosphates, polyphosphonates, polyphosphoesters, phosphonated poly(meth)acrylates, etc.) has been accelerat-
ing in the recent past, as they are biodegradable (by enzymatic digestion of phosphate
linkages under physiological conditions), are compatible with blood compounds, present
structural similarities to the naturally occurring nucleic and teichoic acids, exhibit
reducing protein adsorption, and create strong interactions with dentin or bones [11].
In this context, they play an important role in different biomedicine applications such
as drug delivery, dental applications, tissue engineering, or protein adsorption. Other
specific properties of these functionalized polymers make them suitable for application as carriers for biologically active substances [12]. Besides biomedical domains,
phosphorus-containing polymers are successfully used in several industrial and environmental developments, which make them really attractive for interdisciplinary
research—chemistry, medicine, physics, biochemistry, medical bioengineering, and
medical physics (Figure 5.1). Likewise, the biomimetic structure of some phosphorus-
containing polymers with phospholipid groups is preferred to the classical systems
already used in biomedical fields.

Literature has mentioned intensive studies of polymers containing phosphorus
in the backbone, mainly due to their excellent fire resistance and good mechanical
properties [13,14]. Starting from them, *polyphosphoesters* have been developed as
biomaterials with good physicochemical and film-forming properties; for example,
they can form a cross-linking matrix with mechanical properties close to a natural
trabecular bone and represent a potential injectable tissue engineering scaffold material with excellent characteristics. Recent trends in this area highlight new methods
of nanocomposites preparation, based on hydroxyapatite-polyvinyl alcohol modified with phosphate groups [15], which show excellent hemocompatibility, successfully used as bone implants. Phosphate-grafted polymers are also used as selective

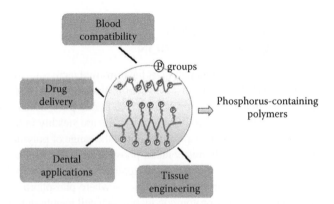

FIGURE 5.1   Main applications of the phosphorus-containing polymers.

materials in *craniofacial implants*; for this, an increase of their surface hydrophilicity had to be made previously. On the other hand, biodegradable polyphosphoesters used for obtaining some polymer microspheres were evaluated in the context of controlled delivery of neurotrophic proteins to a target tissue, to treat various diseases of the nervous system. In this context, it was demonstrated that sustained release of nerve growth factor for a prolonged period of time from microspheres loaded into synthetic nerve guide conduits might improve peripheral nerve regeneration [16,17], recommending these polymers for *antitumor drug delivery applications*.

Moreover, polymeric *phosphate* and *phosphonates* evidenced an increased commercial interest, because of their flame-retardant characteristics and their utilization as high-performance plastics [18]. At the same time, they exhibit good biodegradability, blood compatibility, reduced protein adsorption, and strong interaction with bones, which make them applicable in medical domains. In *dental applications*, this polymer class assured an improved adhesion on the tooth surface, because of the incorporation of phosphonic functions and the formation of calcium complexes from bone structure [19]. The previously mentioned property was also important for the employment of these functionalized polymers in bone *tissue engineering*— especially for scaffold design. Polyphosphates have been investigated as biomaterials in gene delivery, drug delivery, tissue engineering, and agriculture as well. Recently, more attention has been paid to environmental protection and ecological balance, the absence of catalysts, and the avoidance of organic solvents, becoming the main goals in using these types of polymers as eco-friendly compounds [20,21].

In response to the need of developing phosphorus-containing polymers as biodegradable and flame-retardant materials, systematic studies on the synthesis and characterization of such polymers were performed. Thus, reduction and/or optimization of the undesirable side reactions of classical methods can be applied to the broad areas of chemistry, including synthesis, catalysis, reaction conditions, separations, and analysis. These methods follow the trend of green chemistry, yielding reduction of environmental pollution and recent achievements of chemistry.

This chapter is structured into two parts: the first highlights the state of art on phosphorus-containing polymers (new conventional and unconventional synthetic strategies for the preparation of polymers), whereas the second discusses recent developments—including relevant properties and applications—of phosphorus-containing polysulfones. Moreover, significant researches, made by the author in the synthesis and characterization of phosphorus-modified polysulfones for applications in the electrotechnical industry and biomedical domains, are evidenced.

5.2   SYNTHESIS, PROPERTIES, AND APPLICABILITY CORRELATIONS OF PHOSPHORUS-CONTAINING POLYMERS

Phosphorus-containing polymers represent a relatively new family compared with other polymer classes that, besides their excellent properties (e.g., fire resistance), may disrupt—by means of their phosphonyl link group—the molecular symmetry, thus making them amorphous and soluble in common organic solvents.

The most important phosphorus-containing polymers synthesized in the literature are polyphosphazenes [22,23], polyphosphonites [24,25], polyphosphonates

[26,27], poly(phosphorus amide) [28,29], and polyphosphines [30,31]. Among them, the phosphorus-containing high-performance polymers, such as poly(arylene ether)s, epoxy, and cyanate, are the most important ones, due to their good thermal and chemical stability and excellent mechanical properties.

Phase-transfer catalysis is a very convenient and well-known technique used for organic synthesis. This method is preferred because, by the chemical modification of polymers, it permits the synthesis of diverse functional polymers [32,33], with the functionality being introduced as side groups, chain-end, in-chain, block, or graft structures [34].

Due to their biodegradable characteristics given by the hydrolyzable ester groups or P(O)—O—C bond from the backbone, *polyphosphoesters* have provided the reason to further develop the synthesis of phosphorus-containing polymers, in order to obtain new polymers applicable to interdisciplinary domains [35]. The phase transfer catalysis method has attracted much interest due to the simplicity of the operations and technological devices required, economy of energy and raw materials, and new perspectives available in the modern organic synthesis. The latest advances in this domain are based on the development of a new synthesis technique—inverse phase-transfer catalysis [36], in which the organic reagent reacts with the catalysts and forms an intermediate water-soluble product, which subsequently reacts with the aqueous surfactant for obtaining the desired product. The new method of phosphorus-containing polymer synthesis is based on the different chemical composition of the phosphorylating and bisphenol agents; the alternative technique consists of inversion in the addition order, considering the addition of one reaction phase to another (i.e., adding the aqueous phase to the organic one). The main advantage of this new method is that it requires no reagent purification and allows a high efficiency of the obtained polymers, without the formation of unwanted by-products. Also, this procedure eliminates the major shortcomings of the classical methods caused by high temperatures, corrosion, and high stirring speed. By this method, polyphosphates, polyphosphonates, polyarylazophosphonates, polyphosphoesters, and polyarylazophosphates with high yields and inherent viscosities [37–41] were obtained.

More recently, *organophosphorus* polymers have aroused researchers' interest as polymer electrolytes that appear as promising materials for electrochemical devices, such as fuel cells or high-energy density rechargeable batteries. In this context, polyphosphoester electrolytes were obtained by the polycondensation reaction, for improving ionic conductivity at environmental temperature for polymeric membrane applications [42,43]. Synthesis by phase-transfer catalysis also presents some disadvantages, determined by water presence, which may induce side reactions (hydrolysis of the phosphorus-chloride bond of the reagent or chain end groups of the polymer).

The conversion of gas–liquid or liquid–liquid into solid–liquid phase-transfer catalysis appears ideal for the elimination of the side reactions and for obtaining a polymer electrolyte with no impurities and moisture. Thus, the application of this new method in a solid–liquid system for the synthesis of phosphorus solid polymer electrolytes as an environmentally friendly and economical procedure leads to a safe and nonflammable material. The novelty of this method consists in the improvement of polyphosphonate membranes safety for lithium batteries, and, also, in the presence of the phosphonate group, which assures a low flammability of both polymers and membranes [37].

Other literature data presented a modern synthetic methodology applied to produce polyphosphates by gas–liquid interfacial polycondensation of arylphosphoric dichlorides with bisphenol A [44]. The main advantage of this method refers to organic solvent-free synthesis, for environmental protection and maintaining the ecological balance, that represents important goals in green chemistry. Water is the solvent preferred in modern chemistry because it is inexpensive, safe to use, and environmentally friendly. The efficiency of this technique is given by the lower number of reaction components and by solving any solvent recycling requirements [45].

Poly(organo)phosphazenes are a specific class of phosphorus-containing polymers, extremely versatile, that can be used in a wide range of biomedical applications, including tissue engineering and drug delivery; moreover, in some recent advanced studies, polyphosphazenes were designed for gene delivery [19]. This class of phosphorus-functionalized polymers possesses significant advantages as carriers for bioconjugates, being prepared with controlled molecular masses and self-assembled supra-molecular structures. An important step in biomedical application is represented by the establishment of the desired degradation/hydrolysis rate of the polymers. The laws that govern the delivery of small-molecules via polymer conjugates aim at obtaining a polymer with a proper molecular weight, solubility, and biocompatibility [46]. The most widely applied method for the synthesis of polyphosphazenes is thermal ring-opening polymerization, which can be carried out either in vacuum or in solvents with high boiling points [47,48]. Several promising *in vitro* and *in vivo* studies developed for a large range of therapies show the potential of poly[(organo)phosphazene] in drug and gene delivery applications.

Other important applications of phosphorus-containing polymers are as antibacterial agents or biocides [49], for plant protection against fungi, bacteria, viruses, and other pathogenic agents. In this context, phytotoxicity studies evidence more advantages than common toxicity analyses, especially because of their improved sensitivity and low cost [50]. As an example, polyethylene functionalized with diphenyl vinylphosphonium is preferred due to its lipophilic and cationic salt character, which permits easier transport through plasma membrane or cell wall. Polymer functionalization degree becomes an extremely important factor for its frequent utilization as an antibacterial agent, as well as the concentration of the complex formed with phosphorus salts [51].

Studies developed on phosphorus-containing polymers, devoted to polymer diversification and their applications in various domains, are in development. One of the most intense preoccupation in this domain lies in the intensification of fire proofing of macromolecular compounds as ignifugation agents, accent being laid on their technical and economical advantages.

Polyphosphonates have a commercial interest due to their flame-retardant characteristics [52,53] and potential use as high-performance plastic materials. In recent years, the synthesis of polyphosphonates and polyphosphates by liquid–liquid interfacial polycondensation and gas–liquid interfacial polycondensation was performed [44,45,54]. The advantages of gas–liquid polycondensation permit to obtain low-molecular-weight polymers in the absence of solvent and catalysts (whereas the presence of aqueous alkali may prevent obtaining high-molecular-weight polymers). The simultaneous influence of various parameters—temperature, sodium hydroxide

(NaOH) concentration, reaction time, and molar ratio of reactants—was studied for the minimization of undesirable side reaction and the optimization of the quality of synthesis [55]. This method represents an alternative to the classical method, in which many parameters can be varied simultaneously, although the working time and costs needed for synthesis optimization are lower. The statistical analyses performed in this respect led to the development of a mathematical model on the interactions of process parameters. The obtained results indicated that high values of reaction time and temperature, together with minimum values of NaOH concentration, induce maximum quality of polyphosphonates.

The α-*hydroxyphosphonates* with specific properties have been studied for some biological applications, as well as synthetic intermediates for other important α-substituted phosphorus compounds. The literature mentions different types of ion exchangers resins used in the removal, preconcentration, and the determination of various metal ions in aqueous solutions [56]. Thus, resins functionalized with phosphonate [57], phosphinic [58,59], and phosphonic [60] groups are reported and characterized as to their catalytic and ion-exchange properties. Obtaining a styrene-divinylbenzene copolymer grafted with aldehyde side groups by the phase-transfer catalysis method is detailed [61], and its use for the preparation of the new α-hydroxyphosphonic acid grafted on polymeric backbone is presented [62]. New chelating polymers are characterized by the presence of reactive functional groups containing oxygen and phosphorus as donor atoms. As a possible application of functionalized resins, one can mention decoloration of textile wastewater under optimal conditions (minimum temperature of 45°C and pH 4.0); the process was not expensive and environmentally friendly.

A special class of phosphorus-containing polymers with specific applications is represented by *homo and copolymeric hydrogels*—three-dimensional hydrophilic polymer networks capable of swelling in water or biological fluids. Hydrogel-based network complexes have been designed and produced to meet the needs of pharmaceutical and medical fields for peptides, proteins, and drug delivery applications. Two classes of phosphorus-containing hydrogels were currently under investigation: one contains phosphorus in the main chain, whereas the other contains phosphorus–nitrogen bonds in the side chain. The most important properties of these compounds recommend them in tissue engineering and nanotechnology applications. At the same time, *in vitro* experiments also revealed some limitations on their use in medical application, being essential to determine the typical interactions that appear between all polymer components once inside the body. Therefore, the advances in synthetic organic chemistry permit the development of new classes of hydrogels-containing phosphorus that may improve their compatibility with biological fluids, augment the therapeutic effect by releasing the drug into the specific site, and sustain the therapeutic effect in the target site [63]. As hydrogels have also shown great potential as scaffolds for tissue engineering, due to their tissue-like water contents, they may be used *in situ* for easy implantation. Phosphate-containing and photo-cross-linkable polymers containing poly(ethylene glycol) and methacrylate segments have been analyzed [64], connected by the phosphate linker and photopolymerized hydrogels used in marrow-derived mesenchymal stem cell encapsulation and tissue engineering of bones [65].

Polyphosphazenes and some *polyphosphoesters* having unsaturated linkages in the molecule have been frequently used for several medical devices, contact lenses, drug controlled release, and for certain tissue engineering applications. Due to the correlation between their properties and their specific applications—biological compatibility, degradability, and good swelling properties—these types of polymers were recommended for medical uses and pharmaceutical formulations. The *in vitro* and *in vivo* studies highlighted the antitumor drug release capacity (e.g., 5-Fluorouracil and Paclitaxel) [66,67]. Complexes based on polyphosphazenes and microspheres cross-linked with aluminum ions were used as vaccine delivery vehicles [68], whereas polyphosphazenes functionalized with carboxyl groups were useful for controlled drug delivery, including intestine-specific oral delivery systems [69–71]. The unsaturated polyphosphoester polymers exhibited specific properties that qualify them as biodegradable and injectable systems for alveolar bone repair in the treatment of periodontal diseases [72].

Other systems that correlate unique properties with specific applications are represented by the novel thermoresponsive block copolymers of *polyphosphoester* and *poly(ethylene glycol)*. Self-assembly, biocompatibility, and hydrolytic degradation behavior [73] evidenced the absence of local acute inflammatory response in the muscle following intramuscular injection. Therefore, these biodegradable block copolymers with good biocompatibility represent promising stimuli-responsive materials for biomedical applications.

5.3   POLYSULFONES AS HIGH-PERFORMANCE POLYMERS

Polymer properties are influenced by their chemical composition, molecular mass, and specific molecular architecture. There are similarities between polymers and other molecules, the structure of the better ones conditioning essentially the property–structure relationships and specific uses, making them suitable for theoretical studies and modern applications.

High-performance polymers with specific macromolecular structures, similar to the naturally occurring systems, have been the subject of extensive research; their various environmental and biological applications make them highly attractive materials. Complex polymer systems with applications in modern nano and biotechnology have raised interest because of their special macromolecular structures, with unique morphologies and specific properties, given by the functional groups from the side chain. Literature pays special attention to some special polysulfones with versatile reactivity that makes them suitable for a wide range of technological applications. These high-performance thermoplastic polymers contain a phenyl and $-SO_2$ group (aryl$-SO_2-$aryl) and are used in different application fields, being characterized by good optical properties, high thermal and chemical stability, mechanical strength, and resistance to extreme pH values [74–78]. Also, polysulfones can contain different groups in their structure: substituted or unsubstituted aryl groups (phenyl, diphenyl, and bisphenol), aryl groups with aromatic hydrocarbon, and aromatic cycle or diaryl sulfone groups ($HO-(C_6H_4)-(C_6H_4)-OH$). Commercial polysulfones mainly contain only one type of diaryl sulfone group and diphenol (diphenol or bisphenol A). Chain rigidity is derived from the relatively inflexible phenyl and $-SO_2$ groups, whereas their toughness is generated by the connecting ether oxygen [79].

The most common polysulfones studied in the literature are as follows:

- PSFs with diphenyl sulfone and bisphenol A—Udel® polysulfone—obtained by condensation of bisphenol A with 4,4′-dichlorodiphenyl sulfone
- Radel R® polysulfone—obtained by 4,4′-bisphenol A with 4,4′-dichlorodiphenyl sulfone; the most used is Radel A® that contains interlinked groups: $(-aryl-SO_2-aryl-O-)_n$ and a relatively small segment—polyether ether sulfone $(-aryl-SO_2-aryl-O-aryl'-O-)_m$

5.3.1 FUNCTIONALIZED POLYSULFONES—GENERAL CHARACTERISTICS AND APPLICATIONS

Polysulfones have been the first materials used for a long time at temperatures higher than 160°C, offering a unique combination of properties, making them the most frequently used thermoplastic materials that can resist at this temperature. The main characteristics that recommend them for different applications are as follows:

- *High thermal stability*—the maximum temperature for using polysulfones is 160°C for 20 h in environmental medium.
- *Hydrolytic stability*—stability to steam and hot water (the pH having no effect on hydrolysis degree).
- *Chemical resistance*—extremely efficient in acid and alkaline solutions, alcohols, detergents, oils, and salt solutions.
- *Transparency*—pristine polysulfones are transparent materials, allowing a transmission of about 80%–85% light rays.
- *Low dielectric constants and loss parameters*—good insulators, due to these properties being maintained over large frequency and temperature domains.

Also known is that polysulfones possessing superior properties, such as electrical, mechanical, and flame retardancy, represent good candidates for applications in the biomedical, electronic, and electrotechnical industry. Their uses, restricted by intrinsic hydrophobicity, may be improved by modification through different processes. Thereby, the desirable combination between the properties of polysulfones and their availability makes them attractive materials for specific applications [80–82]. To improve their performance, polysulfones can be modified by chloromethylation, amination, or phosphorylation; all these procedures are being accounted for the recent advances recorded in functionalized polysulfones for special applications in industry and medicine. These modifications aim at obtaining precursors for new complex polymer systems used in different applications, such as ion change resins, selectively permeable membranes, and coatings [83–85].

The specific structure, composition, and types of derivatives of functionalized polysulfones—chloromethylated, quaternized with ammonium pendant groups, or obtained by phosphorylation (PSFP)—have challenged interesting investigations on their properties and possible applications, for example, bio and nanotechnology, medicine, and food and environmental industry [86–89]. Quaternization with ammonium groups represents an efficient method for enhancing the hydrophilic properties of pristine polysulfones; the obtained quaternized polysulfones are subsequently used as biomaterials and semipermeable membranes. Literature mentions that the thermal properties of modified polysulfones are weaker than those of the unmodified ones [90]. On the other hand, particular physical and chemical properties of polysulfones—chemical and thermal stabilities, mechanical resistance, and excellent resistance to oxidation—explain the selection of these materials as membrane substrates. The special morphology of polysulfones (smooth layers, porous, and hollow structures) makes them suitable for filtration membrane applications. Also, polysulfones are used as ion-exchange resin membranes in electromembrane processes, such as electrodialysis and membrane electrolysis with polyelectrolytes [91–96].

The use of these polymers as chelating agents in hydrophilic medium, for heavy metals contamination or in certain separation techniques, is restricted by their hydrophobicity and may be improved by chemical modification through different processes. In this context, the synthesis and application of such new functionalized polysulfones allow future scientific research, which meets the industrial requirements.

The most important applications of functionalized polysulfones are summarized further, highlighting the latest advances recorded in the field:

- As *membranes*—asymmetric capillary membranes made of polysulfones were used as starting materials in gas separation processes from chemical industry. Due to their high hydrogen permeability, polysulfone membranes are used as an efficient energetic alternative, including distillation at low temperatures. At the same time, polysulfone membranes were studied as an alternative to cellulose membrane in separation processes, considering their good strength under extreme pH conditions and excellent thermal stability. Polysulfone membranes are easy to obtain by inverse phase-transfer catalysis, because of their good solubility in chloroform ($CHCl_3$) and N,N-dimethylformamide (DMF). Due to their porosity, polysulfone membranes are used in processes such as microfiltration, nanofiltration, and inverse osmosis, and in composite membranes for facilitated transport [97].
- In the *electrical and electronic industry*—because of their excellent mechanical properties and radiation resistance. Also, the heat stability of polysulfone is quite high compared with that of other polymeric materials, which makes it a suitable candidate for applications in automotive industry. Due to their excellent electrical properties, polysulfones are used as dielectrics in capacitors [98].
- In the *medical field*—they appear as a viable alternative to stainless steel or glass. For these applications, polysulfones must combine high strength, display unique long life under sterilization procedures, should be biologically inert, and resistant to most common hospital chemicals. At the same time, in the case of an implant material, the replacement polymer should mimic the living tissue: mechanically, chemically, biologically, and functionally. Likewise, the polymeric materials must exhibit the ability to be repeatedly sterilized without hydrolytic degradation or color change [99,100].

- Udel polysulfones were tested versus acids, alkalis, alcohols (knowing their high resistance to these substances), biocides, and equipment and devices for inhalation. The obtained results prove that this type of polysulfones possesses strength and rigidity at elevated temperatures, long-term heat resistance, dimensional stability, and outstanding resistance to acidic and basic environments. At the same time, to simulate physiological conditions, various levels of stress were applied and, where appropriate, temperatures were elevated; in certain cases, proper design and processing techniques prevent the appearance of higher stress levels. All these characteristics account for polysulfones suitability as *separation membranes in pharmaceutical and biological purification applications.* Also, the successful results recorded by Udel polysulfone during biological tests recommend their utilization for containers and accessories for parenteral preparations. Cytotoxicity tests have proved no adverse tissue responses with Udel polysulfone implants in rats, rabbits, and dogs; no carcinogenic effect of the polymer on these lab animals was observed.

- The literature also mentions the preparation of polysulfone hollow-fiber membranes with a developed inner wall structure for cell cultivation and utilization as a synthetic carrier playing a supporting role for biological components (e.g., hepatocytes); however, several tests are still to be performed in view of their application in the design of bioartificial organs [101].

- Some initial tests reported the application of polysulfone capillary fibers for intraocular drug delivery [102]; in recent years, researchers have shown interest in developing polysulfones for porous coatings in targeted drug delivery applications [103]. To this end, a porous, biocompatible, and nontoxic polymer coating of polysulfone was prepared by selectively dissolving $CaCO_3$ nanoparticles embedded in it. (Rhodamine B was utilized as a model drug.) Cell viability tests with human fibroblast cells demonstrated a similar behavior with other commonly used biocompatible coatings such as gold, and a low level of adhesion on the porous polysulfone coatings, making them suitable for intraocular drug delivery.

- Polysulfones also found their use in different lab medical devices, the most frequent ones being *microsurgical knives*, designed as integral units or as tips in various configurations [104]. At the same time, *polysulfone medical bottles* were transparent and theoretically unbreakable, resistant to the vacuum pressure applied during the removal of unwanted body fluids; also they withstand to high cleaning temperature, without losing their clear aspect. They are used as lab equipments for health services in hospitals. Biomedical researchers have discovered a new alternative to the tissue culture roller bottles, now available. Competing with glass bottles, polysulfones—preferred for their high purity—offer an important utility as a *substrate for tissue culture cell attachment and growth,* with no breakage problems [105].

5.4 RECENT TRENDS IN TECHNOLOGICAL AND BIOMEDICAL APPLICATIONS OF PHOSPHORUS-CONTAINING POLYSULFONES

Polysulfones with phosphorus in their chain represent an important class of polymers with specific properties; this type of polysulfone has not been extensively studied so far, for optimizing product performance. Nevertheless, an initial study was proposed to incorporate phosphorus-containing diols into the polymer to further improve its fire behavior, and thus to use these new materials not only as toughness modifiers, but concomitantly as flame retardants [106,107]. The novel phosphorus compound has high thermal stability and very high glass transition temperature, as well as modified flame retardancy—depending on the type of diol incorporated (Figure 5.2).

As a result of the increasing usage of this type of polymer, as well as of the current trend toward a sustainable conservation of resources, the thermal stability, flame resistance, and toxicological consequences of flame-retarded epoxies have recently become a subject of considerable attention. Thus, a recent study has shown that an epoxy resin can be simultaneously equipped with both enhanced toughness and improved flame retardancy by the addition of a new type of polysulfone containing phosphorus in the backbone [108]. Such a blend was found to have an increased glass transition temperature and particular microstructures. A combination of these characteristic properties might efficiently improve the flame retardancy of thermosetting materials for modern-day applications.

Polysulfones functionalized with chlorophosphonic acid esters, obtained by a nucleophilic substitution reaction at phosphorus, show good membrane-forming properties and appear as suitable candidates for components in ionomer composite membranes for fuel cells. The substitution degree of the obtained compounds was obtained by a careful selection of the reaction parameters, to avoid cross-linking. Functionalized polysulfones have high thermal stability, a decomposition temperature of approximately 350°C, and good membrane-forming properties. The use of

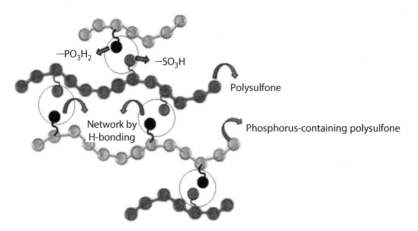

FIGURE 5.2 General structure of the phosphorus-containing polysulfones.

these polymers as components in composite membranes for fuel cells is currently under investigation [109].

Other new polysulfones-based dialylaminophosphonium salts have been synthesized, their structure being identified by specific analyses (UV-VIS and NMR spectra). Microbiological tests performed have shown their good antimicrobial activity against Gram-positive bacteria [110,111], emphasizing possible biological applications.

In other research studies, 9,10-dihydro-9-oxa-10-phosphophenanthrene-10-oxide (DOPO)-based compounds have attracted attention because of the flame retardancy of epoxies; their use has been shown to induce important improvements of epoxy resins and to avoid many disadvantages, such as poor compatibility or release of toxic gases upon burning, in comparison with other commonly used flame retardants. Using DOPO-based compounds reduces processing difficulties and, sometimes, the degradation of the resulting physical and mechanical properties of the base resin, by adjusting the phosphorus content (until 3 wt% phosphorus) [112]. Thus, the effectiveness of a novel organophosphorus compound as an efficient, nonreactive flame retardant for modern epoxy systems was demonstrated, as well as the potential of the DOPO compound to provide a polyfunctional system with high flame retardancy, without deteriorating the overall performance of the resulting material [113]. Another study analyzed chloromethylated polysulfones (CMPSF) with different substitution degree that reacted with a phosphorus compound with a reactive P—H bond (e.g., DOPO) [114]. The structural characteristics of phosphorus-modified polysulfones evidenced an amorphous morphology and a thermal stability higher than that of CMPSF, a slight decrease being observed with the increase of substitution degree. The morphology of these polysulfones is quite different from those of pristine polysulfone or CMPSF, a nonsmooth surface with larger pores size being observed. Thereby, this phosphorus-modified polysulfone with its new morphology, induced by the attached bulky groups, would represent a promising candidate for the preparation of membrane with different permeability and selectivity.

Chemical modification of polysulfones by chloromethylation and subsequent phosphorus modification influenced their thermal behavior. Thus, thermal stability slightly differs in nitrogen from air atmosphere, a decrease in nitrogen being noticed when the substitution degree is increased. Another observation was that phosphorus-modified polysulfones decomposed in two or four degradation steps, as a function of the atmosphere employed: in an inert atmosphere, the DOPO groups remained mainly in the nonvolatile fraction, whereas in air, the DOPO pendant groups formed a compact char residue that could prevent the heat attack [115].

The appearance of fuel cell technology in modern-day life depends mainly on the development of new multifunctional materials designed to reduce the cost and complexity of these systems and to increase their durability. In recent years, the advances in this domain have been determined by the requirements of automotive industry. In this context, the modern trends in polymer membrane applications, capable of operating at elevated temperatures (over 100°C) and low humidity values, constitute an important scientific and engineering challenge. Consequently, recent researches in this field have focused on the synthesis and structural characterization of phosphorus-containing polysulfones, as well as on relevant membrane properties, to establish their potential use as fuel cell materials. In this respect, polysulfones were grafted with phosphonic acid in a two-step reaction—chloromethylation and phosphonation—at different contents of phosphonic acid per repeating unit. The obtained membranes exhibited higher levels of water uptake in comparison with other phosphonated polymers reported in the literature so far, as a result of the high concentration of phosphonic acid moieties. Also, the synthesized membranes show high thermal stability (up to 252°C in air) and low methanol permeability, which indicate that they are future candidates for proton exchange membrane fuel cells [11,116].

Anion exchange membrane alkaline fuel cells have aroused increased scientific research interest, due to their catalyst electrokinetics, that can be improved in alkaline media and CO_2 contamination [117]. The system used is based on materials containing quaternized group with quaternary nitrogen atom or quaternary phosphorus—an element from the same family as nitrogen. In this context, triphenylphosphine- and tributylphosphine-based quaternary phosphonium polysulfones for anion exchange membranes were successfully prepared. The obtained results highlighted that triphenylphosphine-based quaternary phosphonium polysulfone showed higher alkaline stability than the other one, although its ionic conductivity increased with the chloromethylation degree of CMPSF. Also, thermal analysis, water uptake, and methanol permeability analyses have proved that phosphorus-functionalized polysulfones are promising materials for anion exchange membrane fuel cells.

Hydroxide exchange membrane fuel cells have the potential to solve the problems of catalyst cost and durability toward classical hydrogen proton exchange fuel cells, by switching from an acidic medium to a basic one. Cathode kinetics allows nonprecious metals to be used as catalysts, thus diminishing fuel cell cost. At the same time, this type of fuel cell offers flexibility, due to its lower overpotential for hydrocarbon fuel oxidation and reduced fuel crossover [118]. Also, it has been shown that quaternary phosphonium-containing polysulfones exhibit excellent solubility in methanol, but the strong basicity of the tertiary phosphine shows that quaternary phosphonium hydroxides are strong bases. Taking into account all these assumptions, researchers have synthesized a new quaternary phosphonium-based ionomer that may be dissolved in water-soluble solvents with low boiling point and highly hydroxide conductive. The obtained phosphonium-based polysulfone ionomer has good solubility in pure methanol, ethanol, n-propanol, and their aqueous solutions and is insoluble in pure water, even at elevated temperature (80°C). Besides the excellent solubility and high ionic conductivity, the obtained compound has an outstanding stability. This type of membranes maintained their ionic conductivity after immersion in deionized water or sodium hydroxide under specific conditions (60°C for 48 h), indicating good long-term stability. Therefore, novel phosphorus-based hydroxide conductive ionomers, evidencing excellent solubility, increased hydroxide conductivity and notable alkaline stability, assured an important increase of peak power density and a considerable reduction of internal resistance [118].

Polymer functionalization reactions, especially phosphonation, were studied for the development of ion-exchange membranes for fuel cells, or, more recently, for electrodialysis. In the past, the synthesis of phosphorus-containing polymers was mainly related to the development of flame-retardant materials [106,107], phosphonation also being applied to improve their compatibility with blood [119]. In this context, membranes based on phosphonated polyphenylsulfones with high functionalization degree were compared with sulfonated membranes [120]. The obtained results indicate that phosphorus-based membranes show some advantages over sulfonated polymer membranes, operating under low-humidity conditions at high temperatures. At high water content, the protons were transported through the dynamics of the water; in addition, because of the amphoteric nature of the phosphonic group, it is possible to transport protons through diffusion within hydrogen bonding phosphonic acid networks at low water contents. Moreover, phosphonated polymers showed higher hydrolytic and thermal stability than sulfonated polymers, due to the strength of the C—P bond. The results show that phosphonated polysulfones exhibit better thermal stability than the sulfonated ones, much higher swelling, and increased permeability to water and methanol, all these characteristics being observed for their blends as well. The encouraging results point out the ability of the phosphonated polyphenylsulfone membrane to be used for fuel cell application.

Membranes with high local concentrations of phosphonic acid have been obtained by grafting poly(vinylphosphonic acid) side chains onto polysulfones [121]. The graft copolymers exhibited some interesting features for their utilization as fuel cell membranes. One of the important advantages is that membranes were prepared from an inexpensive starting material, with good solubility and film-forming properties of the solution [122]. The poly(vinylphosphonic acid) side chains formed separate phases in the membranes with high local concentration of phosphonic acid units, large hydrogen-bonded aggregates being obtained—necessary for an efficient proton conduction in dry state. Besides specific properties such as flexibility and strong mechanical properties, another important characteristic of these membranes is their enhanced conductivity, especially at low temperatures. The findings of this study have proved that phosphonated membranes with a proper macromolecular design may show significant advantages in comparison with the commonly studied sulfonated membranes for proton exchange membrane fuel cell applications.

5.4.1 INFLUENCE OF THE PHOSPHORUS SIDE CHAIN GROUPS ON THE FLOW BEHAVIOR OF PS-DOPO AND PSFP

In the previously mentioned context of phosphorus-containing polysulfones with high-performance applications in advanced technologies, our research team has studied the synthesis of new polysulfones containing phosphorus in the side chain, using CMPSF with different values of substitution degrees as a precursor [114,123,124]. The main objective was to evaluate the effect of the chemical structure of this type of polysulfones on the rheological and morphological data, and to establish the relationship among the processing, morphology, and specific properties.

The general chemical structures of polysulfones with bulky phosphorus pendant groups (PSFP)—obtained by the chemical modification of CMPSFs, performed by reacting the chloromethyl group with the P—H bond of the DOPO group—and of quaternary polysulfones with triphenylphosphonium pendant groups (PSFP)—synthesized by reacting CMPSF (6.29% chlorine content) with triphenylphosphine—are presented

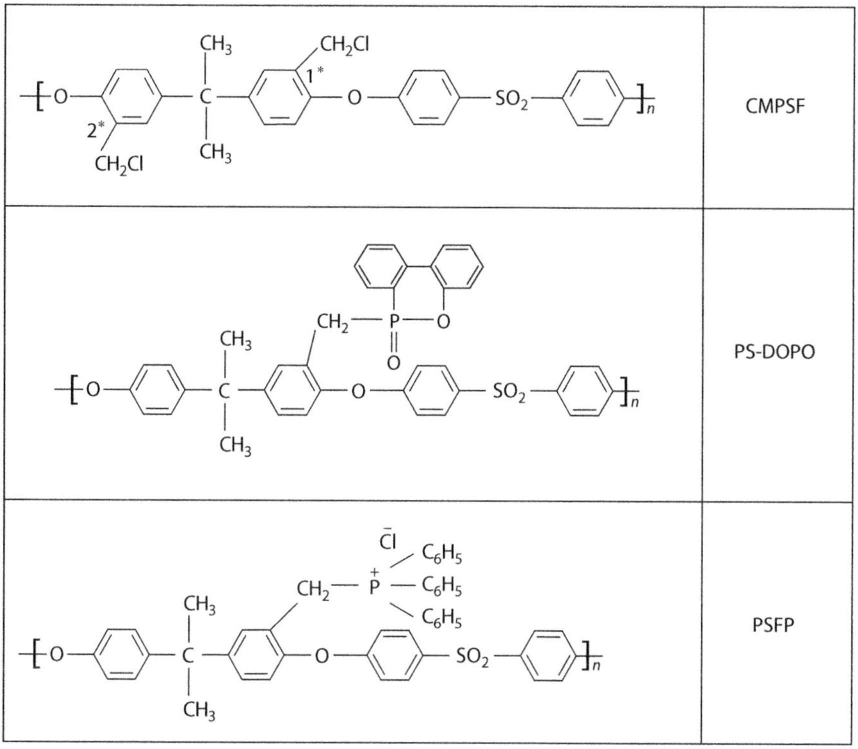

SCHEME 5.1 General structure of different phosphorus-containing polysulfones. (Data from Ioan S. et al., *Polym. Plast. Technol. Eng.*, 50, 36–46, 2011; Buruiana L. I. et al., *J. Appl. Polym. Sci.*, 129, 1752–1762, 2013.)

in Scheme 5.1 (CMPSF, PS-DOPO, and PSFP). For PS-DOPO, the reactive P—H group interacts with the CH_2Cl group of CMPSF; the chloromethylation reaction of polysulfone can occur in position 1* for CMPSF-1 and CMPSF-2, when the substitution degree is lower than 1; for CMPSF-3, when the substitution degree is higher than 1, the chloromethylation reaction occurs in positions 1* and 2*. For PSFP, the quaternization reaction of CMPSF occurred at a transformation degree around 46%.

The flow properties of the studied phosphorus-containing polysulfones in *N,N*-DMF and DMF/water solvent mixtures show different behaviors, influenced by their different chemical structures. Thus, in Figure 5.3, which exhibits the logarithmic plots of viscosity as a function of shear rate for PS-DOPO-1, PS-DOPO-2, and PS-DOPO-3 in DMF, at 30°C, a constant region of viscosity for the studied shear rates and different concentration appears, revealing a Newtonian behavior of the samples—the same characteristics having been observed over the whole range of temperatures (25°C–40°C) [123].

On the other hand, the molecular restructurations—which appear in the case of PSFP—generated by hydrogen bonding, electrostatic interactions, and association phenomena in ternary quaternized polysulfone/*N,N*-DMF (solvent)/water

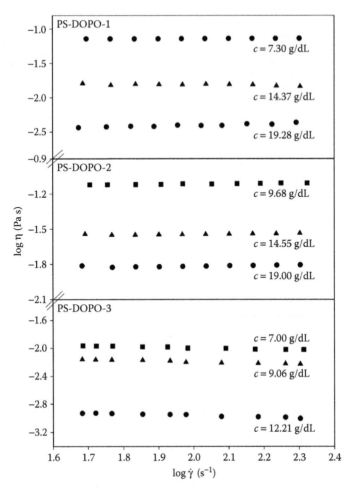

FIGURE 5.3 Logarithmic plots of viscosity as a function of shear rate, for PS-DOPO-1, PS-DOPO-2, and PS-DOPO-3 in DMF, at 30°C.

(nonsolvent) systems were evaluated by rheological investigations. Figure 5.4 exemplifies the logarithmic plots of viscosity as a function of shear rate for PSFP in 100/0 and 75/25 (v/v) DMF/water, at 25°C. This graphical representation shows that the polysulfone that exhibits a shear-thinning profile is a pseudoplastic material, characterized by a decreasing entanglement density, and by oriented segments whose number increases with increasing shear rates. A higher orientation of the polymer chains represents the major cause of the non-Newtonian behavior.

The polyelectrolyte effect of PSFP quaternized polysulfones is due to the expansion of the polyionic chain caused by the progressively enhanced dissociation of ionizable groups, as concentration decreases; consequently, the intensification of the intramolecular repulsive interactions between the ionized groups (i.e., triphenylphosphonium) and a more expanded hydrodynamic volume spread all along the

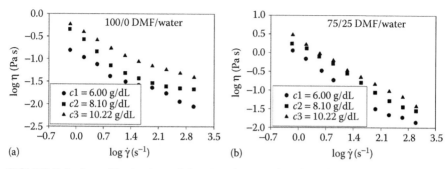

FIGURE 5.4 Logarithmic plots of the viscosity as a function of shear rate for PSFP in (a) 100/0 and (b) 75/25 (v/v) DMF/water, at 25°C.

chain arise. For this reason, at lower concentrations, higher values of viscosities can be expected. In addition, the affinity of the DMF or DMF/water for the quaternized sample depends on the neutral segment and charged groups; the influence of the solvent–mixture composition is illustrated in Figure 5.4 [124]. The shear-thinning behavior of PSFP—which obeys the power–law relationship between shear stress, σ, and shear rate, $\dot{\gamma}$, expressed in Equation 5.1—is also confirmed by the values listed in Table 5.1.

$$\sigma = K\dot{\gamma}^n \tag{5.1}$$

where:

n and K stand for flow behavior index and consistency index, respectively

In this context, the flow behavior indices are lower that the unit, for 8.10 g/dL concentration and all solvent mixtures. On the other hand, for 85/15 and 75/25 v/v DMF/water compositions, the flow behavior indices generally decrease with increasing water content. Solution consistency—induced by the water nonsolvent component from solvent mixtures—takes higher values than in a pure DMF solvent, as a result of the modified interactions in the system, generated by the composition of solvent mixtures and by solution concentrations.

The dependence between polysulfone concentration and viscosity, at a shear rate of approximately 200 s⁻¹, is described by a power law $\eta \propto c^x$, where x increases with temperature and presents a specific behavior at different substitution degrees.

TABLE 5.1

Flow Behavior and Consistency Indices of PSFP in Solvent Mixtures, at 8.10 g dL⁻¹ Concentration

PSFP in Solvent Mixtures (v/v)	n	K
100/0 DMF/water	0.62	0.21
85/15 DMF/water	0.55	1.76
75/25 DMF/water	0.47	1.97

Thereby, the presence of substituted groups in position 1* for the PS-DOPO-1 and PS-DOPO-2 samples, and in positions 1* and 2* for the PS-DOPO-3 sample, influences through their volume in the chemical structure the rheological properties, leading to the modification of slopes in the dependencies of viscosity *versus* concentration and temperature. As an example, one can notice that, at 30°C, for PS-DOPO-3, the slope is higher ($\eta \propto c^{3.760}$) in comparison with that of PS-DOPO-1 ($\eta \propto c^{3.276}$) and PS-DOPO-2 ($\eta \propto c^{2.314}$), and enhances with temperature.

The interactions between chain segments, which imply the size of the energy barrier for the movement of an element in the fluid, can be described by the activation energy, E_a, using the Arrhenius equation [125]:

$$\ln \eta = \ln \eta_0 + \frac{E_a}{RT} \qquad (5.2)$$

where:

η_0 represents a preexponential constant
R is the universal gas constant
T is absolute temperature

The values obtained for the activation energy are influenced by the chemical structure of the phosphorus-containing polysulfones (Table 5.2). Thus, one can observe that an increased substitution degree leads to an increase in the activation energy, which involves a higher energy barrier for the movement of an element from the fluid and, consequently, a more rigid structure of the polymer chain. The energy barrier, related to the interaction between chain segments, can be explained by polymer entanglements; for the PS-DOPO-3 sample with higher chain rigidity, induced by the substitution reaction in positions 1* and 2*, the activation energy exhibits an intense variation with concentration; at the same time, the specific molecular rearrangement of the system at different concentrations, with modification of temperature, can be speculated on different forms of entanglement in polymer solutions.

TABLE 5.2
E_a Values for PS-DOPO-1, PS-DOPO-2, and PS-DOPO-3 at Different Concentrations

Sample	Concentration (g dL^{-1})	E_a (kJ mol^{-1})
PS-DOPO-1	19.28	19.19
	14.37	10.34
	7.30	2.50
PS-DOPO-2	19.00	20.82
	14.55	13.81
	9.68	12.37
PS-DOPO-3	12.21	19.28
	9.06	11.32
	7.00	7.47

TABLE 5.3

Apparent Activation Energy for PSFP Solutions in Different Solvent Mixtures

Concentration of PSFP	DMF/Water Solvent Mixtures (v/v)	E_a (kJ mol^{-1})
6.00 g/dL	100/0	54.04
	85/15	23.45
	75/25	19.68
10.22 g/dL	100/0	57.81
	85/15	42.76
	75/25	−18.31

The Arrhenius plots for the lower shear viscosity ($\dot{\gamma} \approx 0.7\,\text{s}^{-1}$) measured for PSFP in different solvent mixtures are listed in Table 5.3, over the 25°C–40°C temperature range. The linear dependencies between viscosity and reverse temperatures lead to an apparent activation energy, depending on the solvent–nonsolvent composition; positive values of E_a were obtained for all DMF/water compositions at the studied concentrations. An exception was observed for 10.22 g dL^{-1} concentration at a higher water content, 75/25 v/v DMF/water.

In this context, two processes—described by Equation 5.3—that are involved in the apparent activation energy can be discussed:

$$E = E_{dis} + E_{ass} \qquad (5.3)$$

where:

E_{dis} is the positive contribution of disengagement

E_{ass} is the negative contribution of the associated formations

The apparent activation energy for PSFP solutions evidenced no associated chain formation, where the positive contribution of the disengagement process is higher than the negative contribution of the associated chain formation.

The positive contribution of disengagement, E_{dis}, which becomes predominant in comparison with the negative contribution of the associated formations, E_{ass}, leads to positive values of E_a, whereas the negative value is generated by the preponderantly negative contribution of E_{ass}, comparatively with E_{dis}. In this manner, the water content contributes to the specific molecular rearrangement of the system once temperature is modified, facilitating associated molecules formation, at high concentrations and water compositions. Also, the type of pendant groups from quaternized polysulfones influences the solubility process in DMF/water, generating certain molecular restructurations in solution, under the influence of hydrogen bonding, electrostatic interactions, and association phenomena. Thereby, it is obvious that the rheological properties of PSFP are influenced by the small hydrophilic characteristics given by the triphenylphosphonium pendant groups that allow some limitation of the water content in solvent mixtures, and a well-established solubility domain.

At the same time, viscoelastic measurements can significantly contribute to the knowledge and differentiation of polymer systems, completing the rheological studies developed in shear regime. For better comparison between the two studied phosphorus-containing polysulfones, the storage (G') and loss (G'') moduli are plotted as a function of frequency for PS-DOPO-1 solution at 25°C in Figure 5.5 and for PSFP solution in DMF/water at 6.00 g/dL and 25°C in Figure 5.6, respectively.

Gelation kinetics of PS-DOPO is monitored by both moduli, as a function of frequency and concentration from dynamic oscillatory measurements. Gel behavior was established by the $G' \sim G'' \sim f^x$ power law, with $G' > G''$. These features are characteristic for a gel network [126]. The value of x is dependent on the structure and concentration of the modified polysulfones, due to the intramolecular interactions along with intermolecular attractions. Thus, at low substitution degrees, increasing the concentration in the 7.30–19.00 g dL^{-1} range determines an increase of the slope of G' and G'' *versus* frequency, from 2.4 to 3.6; for sample with intermediate substitution degree, increasing the concentration in the 9.68–19.00 g/dL range leads to a lower variation of slope, from 3.2 to 3.8 while, at higher substitution degree, the data showed no slope modification, and a constant value of 3.2 at different concentrations. One can conclude that the gelation process of PS-DOPO is influenced by intramolecular interactions, depending on the substitution degrees, and by the intermolecular attractions, which depend on the concentration in DMF.

For PSFP in DMF/water, at low frequency, the storage and loss moduli are proportional to f^2 and f^1, respectively, whereas, over this frequency range, G' is always higher than G''—a behavior characteristic to viscoelastic fluids. In addition, $G'' > G'$ at lower frequencies, with G' becoming higher once frequency increases, while the frequency corresponding to their overlapping decreases with increasing concentration and the nonsolvent content. Still, at a 10.22 g dL^{-1} concentration of PSFP in

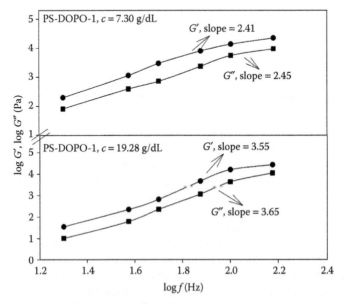

FIGURE 5.5 Storage (G') and loss (G'') moduli as a function of frequency for PS-DOPO-1 solution in DMF, at 25°C.

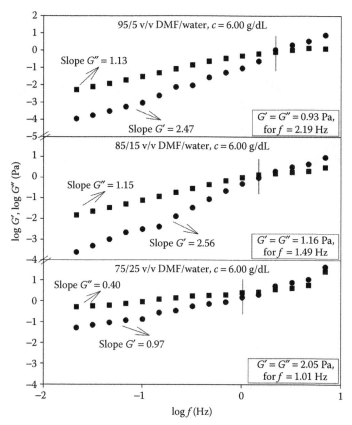

FIGURE 5.6   Storage (G') and loss (G'') moduli as a function of frequency for PSFP solution in DMF/water, at 6.00 g dL^{-1} concentrations and 25°C.

DMF/water, the corresponding exponents of frequency become smaller, due to the association phenomena generated by the addition of water into the system.

5.4.2   MORPHOLOGICAL ASPECTS OF PS-DOPO AND PSFP FILMS

The use of phosphorus-containing polysulfones, restricted by their hydrophobicity, could be improved by the modification of different processes. Thus, the introduction of nonsolvents plays an important role in membrane formation through the occurrence of specific interactions in the three-component systems. Morphological modifications of film surfaces obtained from quaternized polysulfone with triphenylphosphonium pendant groups in 100/0 and 85/15 v/v DMF/water solvent/nonsolvent mixtures were investigated, for obtaining highly porous membranes (Figure 5.7). The results are compared with those obtained from casting solutions of polysulfones with bulky phosphorus pendant groups (Figure 5.8).

The modifications produced in the morphology of PSFP were illustrated by AFM images obtained at different compositions of solvent/nonsolvent mixtures; one can

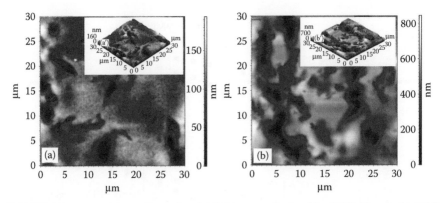

FIGURE 5.7 Bi- and three-dimensional AFM images obtained for PSFP films in (a) 100/0 and (b) 85/15 v/v DMF/water solvent mixtures.

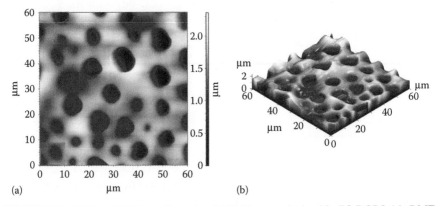

FIGURE 5.8 (a) Bi- and (b) three-dimensional AFM images obtained for PS-DOPO-1 in DMF.

notice that increasing the water content induced a decrease of pores number and an increase in their characteristics (area, average length, depth), as well as their surface roughness parameters (including average roughness and root-mean-square roughness). Association phenomena and increasing interactions due to hydrogen bonding from the casting solutions enhance the pore sizes, while the small hydrophilic characteristics given by the triphenylphosphonium pendant groups—in which the electron-donor interactions exceed the electron-acceptor ones—become important for the understanding of the film rheology/morphology correlation. In the same context, the molecular interactions from the polymer structure were reflected in foreseeable properties of these phosphorus-containing materials. Consequently, surface morphology depends on the history of film preparation, including the characteristics of quaternized polysulfones and the thermodynamic quality of solvents. By comparison, the structure topography of PS-DOPO films emphasized that the bulky phosphorus pendant groups yielded the appearance of domains with pores in an approximately continuous matrix [123], whose dimensions increase while their depth decreases with increasing the substitution degree. On the other hand, AFM studies have confirmed the poor adhesion of modified polysulfones films and have supported the idea that bulky phosphorus pendant groups determine the different forms of entanglement in polymer solutions, influencing membrane morphology.

The presented results have demonstrated that phosphorus-containing polysulfones with a proper macromolecular design provide important advantages that recommend them for specific applications, especially as biomaterials and membranes with enhanced porosity and selectivity.

5.5   CONCLUDING REMARKS

Phosphorus-containing polymers represent an important class of polymers used in different technological applications, such as flame retardants, proton-conducting fuel cell membranes, antistatic agents, biocides, humidity sensors, and water filtration membranes. Also, they possess specific properties, such as biodegradability, compatibility with blood compounds, and structural similarities to the naturally nucleic and teichoic acids; all these characteristics make them suitable for some biomedicine applications such as drug delivery, dental uses, tissue engineering, protein adsorption, or even carriers for biologically active substances [127].

Among the high-performance polymers with specific macromolecular structures, unique morphologies and special properties, polysulfones have drawn attention due to their versatile reactivity and participation in a wide range of technological applications. In this context, polysulfones with superior properties, such as electrical, mechanical, and flame retardancy, are frequently used in biomedicine, electronic, and electrotechnical industry. Their special morphology—smooth layers, porous, and hollow structures—makes this type of polymers suitable for filtration membrane applications and ion-exchange resin membranes in electromembrane processes (i.e., electrodialysis). Among them, phosphorus-containing polysulfones—a special class of functionalized polysulfones—have been employed for high-performance applications such as

- Flame retardancy
- Fuel cell technology—as proton exchange membranes, anion exchange membranes, hydroxide exchange membranes, and ion exchange membranes
- Electrodialysis procedures
- Different biological applications

Recent studies have focused on the synthesis and characterization of new polysulfones containing phosphorus in the side chain, following the effect of the chemical structure on the rheological behavior and topography, and establishing the relation among their processing, morphology, and specific properties. The conclusions of these works may be summarized as follows:

- For polysulfones with bulky phosphorus group in the side chain—PS-DOPO
  - The influence of the substitution degree indicates a Newtonian behavior.
  - Different forms of entanglement are generated by the specific molecular rearrangement of the polysulfone with different substitution degrees, at different concentrations and temperatures.

- Viscoelastic characteristics evidenced the characteristic behavior of an elastic gel at high frequencies, when $G' > G''$, and where both moduli are dependent on frequency.
- AFM images of the films reveal that the bulky phosphorus pendant groups determine the formation of domains with pores whose dimensions increase, although the depth decreases with increasing the substitution degrees; at the same time, it can be seen that increasing the density of the bulky phosphorus pendant groups from the side chain decreases the roughness and, implicitly, confirms the poor adhesion of the modified polysulfone films.
- For polysulfones with triphenylphosphonium in the side chain—PSFP
  - They present a shear-thinning behavior, characterized by a decreased entanglement density, and an enhanced number of oriented segments at increased shear rates.
  - Shear moduli dependence on frequency follows a power law, where the exponents are characteristic to viscoelastic fluids.
  - Surface morphology is characterized by roughness and pore formation, depending on the thermodynamic quality of the solvent; increasing water content leads to a decrease of pore number, whereas their area, depth, average length, and mean width cause a higher hydrophobicity of the samples, thus increasing surface roughness.

To conclude, the shear thinning behavior, good film-forming properties, viscoelastic characteristics, and appropriate surface topography make phosphorus-containing polysulfones suitable materials for applications in medicine. Also, the specific properties of these functionalized polysulfones and the proper macromolecular design, assured by the phosphorus group from the side chain, provide important advantages for their application as membranes with different selectivity and permeability.

REFERENCES

1. Monge S., Canniccioni B., Graillot A., and Robin J. J., Phosphorus-containing polymers: A great opportunity for the biomedical field. *Biomacromolecules*, 12(6), 1973–1982, 2011.
2. Essahli M., Colomines G., Monge S., Robin J. J., Collet A., and Boutevin B., Synthesis and characterization of ionomers based on telechelic phosphonic polyether or aromatic polyesters. *Polymer*, 49(21), 4510–4518, 2008.
3. Canadell J., Hunt B. J., Cook A. G., Mantecon A., and Cadiz V., Flame retardance and shrinkage reduction of polystyrene modified with acrylate-containing phosphorus and crosslinkable spiro-orthoester moieties. *Polym. Degrad. Stab.*, 92(8), 1482–1490, 2007.
4. Chang S., Sachinvala N. D., Sawhney P., Parikh D. V., Jarrett W., and Grimm C., Epoxy phosphonate crosslinkers for providing flame resistance to cotton textiles. *Polym. Adv. Technol.*, 18(8), 611–619, 2007.
5. Singh H. and Jain A. K., Ignition, combustion, toxicity, and fire retardancy of polyurethane foams: A comprehensive review. *J. Appl. Polym. Sci.*, 111(2), 1115–1143, 2009.
6. Bock T., Mülhaupt R., and Möhwald H., Halogen-free polyarylphosphonates and polyelectrolyte membranes for PEMFC by nickel-catalyzed phosphonylation with silylated phosphates. *Macromol. Rapid Commun.*, 27(24), 2065–2071, 2006.

7. Jiang F., Kaltbeitzel A., Meyer W. H., Pu H., and Wegner G., Proton-conducting polymers via atom transfer radical polymerization of diisopropyl-p-vinylbenzyl phosphonate and 4-vinylpyridine. *Macromolecules*, 41(9), 3081–3085, 2008.

8. Zuo Z., Fu Y., and Manthiram A., Novel blend membranes based on acid-base interactions for fuel cells. *Polymers*, 4(4), 1627–1644, 2012.

9. Cheng S., Beyer F. L., Mather B. D., Moore R. B., and Long T. E., Phosphonium-containing ABA triblock copolymers: Controlled free radical polymerization of phosphonium ionic liquids. *Macromolecules*, 44(16), 6509–6517, 2011.

10. Schuster M., Rager T., Noda A., Kreuer K. D., and Maier J., About the choice of the protogenic group in PEM separator materials for intermediate temperature, low humidity operation: A critical comparison of sulfonic acid, phosphonic acid and imidazole functionalized model compounds. *Fuel Cells*, 5(3), 355–365, 2005.

11. Macarie L. and Ilia G., Poly(vinylphosphonic acid) and its derivatives. *Prog. Polym. Sci.*, 35(8), 1078–1092, 2010.

12. Dahiyat B. I., Richards M., and Leong K. W., Controlled release from poly(phosphoester) matrices. *J. Control. Release*, 33(1), 13–21, 1995.

13. Ren H., Sun J., Wu B., and Zhou Q., Synthesis and properties of a phosphorus containing flame retardant epoxy resin based on bis-phenoxy (3-hydroxy) phenyl phosphine oxide. *Polym. Degrad. Stab.*, 92(6), 956–961, 2007.

14. Petreus O., Vlad-Bubulac T., and Hamciuc C., Synthesis and characterization of new polyesters with enhanced phosphorus content. *Eur. Polym. J.*, 41(11), 2663–2670, 2005.

15. Pramanik N., Biswas S. K., and Pramanik P., Synthesis and characterization of hydroxy-apatite/poly(vinyl alcohol phosphate) nanocomposite biomaterials. *Int. J. Appl. Ceram. Technol.*, 5(1), 20–28, 2008.

16. Dordunoo S. K., Vineek W. C., Chaubal M., Zhao Z., Lapidus R., Hoover R., and Dang W. B. In *Polymeric Drug Delivery II: Polymeric Matrices and Drug Particle Engineering*, ed. Svenson S., ACS Symposium Series 924, Washington, DC: American Chemical Society, 2006.

17. Xu X. Y., Yee W. C., Hwang P. Y. K., Yu H., Wan A. C. A., Gao S. J., Boon K. L., Mao H. Q., Leong K. W., and Wang S., Peripheral nerve regeneration with sustained release of poly(phosphoester) microencapsulated nerve growth factor within nerve guide conduits. *Biomaterials*, 24(13), 2405–2412, 2003.

18. Minegishi S., Komatsu S., Kameyama A., and Nishikubo T., Novel synthesis of poly-phosphonates by the polyaddition of bis(epoxide) with diaryl phosphonates. *J. Polym. Sci., Part A Polym. Chem.*, 37(7), 959–965, 1999.

19. Fu B., Sun X., Qian W., Shen Y., Chen R., and Hannig M., Evidence of chemical bonding to hydroxyapatite by phosphoric acid esters. *Biomaterials*, 26(25), 5104–5110, 2005.

20. Zhao Z., Wang J., Mao H. Q., and Leong K. W., Polyphosphoesters in drug and gene delivery. *Adv. Drug Deliv. Rev.*, 55(4), 483–499, 2003.

21. Sen Gupta A. and Lopina S. T., Synthesis and characterization of l-tyrosine based novel polyphosphates for potential biomaterial applications. *Polymer*, 45(14), 4653–4662, 2004.

22. Eng N. F., Garlapati S., Gerdts V., Potter A., Babiuk L. A., and Mutwiri G. K., The potential of polyphosphazenes for delivery of vaccine antigens and immunotherapeutic agents. *Curr. Drug. Deliv.*, 7(1), 13–20, 2010.

23. Teasdale I. and Brüggemann O., Polyphosphazenes: Multifunctional, biodegradable vehicles for drug and gene delivery. *Polymers*, 5(1), 161–187, 2013.

24. Vallée M. R. J., Artner L. M., Dernedde J., and Hackenberger C. P. R., Alkyne phospho-nites for sequential azide–azide couplings. *Angew. Chem. Int. Ed.*, 52(36), 9504–9508, 2013.

25. Corbin W. C., Mai K. M., Freeman J. L., Hastings S. D., and Gray G. M., The coordination chemistry of phosphonites. *Inorg. Chim. Acta*, 407, 223–230, 2013.

26. Chen L. and Wang Y. Z., Aryl polyphosphonates: Useful halogen-free flame retardants for polymers. *Materials*, 3(10), 4746–4760, 2010.

27. Hamdona S. K., Hamza S. M., and Mangood A. H., The influence of polyphosphonates on the precipitation of strontium sulfate (celestite) from aqueous solutions. *Desalin. Water Treat.*, 24(1–3), 55–60, 2010.

28. Agrawal S. and Kumar Narula A., Synthesis and characterization of phosphorus containing aromatic poly(amide-imide)s copolymers for high temperature applications. *Polym. Bull.*, 70(12), 3241–3260, 2013.

29. Xie X., Wang Z., Zhang K., and Xu J., Synthesis, characterization and thermal degradation of phosphorus–nitrogen containing poly(aryl ether ketone)s. *High Perform. Polym.*, 24(6), 521–529, 2012.

30. Ni Q. L., Jiang X. F., Huang T. H., Wang X. J., Gui L. C., and Yang K.G., Gold(I) chloride complexes of polyphosphine ligands with electron-rich arene spacer: Gold–arene interactions. *Organometallics*, 31(6), 2343–2348, 2012.

31. Chen J. L., Zhang L. Y., Shi L. X., Ye H. Y., and Chen Z. N., Synthesis, characterization and redox properties of di- and poly-phosphine linked oligomeric complexes of oxo-centered triruthenium clusters. *Inorg. Chim. Acta*, 359(5), 1531–1540, 2006.

32. Tagle L. H., Diaz F. R., Nuñez M., and Canario F., Polymerization by phase transfer catalysis. 27. Synthesis of polyesters containing silicon or germanium. Influence of the base concentration. *Int. J. Polym. Mater. Polym. Biomater.*, 52(4), 287–294, 2003.

33. Murugan E. and Tamizharasu G., Synthesis and characterization of new soluble multisite phase transfer catalysts and their catalysis in free radical polymerization of methyl methacrylate aided by ultrasound—A kinetic study. *J. Appl. Polym. Sci.*, 125(1), 263–273, 2012.

34. Mustaque K. M., Jayakumar S., and Shabeer T. K., Phase transfer catalysis: Kinetics of acrylonitrile polymerization initiated by potassium peroxomonosulfate-cetylpyridinium chloride system. *J. Chem. Bio. Phy. Sci.*, 2(2), 601–607, 2012.

35. Iliescu S., Pascariu A., Plesu N., Popa A., Macarie L., and Ilia G., Unconventional method used in synthesis of polyphosphoesters. *Polym. Bull.*, 63(4), 485–495, 2009.

36. Iliescu S., Ilia G., Pascariu A., Popa A., and Plesu N., Novel synthesis of phosphorus containing polymers under inverse phase transfer catalysis. *Polymer*, 47(19), 6509–6512, 2006.

37. Roy S. and Maiti S., Synthesis and characterization of a new polyphosphonate for structure-flammability relationship towards group contribution approach. *J. Polym. Mater.* 21(1), 39–48, 2004.

38. Narendran N. and Kishore K., Hydrolytic degradation studies on poly(phosphate ester)s. *J. Appl. Polym. Sci.*, 87(4), 626–631, 2003.

39. Ranganathan T., Zilberman J., Farris R. J., Coughlin E. B., and Emrick T., Synthesis and characterization of halogen-free antiflammable polyphosphonates containing 4,4′-bishydroxydeoxybenzoin. *Macromolecules*, 39(18), 5974–5975, 2006.

40. Iliescu S., Avram E., Visa A., Plesu N., Popa A., and Ilia G., New technique for the synthesis of polyphosphoesters. *Macromol. Res.*, 19(11), 1186–1191, 2011.

41. Iliescu S., Augusti M. G., Fagadar-Cosma E., Plesu N., Fagadar-Cosma G., Macarie L., Popa A., and Ilia G., Synthesis of new phosphorus-containing (co)polyesters using solid-liquid phase transfer catalysis and product characterization. *Molecules*, 17(8), 9090–9103, 2012.

42. Morris S. R. and Dixon B. G., A novel approach for development of improved polymer electrolytes for lithium batteries. *J. Power Sources*, 119–121, 487–491, 2003.

43. Dixon B. G., Morris R. S., and Dallek S., Non-flammable polyphosphonate electrolytes. *J. Power Sources*, 138(1/2), 274–276, 2004.

44. Iliescu S., Ilia G., Plesu N., Popa A., and Pascariu A., Solvent and catalyst-free synthesis of polyphosphates. *Green Chem.*, 8(8), 727–730, 2006.

45. Iliescu S., Ilia G., Pascariu A., Popa A., and Plesu N., Organic solvent-free synthesis of phosphorus containing polymers. *Pure Appl. Chem.*, 79(11), 1879–1884, 2007.

46. Edinger D. and Wagner E., Bioresponsive polymers for the delivery of therapeutic nucleic acids. *WIREs Nanomed. Nanobiotechnol.*, 3(1), 33–46, 2011.

47. Andrianov A. K., Chen J., and LeGolvan M. P., Poly(dichlorophosphazene) as a precursor for biologically active polyphosphazenes: Synthesis, characterization, and stabilization. *Macromolecules*, 37(2), 414–420, 2004.

48. Carriedo G. A., Garcia Alonso F. J., and Presa-Soto A., High molecular weight phosphazene copolymers having chemical functions inside chiral pockets formed by (R)-(1,1′-binaphthyl-2,2′- dioxy)phosphazene units. *Eur. J. Inorg. Chem.*, 24, 4341–4346, 2003.

49. Ilia G., Plesu N., Sfirloaga P., Vasile M., Popa A., and Iliescu S., Polyvinylphosphonic acid used in synthesis of organic inorganic hybrids by sol-gel method. *Optoelectron. Adv. Mater. Rapid Commun.*, 3(12), 1253–1258, 2009.

50. Wang X., Sun C., Gao S., Wang L., and Shuokui H., Validation of germination rate and root elongation as indicator to assess phytotoxicity with *Cucumis sativus*. *Chemosphere*, 44(8), 1711–1721, 2001.

51. Popa A., Crisan M., Visa A., and Ilia G., Effect of a phosphonium salt grafted on polymers on cucumber germination and initial growth. *Braz. Arch. Biol. Technol.*, 54(1), 107–112, 2011.

52. Huang X., Li B., Shi B., and Li L., Investigation on interfacial interaction of flame retarded and glass fiber reinforced PA66 composites by IGC/DSC/SEM. *Polymer*, 49(4), 1049–1055, 2008.

53. Lyon R. E., Takemori M. T., Safronava N., Stoliarov S. I., and Walters R. N., A molecular basis for polymer flammability. *Polymer*, 50(12), 2608–2617, 2009.

54. Popa A., Ilia G., Iliescu S., Dehelean G., Pascariu A., Bora A., and Davidescu C. M., Mixed quaternary ammonium and phosphonium salts bound to macromolecular supports for removal bacteria from water. *Mol. Cryst. Liq. Cryst.*, 418(1), 195–203, 2004.

55. Iliescu S., Grozav I., Funar-Timofei S., Plesu N., Popa A., and Ilia G., Optimization of synthesis parameters in interfacial polycondensation using design of experiments. *Polym. Bull.*, 64(3), 303–314, 2010.

56. Popa A., Davidescu C. M., Negrea P., Ilia G., Katsaros A., and Demadis K. D., Synthesis and characterization of phosphonate ester/phosphonic acid grafted styrene-divinylbenzene copolymer microbeads and their utility in adsorption of divalent metal ions in aqueous solutions. *Ind. Eng. Chem. Res.*, 47(6), 2010–2017, 2008.

57. Popa A., Parvulescu V., Tablet C., Ilia G., Iliescu S., and Pascariu A., Heterogeneous catalysts obtained by incorporation of polymer-supported phosphonates into silica used in oxidation reactions. *Polym. Bull.*, 60(1), 149–158, 2008.

58. Mohandas J., Kumar T., Rajan S. K., Velmurugan S., and Narasimhan S. V., Introduction of bifunctionality into the phosphinic acid ion-exchange resin for enhancing metal ion complexation. *Desalination*, 232(1–3), 3–10, 2008.

59. Trochimczuk A. W. and Czerwińska S., In(III) and Ga(III) sorption by polymeric resins with substituted phenylphosphinic acid ligands. *React. Funct. Polym.*, 63(3), 215–220, 2005.

60. Pilsniak M. and Trochimczuk A. W., Synthesis and characterization of polymeric resins with aliphatic and aromatic amino ligands and their sorption behavior towards gold from ammonium hydroxide solutions. *React. Funct. Polym.*, 67(12), 2007, 1570–1576.

61. Popa A., Ilia G., Davidescu C. M., Iliescu S., Plesu N., Pascariu A., and Zhang Z., Wittig-Horner reactions on styrene-divinylbenzene supports with benzaldehyde side-groups. *Polym. Bull.*, 57(2), 2006, 189–197.

62. Popa A., Muntean S. M., Paska O. M., Iliescu S., Ilia G., and Zhang Z., Resins containing α-hydroxyphosphonic acid groups used for adsorption of dyes from wastewater. *Polym. Bull.*, 66(3), 419–432, 2011.

63. Ilia G., Phosphorus containing hydrogels. *Polym. Adv. Technol.*, 20(9), 707–722, 2009.
64. Wang D. A., Williams C. G., Li Q., Sharma B., and Elisseeff J. H., Synthesis and characterization of a novel degradable phosphate-containing hydrogel. *Biomaterials*, 24(22), 3969–3980, 2003.
65. Wang D. A., Williams C. G., Yang F., Cher N., Lee H., and Elisseeff J. H., Bioresponsive phosphoester hydrogels for bone tissue engineering. *Tissue Eng. A*, 11(1/2), 201–213, 2005.
66. Wang Y. C., Tang L. Y., Sun T. M., Li C. H., Xiong M. H., and Wang J., Self-assembled micelles of biodegradable triblock copolymers based on poly(ethyl ethylene phosphate) and poly(∈-caprolactone) as drug carriers. *Biomacromolecules*, 9(1), 388–395, 2008.
67. Chun J. C., Lee S. M., Kim S. Y., Yang H. K., and Song S. C., Thermosensitive poly(organophosphazene)–paclitaxel conjugate gels for antitumor applications. *Biomaterials*, 30(12), 2349–2360, 2009.
68. Rahimi A., Inorganic and organometallic polymers: A review. *Iran. Polym. J.*, 13(2), 149–164, 2004.
69. Qiu L., Novel degradable polyphosphazene hydrogel beads for drug controlled release. *J. Appl. Polym. Sci.*, 87(6), 986–992, 2003.
70. Chang Y., Bender J. D., Phelps M. V. B., and Allcock H. R., Synthesis and self-association behavior of biodegradable amphiphilic poly[bis(ethyl glycinat-N-yl)phosphazene]–poly(ethylene oxide) block copolymers. *Biomacromolecules*, 3(6), 1364–1369, 2002.
71. Qiu L., Preparation and evaluation of chitosan-coated polyphosphazene hydrogel beads for drug controlled release. *J. Appl. Polym. Sci.*, 92(3), 1993–1999, 2004.
72. Zhang Z., Feng X., Mao J., Xiao J., Liu C., and Qiu J., *In vitro* cytotoxicity of a novel injectable and biodegradable alveolar bone substitute. *Biochem. Biophys. Res. Commun.*, 379(2), 557–561, 2009.
73. Wang Y. C., Tang L. Y., Li Y., and Wang J., Thermoresponsive block copolymers of poly(ethylene glycol) and polyphosphoester: Thermo-induced self-assembly, biocompatibility, and hydrolytic degradation. *Biomacromolecules*, 10(1), 66–73, 2009.
74. Wei X., Wang Z., Wang J., and Wang S., A novel method of surface modification to polysulfone ultrafiltration membrane by preadsorption of citric acid or sodium bisulfite. *Membr. Water Treatment*, 3(1), 35–49, 2012.
75. Jang I. Y., Kweon O. H., Kim K. E., Hwang G. J., Moon S. B., and Kang A. S., Application of polysulfone (PSf)—and polyether ether ketone (PEEK)—tungstophosphoric acid (TPA) composite membranes for water electrolysis. *J. Membr. Sci.*, 322(1), 154–161, 2008.
76. Hu Z. A., Ren L. J., Feng X. J., Wang Y. P., Yang Y.Y., Shi J., Mo L. P., and Lei Z. Q., Platinum-modified polyaniline/polysulfone composite film electrodes and their electrocatalytic activity for methanol oxidation. *Electrochem. Commun.*, 9(1), 97–102, 2007.
77. Mano J. F., Sousa R. A., Boesel L. F., Neves N. M., and Reis R. L., Bioinert, biodegradable and injectable polymeric matrix composites for hard tissue replacement: State of the art and recent developments. *Compos. Sci. Technol.*, 64(6), 789–817, 2004.
78. Kim S., Chen L., Johnson J. K., and Marand E., Polysulfone and functionalized carbon nanotube mixed matrix membranes for gas separation: Theory and experiment. *J. Membr. Sci.*, 294(1/2), 147–158, 2007.
79. Barikani M. and Mehdipour-Ataei S., Synthesis, characterization, and thermal properties of novel arylene sulfone ether polyimides and polyamides. *J. Polym. Sci. A Polym. Chem.*, 38(9), 1487–1492, 2000.
80. Camacho-Zuniga C., Ruiz-Trevino F. A., Hernandez-Lopez S., Zolotukhin M. G., Maurer F. H. J., and Gonzalez-Montiel A., Aromatic polysulfone copolymers for gas separation membrane applications. *J. Membr. Sci.*, 340(1/2), 221–226, 2009.
81. Wang L., Yi B. L., Zhang H. M., and Xing D. M., Pt/SiO$_2$ as addition to multilayer SPSU/PTFE composite membrane for fuel cells. *Polym. Adv. Technol.*, 19(12), 1809–1815, 2008.

82. Chang J. J., Lin P. J., Yang M. C., and Chien C. T., Removal of lipopolysaccharide and reactive oxygen species using sialic acid immobilized polysulfone dialyzer. *Polym. Adv. Technol.*, 20(12), 871–877, 2009.

83. Li J. F., Xu Z. L., and Yang H., Microporous polyethersulfone membranes prepared under the combined precipitation conditions with non-solvent additives. *Polym. Adv. Technol.*, 19(4), 251–257, 2008.

84. Higuchi A., Shirano K., Harashima M., Yoon B. O., Hara M., Hattori M., and Imamura K., Chemically modified polysulfone hollow fibers with vinylpyrrolidone having improved blood compatibility. *Biomaterials*, 23(13), 2659–2666, 2002.

85. Tomaszewska M., Jarosiewicz A., and Karakulski K., Physical and chemical characteristics of polymer coatings in CRF formulation. *Desalination*, 146(1–3), 319–323, 2002.

86. Savariar S., Underwood G. S., Dickinson E. M., Schielke P. J., and Hay A. S., Polysulfone with lower levels of cyclic dimer: Use of MALDI-TOF in the study of cyclic oligomers. *Desalination*, 144(1–3), 15–20, 2002.

87. Sotiriou K., Pispas S., and Hadjichristidis N., Effect of the end-positioning of a lithium sulfonate group on the aggregation and micellization behavior of ω-lithium sulfonate polystyrene-block-polyisoprenes. *Macromol. Chem. Phys.*, 205(1), 55–62, 2004.

88. Ismail A. F. and Hafiz W. A., Effect of polysulfone concentration on the performance of membrane-assisted lead acid battery. *Songklanakarin J. Sci. Technol.*, 24(Suppl), 815–821, 2002.

89. Abuin G. C., Nonjola P., Franceschini E. A., Izraelevitch F. H., Mathe M. K., and Corti H. R., Characterization of an anionic-exchange membranes for direct methanol alkaline fuel cells. *Int. J. Hydrogen Energy*, 35(11), 5849–5854, 2010.

90. Mukherjee S., Roy D., and Bhattacharya P., Comparative performance study of polyethersulfone and polysulfone membranes for trypsin isolation from goat pancreas using affinity ultrafiltration. *Sep. Purif. Technol.*, 60(3), 345–351, 2008.

91. Ismail A. F. and Lai P. Y., Effects of phase inversion and rheological factors on formation of defect-free and ultrathin-skinned asymmetric polysulfone membranes for gas separation. *Sep. Purif. Technol.*, 33(2), 127–143, 2003.

92. Camacho-Zuniga C., Ruiz-Trevino F. A., Zolotukhin M. G., del Castillo L. F., Guzman J., Chavez J., Torres G., Gileva N. G., and Sedova E. A., Gas transport properties of new aromatic cardo poly(aryl ether ketone)s. *J. Membr. Sci.*, 283(1/2), 393–398, 2006.

93. Abu Seman M. N., Khayet M., and Hilal N., Nanofiltration thin-film composite polyester polyethersulfone-based membranes prepared by interfacial polymerization. *J. Membr. Sci.*, 348(1/2), 109–116, 2010.

94. Abu Seman M. N., Johnson D., Al-Malek S., and Hilal N., Surface modification of nanofiltration membrane for reduction of membrane fouling. *Desalin. Water Treat.*, 10(1–3), 298–305, 2009.

95. Van der Bruggen B., Chemical modification of polyethersulfone nanofiltration membranes: A review. *J. Appl.Polym. Sci.*, 114(1), 630–642, 2009.

96. Susanto H. and Ulbricht M., Characteristics, performance and stability of polyethersulfone ultrafiltration membranes prepared by phase separation method using different macromolecular additives. *J. Membr. Sci.*, 327(1/2), 125–135, 2009.

97. Macanas J. and Munoz M., Mass transfer determining parameter in facilitated transport through di-(2-ethylhexyl) dithiophosphoric acid activated composite membranes. *Anal. Chim. Acta*, 534(1), 101–108, 2005.

98. Saxena P., Gaur M. S., Shukla P., and Khare P. K., Relaxation investigations in polysulfone: Thermally stimulated discharge current and dielectric spectroscopy. *J. Electrostat.*, 66(11/12), 584–588, 2008.

99. Wang D., Teo W. K., and Li K., Preparation and characterization of high-flux polysulfone hollow fibre gas separation membranes. *J. Membr. Sci.*, 204(1/2), 247–256, 2002.

100. Yoo J. E., Kim J. H., Kim Y., and Kim C. K., Novel ultrafiltration membranes prepared from the new miscible blends of polysulfone with poly(1-vinylpyrrolidone-co-styrene) copolymers. *J. Membr. Sci.*, 216(1/2), 95–106, 2003.

101. Chwojnowski A., Wojciechowski C., Dudziński K., Łukowska E., and Granicka L., New type of hollow fiber membrane for cell and microorganisms cultivation and encapsulation. *Desalination*, 240(1–3), 9–13, 2009.

102. Rahimy M. P., Chin S., Golshani R., Aras C., Borhani H., and Thompson H., Polysulfone capillary fiber for intraocular drug delivery: *In vitro* and *in vivo* evaluations. *J. Drug Target.*, 2(6), 2455–2480, 1994.

103. Sivaraman K. M., Kellenberger C., Pané S., Ergeneman O., Lühmann T., Luechinger N. A., Hall H., Stark W. J., and Nelson B. J., Porous polysulfone coatings for enhanced drug delivery. *Biomed. Microdevices*, 14(3), 603–612, 2012.

104. Mano J. F., Sousa R. A., Boesel L. F., Neves N. M., and Reis R. L., Bioinert, biodegradable and injectable polymeric matrix composites for hard tissue replacement: State of the art and recent developments. *Composites Sci. Technol.*, 64(6), 789–817, 2004.

105. Shintani H., Study on radiation sterilization-resistant polysulfones fabricated free from bisphenol A. *Trends Biomater. Artif. Organs*, 18(1), 36–40, 2004.

106. Hoffmann T., Pospiech D., Häußler L., Komber H., Voigt D., Harnisch C., Kollann C., Ciesielski M., Döring M., Perez-Graterol R., Sandler J., and Altstädt V., Novel phosphorous-containing aromatic polyethers-synthesis and characterization. *Macromol. Chem. Phys.*, 206(4), 423–431, 2005.

107. Braun U., Knoll U., Schartel B., Hoffmann T., Pospiech D., Artner J., Ciesielski M., Döring M., Perez-Graterol R., Sandler J. K. W., and Altstädt V., Novel phosphorus-containing poly(ether sulfone)s and their blends with an epoxy resin: Thermal decomposition and fire retardancy. *Macromol. Chem. Phys.*, 207(16), 1501–1514, 2006.

108. Perez R. M., Sandler J. K. W., Altstadt V., Hoffmann T., Pospiech D., Ciesielski M., Döring M., Braun U., Balabanovich A. I., and Schartel B., Novel phosphorus-modified polysulfone as a combined flame retardant and toughness modifier for epoxy resins. *Polymer*, 48(3), 778–790, 2007.

109. Lafitte B. and Jannasch P., Phosphonation of polysulfones via lithiation and reaction with chlorophosphonic acid esters. *J. Polym. Sci., Part A Polym. Chem.*, 43(2), 273–286, 2005.

110. Gorbunova M. N. and Vorobeva A. I., Polysulfones on the base of new diallylamino-phosphonium salts. *Macromol. Symp.*, 298(1), 160–166, 2010.

111. Laoutid F., Bonnaud L., Alexandre M., Lopez-Cuesta J. M., and Dubois P., New prospects in flame retardant polymer materials: From fundamentals to nanocomposites. *Mat. Sci. Eng., R*, 63(3), 100–125, 2009.

112. Perez R. M., Sandler J. K. W., Altstädt V., Hoffmann T., Pospiech D., Ciesielski M., and Döring M., Effect of DOPO-based compounds on fire retardancy, thermal stability, and mechanical properties of DGEBA cured with 4,4'-DDS. *J. Mater. Sci.*, 41(2), 341–353, 2006.

113. Perez R. M., Sandler J. K. W., Altstädt V., Hoffmann T., Pospiech D., Artner J., Ciesielski M., Döring M., Balabanovich A. I., and Schartel B., Effective halogen-free flame retardancy for a monocomponent polyfunctional epoxy using an oligomeric organophosphorus compound. *J. Mater. Sci.*, 41(24), 8347–8351, 2006.

114. Petreus O., Avram E., and Serbezeanu D., Synthesis and characterization of phosphorus-containing polysulfone. *Polym. Eng. Sci.*, 50(1), 48–56, 2010.

115. Lafitte B. and Jannasch P., Polysulfone ionomers functionalized with benzoyl(difluoromethylenephosphonic acid) side chains for proton-conducting fuel-cell membranes. *J. Polym. Sci., Part A Polym. Chem.*, 45(2), 269–283, 2007.

116. Peighambardoust S. J., Rowshanzamir S., and Amjadi M., Review of the proton exchange membranes for fuel cell applications. *Int. J. Hydrogen Energy*, 35(17), 9349–9384, 2010.

117. Varcoe J. R. and Slade R. C. T., Prospects for alkaline anion-exchange membranes in low temperature fuel cells. *Fuel Cells*, 5(2), 187–200, 2005.
118. Gu S., Cai R., Luo T., Chen Z., Sun M., Liu Y., He G., and Yan Y., A soluble and highly conductive ionomer for high-performance hydroxide exchange membrane fuel cells. *Angew. Chem. Int. Ed.*, 48(35), 6499–6502, 2009.
119. Nho Y. C., Kwon O. H., and Jie C., Introduction of phosphoric acid group to polypropylene film by radiation grafting and its blood compatibility. *Radiat. Phys. Chem.*, 64(1), 67–75, 2002.
120. Parcero E., Herrera R., and Nunes S. P., Phosphonated and sulfonated polyhphenylsulfone membranes for fuel cell application. *J. Membr. Sci.*, 285(1/2), 206–213, 2006.
121. Steininger H., Schuster M., Kreuer K. D., Kaltbeitzel A., Bingol B., Meyer W. H., Schauff S., Brunklaus G., Maier J., and Spiess H. W., Intermediate temperature proton conductors for PEM fuel cells based on phosphonic acid as protogenic group: A progress report. *Phys. Chem. Chem. Phys.*, 9(15), 1764–1773, 2007.
122. Parvole J. and Jannasch P., Polysulfones grafted with poly(vinylphosphonic acid) for highly proton conducting fuel cell membranes in the hydrated and nominally dry state. *Macromolecules*, 41(11), 3893–3903, 2008.
123. Ioan S., Buruiana L. I., Petreus O., Avram E., Stoica I., and Ioanid G. E., Rheological and morphological properties of phosphorus-containing polysulfones. *Polym. Plast. Technol. Eng.*, 50(1), 36–46, 2011.
124. Buruiana L. I., Avram E., Popa A., Stoica I., and Ioan S., Influence of triphenylphosphonium pendant groups on the rheological and morphological properties of new quaternized polysulfone. *J. Appl. Polym. Sci.*, 129(4), 1752–1762, 2013.
125. de Vasconcelos C. L., Martins R. R., Ferreira M. O., Pereira M. R., and Fonseca J. L. C., Rheology of polyurethane solutions with different solvents. *Polym. Int.*, 51(1), 69–74, 2002.
126. Tsitsilianis C. and Iliopoulos I., Viscoelastic properties of physical gels formed by associative telechelic polyelectrolytes in aqueous media. *Macromolecules*, 35(9), 3662–3667, 2002.
127. Buruiana, L. I., Mathematical modeling and theories applied in characterization of some complex polymer structures. PhD Thesis, "Petru Poni" Institute of Macromolecular Chemistry, Romanian Academy, Iasi, Romania, Supervisor Ioan., S, 2012.

6 Origin of Dielectric Response and Conductivity of Some Functionalized Polysulfones

Silvia Ioan

CONTENTS

6.1   INTRODUCTION

In recent years, the application of modified polysulfones (PSFs) in pharmaceutical, chemical, and food industries, as well as in biotechnology, has become a topic of special scientific interest. Modification of PSFs is mostly based on the addition of carboxylic, chloromethylic, or chlorosulfonic groups to the aromatic ring [1–7]. PSFs fit well into the category of super engineering plastics, due to their excellent thermal stability, good resistance to inorganic acids and bases, and an outstanding hydrolytic stability against hot water and steam sterilization. Chain rigidity is derived from the relatively inflexible and immobile phenyl and SO_2 groups, whereas their toughness is derived from the connecting ether oxygen. The presence of these groups enhances their electrical and thermal stability, oxidation resistance, and rigidity even at high temperatures. Thus, their derivatives appear as important topics of scientific research from both theoretical and practical viewpoints, with special reference to their applications areas [8,9].

Quaternization of the PSF backbone with tertiary amines represents a useful way to modify some properties of the material, such as solubility [10–13] and hydrophilicity (which is of special interest for biomedical applications) [3,14,15], allowing higher water permeability and better separation [16,17]. Literature [18] also shows that the membranes made of sulfonated PSF may be applied in separation processes, biotechnology, energy industry (fuel cell), as well as in biomedical engineering. The sulfonating factors are described in different publications by cyclic trimethyl sulfate [$(CH_3)_3SO_3$] [19], and trimethylsilyl chlorosulfate [$(CH_3)_3SiSO_3Cl$] [20], a complex of sulfur trioxide (SO_3) with triethylphosfate [$TEP(SO_3)$] [21] and chlorosulfonic acid [22,23]. PSFs modified by different reagents, used as substrates for enzyme immobilization, improve filtration stability [23]. In addition, Nayac et al. [24] show that PSF nanocomposites with conductive nanofillers (e.g., carbon nanofibers and carbon nanotubes with improved mechanical properties—due to fewer microstructural defects, smaller diameter, and lower density) have important technological applications as materials for electrostatic discharge, electromagnetic interference shielding, fuel cell, and embedded capacitors. The biological materials can be selected to satisfy certain analytic needs, as they operate at specific levels. They can be highly selective, specific to a narrow margin of the compound, or they show a wide specificity spectrum as a sensitive biosensor, for example, only to one antibiotic (for instance, gentamicin), or, later on, to all antibiotics.

On the other hand, the immunoassay methods, based on analytical electrochemical detection of the environmental samples or on medical diagnosis, play an important role in the improvement of public health, providing applications in clinical chemistry, food quality, and environmental monitoring. Technological aspects related to the development of immunosensors include biomolecular interaction kinetics, immobilization techniques, and catalytic studies. Integration of these technologies makes possible diversification in the production of immunosensors applicable for a wide variety of detection and monitoring issues [25].

The literature reports different immobilization techniques for preparing PSF composites based on electrochemical sensors and biosensors [26]. These compounds act not only as membranes but also as reservoirs for immunological materials.

In this context, the optical (transmittance and refractivity) and electrical (dielectric spectrum, relaxation process, or electrical conduction) properties manifested in different complex forms of PSFs are very important for the investigation of molecular motion and induced polarization, in correlation with the different complex structures of modified PSFs, thus orienting their possible applications. Applications of such different and complex structures, including functionalized PSFs, require knowledge of their electrical properties, such as the cooperative phenomena and primary (intrachain) and secondary (i.e., ionic bonding, hydrogen bonding, dipolar, and van der Waals interactions) forces, of temperature (which develops a dissociation energy), or of the applied frequency.

Dielectric spectroscopy is the most commonly employed investigation method, due to the particularly large dynamic range permitting access to it. Conventional dielectric studies are often completed by investigations developed other techniques, as mechanical shear spectroscopy and rheology, offering alternative perspectives on relaxation phenomena [27]. Such a combined approach provides information on the molecular dynamics, by comparing not only the time scale of the structural fluctuations but also the spectral shape probed with different methods. Depolarized light scattering and nuclear magnetic resonance are among the techniques often employed to such ends as, similarly with dielectric spectroscopy, they provide access to molecular orientational correlation functions.

6.2 DIELECTRIC RELAXATION PHENOMENA IN COMPLEX SYSTEMS

Generally, when an electrical field is applied, the atomic and molecular charges of the dielectric materials are displaced from the equilibrium positions because of the polarization effect. The major polarization mechanisms in the polymeric materials studied by dielectric spectroscopy are due to charge migration—which gives rise to conductivity and orientation of permanent dipoles, correlated with induced dipoles—oriented in the direction of the applied field. Unlike the electronic and atomic polarization, considered instantaneous by dielectric spectroscopy, the cooperative molecular motions are caused by the polarization of the permanent dipoles. Thus, upon the removal of the electrical field, dipole relaxation occurs from the time-dependant loss of polarization.

Definition of dielectric permittivity or dielectric constant starts from the understanding of the phenomenon of sample polarization. A dielectric sample acquires a nonzero macroscopic dipole moment, becoming polarized under the influence of an external electric field, E. Polarization of the polymers is defined by the following:

- The dipole moment, P, of the sample is dependent on the macroscopic dipole moment, $\overline{M}$, of the whole sample volume, V (Equation 6.1).
- The strength of the applied external electric field is dependent on the tensor of dielectric susceptibility of the polymer, χ_{ik}, and dielectric permittivity of the vacuum, $\varepsilon_0 = 8.854 \cdot 10^{-12}$ F·m^{-1} (Equation 6.2).

$$P = \frac{\overline{M}}{V} \tag{6.1}$$

$$P_i = \varepsilon_0 \cdot \chi_{ik} \cdot E_k \tag{6.2}$$

According to the macroscopic Maxwell approach, the electrical displacement (induction) vector, D, is correlated with the following:

- The field within the matter considered as a continuum (Equation 6.3)
- The isotropic dielectric medium (when vectors D, E, and P have the same direction, and susceptibility is coordinate independent) (Equations 6.4 and 6.5)

$$D = \varepsilon_0 \cdot E + P \tag{6.3}$$

$$D = \varepsilon_0(1+\chi)E = \varepsilon_0 \cdot \varepsilon \cdot E \tag{6.4}$$

where:

$$\varepsilon = 1 + \chi \text{ (relative dielectric permittivity)} \tag{6.5}$$

On the other hand, the applied electrical field generates a dipole density through deformation (electron and atomic polarizations), orientation (strongly dependent on the applied electrical field, frequency, and temperature), and ionic (where the dipole moment of the whole sample is a resultant of the positive ions that move in the direction of an applied electrical field and the negative ions, which move in opposite direction) polarization mechanisms.

Thus:

- Electron polarization is due to the displacement of nuclei and electrons inside the atom under the influence of an external electric field. As the electrons have low weights, they can be influenced even in the field of optical frequencies.
- Atomic polarization results from the displacement of atoms inside the molecule under the influence of an applied electrical field.
- Orientation polarization is counteracted by molecules thermal motion.
- Ionic polarization depends only slightly on temperature, being correlated with the interface where ions can be accumulated, and influences the cooperative processes in heterogeneous systems.

Generally, the literature shows the influence of both induced (P_α, caused by translation effects) and dipole polarizations (P_μ, caused by the orientation of the permanent dipoles)—(Equation 6.6) and defines a polar dielectric structure (the individual molecules have a permanent dipole moment, even in the absence of an applied field), a nonpolar dielectric structure (the molecules possess a dipole moment only subjected to an electric field), and a mixture of these two types of dielectric structures for complex materials.

$$P_\alpha + P_\mu = \varepsilon_0(\varepsilon - 1)E \tag{6.6}$$

In the statistical mechanics used by Frohlich, the dielectric constants of the polarizable molecules with a permanent dipole moment are evaluated considering that dipole moment, μ_d, has the same nonelectrostatic interactions with other point dipoles, and that the polarizability of molecules is imagined as a continuum with dielectric constant, ε_∞, so that the induced polarization is as follows:

$$P_\mu = \varepsilon_0(\varepsilon_\infty - 1)E \tag{6.7}$$

The orientation polarization for a sphere containing i dipoles with volume V is given by

$$P_\mu = \frac{1}{V}\sum_{i=1}^{N}(\mu_d)_i \tag{6.8}$$

In the same context, Kirkwood considered a correlation factor g (very important for understanding the short-range molecular mobility and the interactions occurring in complex systems), for introducing the correlation between molecules with different orientations (Equation 6.9), while Kirkwood and Froehlich established the relation between the dielectric constant, ε, and the dielectric constant of induced polarization (Equation 6.10):

$$g = \sum_{j=1}^{N} <\cos\theta_{ij}> = 1 + z \cdot <\cos\theta_{ij}> \tag{6.9}$$

where:
θ_{ij} is the angle between the orientation of the ith and jth dipole
z is the nearest neighbor:

$$g\mu_d^2 = \frac{\varepsilon_0 9k_B TV(\varepsilon - \varepsilon_\infty)(2\varepsilon + \varepsilon_\infty)}{\varepsilon(\varepsilon_\infty + 2)^2} \tag{6.10}$$

where:
$k_B = 1.381 \cdot 10^{-23}$ J·K^{-1} is the Boltzmann constant
t is the absolute temperature

Sample polarization under the influence of an external field reaches a steady state after a certain time, whereas the interruption of an abrupt electric field causes time-dependent polarization cancelation. The dielectric response can be interpreted as a function of frequency and time in the complex dielectric permittivity. In addition, the Debye equation (Equation 6.11) includes the relaxation time, τ_m, and the macroscopic linear function, $\phi(t)$ (Equation 6.12) [28]:

$$\frac{\varepsilon^*(\omega) - \varepsilon_\infty}{\varepsilon_s - \varepsilon_\infty} = \frac{1}{1 + i\omega\tau_m} \tag{6.11}$$

where:
ε_s and ε_∞ are the low- and high-frequency limits of dielectric permittivity, respectively

$$\phi(t) = \exp\left(\frac{-t}{\tau_m}\right) \tag{6.12}$$

where:
τ_m is the characteristic relaxation time
$\phi(t)$ is the macroscopic linear function

On the other hand, the non-Debye dielectric behavior is correlated with the continuous distribution of relaxation time by means of the Havriliak–Negami (HN) relationship [29]:

$$\varepsilon^*(\omega) = \varepsilon_\infty + \frac{\varepsilon_s - \varepsilon_\infty}{\left[1 + (i\omega\tau_m)^\beta\right]} \tag{6.13}$$

The empirical exponents α and β involve different interpretations:

$\alpha = 1$ and $\beta = 1$—correspond to the Debye relaxation law.
$\alpha \neq 1$ and $\beta = 1$—correspond to the Cole–Cole equation [30].
$\alpha = 1$ and $\beta \neq 1$—correspond to the Cole–Davidson equation [31].

Asymptotic relaxation processes at both high and low frequencies are analyzed with the Jonscher power law (Equation 6.14), considering $(i\omega)^{n-1}$ and $(i\omega)^m$, where $n > 0$ and $m \leq 1$ are Jonscher stretch parameters [32]:

$$\varepsilon^* = \varepsilon' - i\varepsilon'' = \varepsilon_\infty + \frac{\sigma}{i\varepsilon_0\omega} + \left[\frac{a(T)}{\varepsilon_0}\right]\left[i\omega^{n(T)-1}\right] \tag{6.14}$$

where:
$n(T)$ is the temperature-dependent exponent
$a(T)$ determines the strength of the arising polarizability

The real and imaginary parts of the complex dielectric constant are given by the following relations:

$$\varepsilon' = \varepsilon_\infty + \sin\left(\frac{n(T)\pi}{2}\right)\omega^{n(T)-1}\left[\frac{a(T)}{\varepsilon_0}\right] \tag{6.15}$$

where:
the first term determines the lattice response
the second one reflects the charge carrier contribution to the dielectric constant

$$\varepsilon'' = \frac{\sigma}{i\varepsilon_0\omega} + \cos\left(\frac{n(T)\pi}{2}\right)\omega^{n(T)-1}\left[\frac{a(T)}{\varepsilon_0}\right] \tag{6.16}$$

where:
the first term corresponds to the conduction part
the second one reflects the charge carrier contribution to dielectric permittivity

The temperature and frequency dependencies of dielectric constant ε' are explained by Equation 6.16 [33]. Special mention should also be made of the following proportionality:

- The real part $\varepsilon'(\omega)$ of the complex dielectric permittivity is proportional to the imaginary part $\sigma''(\omega)$ of the complex AC conductivity: $\varepsilon'(\omega) \propto -\sigma''(\omega)/\omega$.
- The dielectric losses $\varepsilon''(\omega)$ are proportional to the real part $\sigma'(\omega)$ of the AC conductivity: $\varepsilon''(\omega) \propto \sigma'(\omega)/\omega$.

The asymptotic power law for $\sigma^*(\omega)$ appears in many types of disordered systems [34]. Generally, in relation with the dynamic molecular properties of a material, the fluctuations of polarization caused by the thermal motion are the same as for the macroscopic rearrangements induced by the electric field [35,36]. Literature presents the macroscopic dipole correlation function as follows:

$$\phi(t) \cong \frac{<M(t)M(0)>}{<M(0)M(0)>} \tag{6.17}$$

where:

$M(t)$ is the macroscopic fluctuating dipole moment of the sample volume unit, which is equal to the vector sum of all molecular dipoles entering it

The rate and laws governing the macroscopic dipole correlation function are directly related to the structural and kinetic properties of the sample and characterize the macroscopic properties of the system under study. Mathematical evaluations show that the macroscopic function can be expressed by a simple exponential law. In this context, different systems deviate from the classical exponential Debye model, so that $\phi(t)$ can be expressed by Equations 6.18 through 6.20 in the Kohlrausch–Williams–Watts (KWW, stretched exponential) law:

$$\phi(t) = \exp\left[-\left(\frac{t}{\tau_m}\right)^{\upsilon}\right] \tag{6.18}$$

where:

τ_m is the characteristic relaxation time and $0 < \upsilon \le 1$

For $\upsilon = 1$, this relation coincides with Equation 6.12 in the asymptotic power law:

$$\phi(t) = A\left(\frac{t}{\tau_l}\right)^{-\mu}, \quad t \ge \tau_l \tag{6.19}$$

where:

A is the amplitude

μ is an exponent higher than 0

τ_l is the characteristic time associated with the effective relaxation time of the microscopic structural unit for a phenomenological decay function with different short- and long-time asymptotic forms, and different characteristic times

$$\phi(t) = \exp\left[-\left(\frac{t}{\tau_m}\right)^{\upsilon}\right]\exp\left[-\left(\frac{t}{t_m}\right)^{\upsilon}\right] \tag{6.20}$$

To describe the relaxation time as a temperature-dependent parameter, $\tau(\propto 1/k)$, the literature presents the Arhenius and Eyring laws (Equations 6.21 and 6.22, respectively) [37–39].

- Arrhenius law [48], where E_a is the activation energy and k_0 is the exponential factor corresponding to $T \rightarrow \infty$:

$$k = k_0 \left(-\frac{E_a}{k_0 T} \right) \qquad (6.21)$$

- Eyring law [49–51], where ΔS and ΔH symbolize the activation entropy and enthalpy, respectively, and $\hbar = 6.626 \cdot 10^{-34}$ J s^{-1} is the Plank constant:

$$k = \frac{k_B T}{\hbar} \exp \left(\frac{\Delta S}{k_B} - \frac{\Delta H}{k_B T} \right) \qquad (6.22)$$

Besides these equations, the literature presents some particular cases of relaxation kinetics, such as the Vogel–Fulcher–Tammann [40] or Fox and Flory [41] laws (for amorphous materials), Turnbull and Cohen [42] (introducing the free volume concept to some disorder solids), and Gotze and Sjögren mode-coupling theories [43].

Investigation of the relaxation phenomena, which intensify and monitor cooperative processes in different materials, especially in those with intermolecular contributions, can be performed by the dielectric spectroscopy method.

6.3 OPTICAL PROPERTIES IN COMPLEX SYSTEMS

The refractive index is one of the parameters used for optically classifying clear materials. It expresses the ratio of the velocity of light in a vacuum to its velocity in the material under study; moreover, it can be defined as a relationship between the sine of the angle of incidence and the sine of the angle of refraction when a ray of light passes from air into the studied medium. Like luminous transmittance, the refractive index is an important property to be considered in the design of optical systems. Thus, for multiple applications, knowledge of the optical properties before the synthesis process is necessary. The optical properties depend on the molar volume and molar refraction of the polymer repeating units. Also, accurate values of the specific refractive index increment, dn/dc, of the polymer solutions must be determined to obtain the average molecular weight, M_w, by light scattering or for the estimation of molecular weight distribution by size exclusion chromatography. Literature shows that the theoretical values of refractive index and the specific refractive index increments can be calculated based on the assumption that the molar volume, V_u, and the molar refraction, R_u, of the chain-repeating unit are additive functions of the composition (Equations 6.23 and 6.24) [44–46]:

$$V_u = \sum_i a_i V_i \qquad (6.23)$$

$$R_u = \sum_i a_i R_i \qquad (6.24)$$

where:
V_i and R_i are the contributions of groups
a_i is the number of groups i in the repeating unit

Huglin [47] presents Equations 6.25 through 6.28 by relating the specific refractive index increments, dn/dc, to the refractive index of polymers, n_2, and solvent n_1; in Equations 6.25 and 6.27, n_2 can be calculated from Equations 6.26, proposed by Lorenz–Lorentz [48,49], and Equation 6.28, proposed by Gladstone–Dale [50], respectively:

$$\frac{dn}{dc} = \bar{v}_2 \left[\frac{\left(n_2^2 - 1\right)}{\left(n_2^2 + 2\right)} - \frac{\left(n_1^2 - 1\right)}{\left(n_1^2 + 2\right)} \right] \frac{\left(n_1^2 + 2\right)^1}{6n_1} \tag{6.25}$$

where:
  $\bar{v}_2$ is the partial specific volume of polymer in solution

$$R_u = \frac{V_u \left(n_2^2 - 1\right)}{\left(n_2^2 + 2\right)} \tag{6.26}$$

$$\frac{dn}{dc} = \bar{v}_2 \left(n_2 - 1\right) - \bar{v}_2 \left(n_1 - 1\right) \tag{6.27}$$

$$R_u = V_u \left(n_2 - 1\right) \tag{6.28}$$

A material with a high refractive index is characterized by high polarizability; thus, the dipole moment per unit volume, induced by the electromagnetic field, tends to a maximal value. The R_i/V_i ratio of different atoms from organic polymers [46], and the increments of some substructures, R_i and V_i, are presented in Tables 6.1 and 6.2, respectively [51,52].

TABLE 6.1
Contribution of Different Atoms to the Refractive Index of a Compound

Atom	R_i/V_i	
	Minimal Values	Maximal Values
H	0.187	0.335
C	0.240	0.561
N	0.451	0.748
O	0.153	0.444
F	0.080	0.153
Cl	0.297	0.410
S	Average value: 0.493	

Source: Groh, W. and Zimmermann, A., *Macromolecules,* 24(25), 6660–6663, 1991.

TABLE 6.2
Increments of Various Substructures R_i (cm³g⁻¹) and V_i (cm³)

				Substructures					
Increments	$-CH_2-$	$p-C_6H_4-$[a]	$\equiv CCH_3$	$-CH_3$	$=CH-$	C_6H_5-[a]	$-O-$	$-SO_2$	C_6H_3-[a]
R_i	4.50	25.24	7.88	5.90	3.41	25.82	1.63	9.63	24.79
V_i	15.53	65.91	22.65	25.81	8.09	74.13	9.05	27.71	53.71

[a] Aromatic group.

It was observed that sulfur has a higher ratio than chlorine, oxygen, and hydrogen. The R_i/V_i ratios have a broad range of values for each atom, depending on the different binding structures and on a varying chemical environment in different organic or inorganic compounds. Starting from theoretical evaluations, the literature provides the following values for PSF [53]: $R_u = 127.6$ cm³g⁻¹, $V_u = 357.9$ cm³, $R_u/V_u = 0.357$, and $n_2 = 1.632$. The theoretical value of the refractive index of PSFs is slightly different from the experimental value given in the literature [54], being situated in the domain of refractive index for optical materials (see Table 6.3).

In addition, Figure 6.1 shows that the experimental values for PSFs and chloromethylated PSFs at 436 nm wavelength agree well with those calculated with the Lorenz–Lorentz equation and are slightly different from those determined by the Gladstone–Dale equation. These slight discrepancies can result from approximation (given in Equation 6.25) of values $\bar{v}_2$ with the specific volume, v_2, of the solid polymer. Figure 6.1 also shows that the specific refractive index increments decrease with increasing the substitution degree.

Similar to refractivity, the dielectric constants depend on the polarizability expressed by the dipole moment per unit volume induced by the electromagnetic field. Generally, the literature shows that the dielectric constant, ε, of polymers decreases gradually with increasing frequency (Figure 6.2).

TABLE 6.3
Typical Refractive Index of Some Transparent Materials

Material	Refractive Index
Polysulfone	1.633
Calibre polycarbonate	1.580
Glass	1.520
Cellulose acetate	1.500
Poly(methyl methacrylate)	1.490

Source: Seferis, J. C., *Polymers Handbook*, Wiley, Toronto, Canada, 1999.

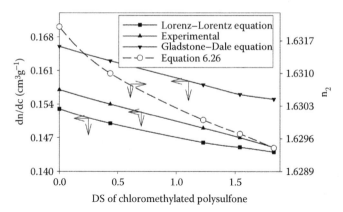

FIGURE 6.1 Variation of refractive index and specific refractive index increment of poly-sulfones and chloromethylated polysulfones with different substitution degree. (Data from Ioan, S. et al., *J. Macromol. Sci. Part B Phys.*, 44, 129–135, 2005.)

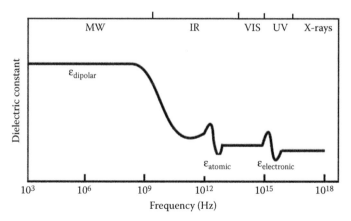

FIGURE 6.2 Frequency responses in a microwave domain on the dielectric mechanisms.

This variation is attributed to the frequency dependence of the polarization mechanisms, which include the dielectric constant. The magnitude of the dielectric constant is dependent on the ability of the polarizable units in a polymer to orient fast enough to keep up with the oscillations of an alternating electric field. The contribution of each polarization mode to the dielectric constant is expressed as follows:

$$\varepsilon = \varepsilon_{electronic} + \varepsilon_{atomic} + \varepsilon_{dipolar} \tag{6.29}$$

where:

$\varepsilon_{electronic}$ is the dielectric constant corresponding to the electronic polarization at high frequencies (10^{15} Hz)

ε_{atomic} is the dielectric constant corresponding to the atomic polarization at lower frequencies (10^{12} Hz)

$\varepsilon_{dipolar}$ is the dielectric constant corresponding to the dipolar polarization occurring at microwave (10^9 Hz)

A comparison between the dielectric constant measured at optical frequency, $\varepsilon_{electronic}$, and the dielectric constant measured at lower frequencies permits a basic understanding of the influence of the molecular structure on the dielectric properties in polymeric materials.

Theoretically, the estimation of the dielectric constant at high frequencies (10^{15} Hz), over the optical range, when only electronic polarization is predominantly manifested, is based on the Maxwell relationship:

$$\varepsilon_{electronic} = n_2^2 \tag{6.30}$$

Theoretical evaluation of the refractive indices starts from the idea that the individual atoms present in organic polymers have a certain contribution to the refractive index and dielectric constant values, respectively. The study is based on the knowledge of molar refractivity, R_u, and molar volume, V_u, of the chain-repeating unit, which are additive functions of the composition (Equations 6.23 and 6.24). A comparison between the optical dielectric constant, $\varepsilon_{electronic}$, or $\varepsilon_{electronic,experimental}$, and the dielectric constant measured at frequencies lower than optical frequency, $\varepsilon_{dipolar}$, may assure a basic understanding on the influence of the molecular structure on the dielectric properties in different materials.

On the other hand, for other complicated structures, such as polysulfonic nanocomposites with metal or semiconductor particles, the literature describes recent progress recorded in the theory of nanoparticle optical properties, particularly the methods for solving Maxwell's equations for light scattering from particles of arbitrary shape in a complex environment [55]. Included is a study on the qualitative features of dipole and quadrupole plasmon resonances for spherical particles and a discussion on the analytical and numerical methods employed for calculating extinction and scattering cross-sections, local fields, and other optical properties for nonspherical particles.

A simple method for obtaining an organic–inorganic nanocomposite involves the mixing of an organic polymer with a metal-oxide nanofiller, followed by the application of the solution grown technique [56]. Thus, PSF/ZnO nanocomposites exhibit drastic changes in their structural and thermal properties with the introduction of a very small quantity of ZnO nanoparticles, rather than of pure PSF. On the other hand, the results on the dispersion of hydrophilic ZnO nanoparticles within hydrophobic polymer matrices have been capitalized to obtain a lower filler content for improving material properties, and to design nano-structured polymer composites [57].

Fundamental knowledge on the nature and optical properties of nanoparticles, including nanocomposites with extremely high or low refractive indices and dichroic nanocomposites, are particularly useful in different electronic applications [58]. The refractive index of polymers can be increased or decreased by the incorporation of inorganic colloids with extreme refractive indices, so that they can cover the range of 1–3—thus exceeding the limits hitherto known for polymers alone. Also, dichroic nanocomposites can be prepared from metal colloids embedded in polymers. These metal aggregates can be deformed by a solid-state drawing into colloid arrays; the maximum absorption wavelength in systems is modified upon variation of the angle between the polarization direction of light and the orientation axis of the particle arrays. Dichroic nanocomposites may find applications in liquid crystal displays.

In addition, the optical properties of complex structures can be modified through the exposure of their thin film to different external conditions, which significantly changes the molecular structure and macromolecular dynamics of the material. In this context, the literature recommends different noninvasive and very high precision methods, such as Brillouin light scattering, particle embedding, dielectric relaxation spectroscopy, buckling instability, positron annihilation spectroscopy, X-ray photon correlation spectroscopy, and spectroscopic ellipsometry [59], for studying the changes produced in film properties, such as density and thickness.

Optical absorption studies, including optical reflection, transmission, adsorption properties, and their relation to the optical constants of films, support the analysis for interpreting various processes of electronic nature—for example, the fundamental gap, electronic transition, trapping levels, and localized states. In an intrinsic system, the fully occupied continuous energy sublevels are the valence bands, and the lowest unoccupied continuous energy sublevels are the conduction bands. Both band types are separated by a forbidden energy bandgap, E_G. In this context, the literature data present different aspects concerning disorder in amorphous materials, which influences band structure and hence the electrical and optical properties of the materials [60]. For semiconductors, the main characteristics of energy distribution of the electronic states density of crystalline solids are as follows:

- A sharp structure of the valence and conduction bands, as well as the abrupt terminations at the maximum band valence and minimum band conduction.
- The sharp edges in the density of states curves produce a well-defined forbidden energy gap.

The amorphous solids

- Do not present structural order.
- Are unstable or metastable and frequently exhibit a gradual or even rapid transition toward an ordered crystalline condition.
- Are characterized by a high-density disorder, yet slightly different from the ideal crystalline structure; the short-range order can be induced by the rigidity of the chemical bonds, and the crystal band structure can be applied for amorphous solids.

To obtain the optical parameters, the approach proposed for amorphous semiconductors by Tauc has been used for polymers with different structures and combinations. Also, it is known that the molecular motion in polymers is subject to primary intrachain and secondary forces (i.e., ionic bonding, hydrogen bonding, dipolar, and van der Waals interactions), the latter ones being more temperature dependent, because of their low values of dissociation energy. Therefore, the knowledge of these properties is important for establishing the electrical characteristics of quaternized PSFs. From this reason, the influence of temperature and electric field on dielectric relaxation and AC conductivity has been investigated by AC-dielectric measurements. Such detailed investigations provide valuable information on the nature of the underlying motional processes responsible for transitions and on their relationship to temperature and frequency.

Besides the refractive index, transmittance spectra provide useful information on the optical properties of PSFs composed of phenylene units in the backbone chain (linked by isopropylidene, ether, and sulfone) and different pendant groups occurring in different complex linkages. These spectra, realized in the visible and near infrared spectral range, reflect the influence of the type of pendant group on the transmission spectra and the position of the absorption edge. To obtain the gap energy and the other energies describing the absorption edge, the method proposed by Tauc for amorphous materials has been applied to polysulfonic compounds [4,61–63]. Some correlations between absorption or transmittance spectra (Equation 6.31) and the molecular structure of polymers, on the one hand, and the history of films preparation, on the other, influence these optical properties.

$$\alpha = \left(\frac{1}{d}\right)\ln\left(\frac{1}{\text{transmittance}}\right) \tag{6.31}$$

where:
d is film thickness

For a typical amorphous semiconductor, three domains are evident in the variation of the absorption coefficient versus photon energy [61–63]:

- In the first region, due to the interband transition near the band gap, the absorption coefficient describes the optical gap energy E_G in amorphous semiconductors.
- In the second region, absorption at the photon energy below the optical gap depends exponentially on the photon energy, which defines the Urbach edge energy, E_U, on knowing that the sharp absorption edge is enlarged by the electric fields produced by charged impurities.
- The third region describes the optical absorption generated by defects appearing at an energy lower than the optical gap; it is sensitive to the structural properties of the materials, being defined as the so-called Urbach tail, E_T. This absorption tail lies below the exponential part of the absorption edge (the second region), and its strength and shape were found to depend on the preparation, purity, and thermal history of the material, varying only slightly with its thickness.

Data exemplified in Figure 6.3 for quaternized PSFs with N-dimethylethylammonium chloride pendant group (PSF-DMEA), and for quaternized PSFs with N-dimethyloctylammonium chloride pendant group (PSF-DMOA) present the absorption edge and Tauc plots as a function of the photon energy. The shape of all edges is very similar to the behavior proposed by Tauc for a typical amorphous semiconductor [64], although the level of absorption is lower than that for amorphous, inorganic thin films. These results and other literature data [65,66] assume that the lower absorption in polymeric materials is due to a lower degree of bonding delocalization. Each of the absorption edges from Figure 6.3 exhibits two different

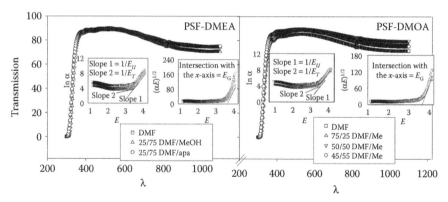

FIGURE 6.3 Typical overall transmission spectra (%) versus wavelength (λ, nm) of PSF-DMOA films obtained from their solutions in DMF, DMF/MeOH, and DMF/water. Small plots represent the absorption coefficient (α, cm^{-1}) and the Tauc dependence [(αE)$^{1/2}$, (eV/cm)$^{1/2}$], respectively, versus the photon energy (E, eV) for the same films. (Data from Albu, R. M. et al., *High Perform. Polym.*, 23, 85–89, 2011.)

exponential regions with different slopes, and a saturation region at higher energy. The exponential parts are described by Equation 6.32 [67,68]:

$$\alpha = \alpha_0 \exp\left(\frac{E}{A}\right) \tag{6.32}$$

where:

α_0 is a constant and E is the photon energy

Parameter A becomes either E_U—in the high-energy exponential region—or E_T—in the low-energy exponential region of the absorption coefficient. For both samples, the absorption edges have been found to follow the Tauc power law (Equation 6.33) in the range over which the photon energy is higher than E_G [64]:

$$\left(\alpha \cdot E\right)^{1/2} = B\left(E - E_G\right) \tag{6.33}$$

where:

B is a constant

Thus, dependencies $(\alpha \cdot E)^{1/2} = f(E)$, illustrated in Figure 6.3, were used to obtain the Tauc optical energy gap, E_G. The approach, typical for amorphous semiconductors, is generally applied to polymeric films [69,70].

The values of the optical parameters show that both quaternized PSFs analyzed here are transparent, having the energy gap values, E_G, between 3.61 and 3.66 eV. These values are insignificantly modified by the different alkyl side groups. On the other hand, apart from their structure, the history of films preparation is generally influenced by the Urbach edge and Urbach tail energy values. These two parameters are related to the localized state induced by the polymer atomic structures. Possible structural defects, such as break, abbreviation, and torsion of the polymer chains, seem to be responsible for the low-energy absorption described by the Urbach tail energy, whereas the electric fields produced by charged impurities influence the Urbach edge energy. Moreover, larger structural disorder may cause an increase in both Urbach edge and Urbach tail energy values. In this context, the literature data show the influence of morphological aspects on film properties obtained by different processes. Thus, energies E_U and E_T are lower for the films obtained from quaternized PSF solutions in N,N-dimethylformamide (DMF)/methanol (MeOH) than for those obtained in DMF/water; their dependence on the composition of solvent mixtures and, implicitly, on the multiple interactions from the system was also being evidenced [69,70]. Generally, the higher values of E_T correspond to the composition of mixed solvents, for which intrinsic viscosity takes lower values. Also, atomic force morphology investigations show that the morphology of these films is modified because of the nonsolvents added in different ratios; consequently, the number of pores and their average size increases, whereas average surface roughness decreases with increasing the nonsolvent content; the Urbach edge energy is being influenced rather by the number and size of pores than by surface roughness.

Consequently, structure appears as a major factor, which influences the physical properties of polymeric films. It has been already shown that these films have different average roughness values and pore characteristics, and that the increase in temperature considerably affects their morphological structure. In addition, the concentration of charged carriers increases with the increase of temperature which, in turn, increases the conductivity of the given sample in a different manner. On the other hand, phenomenologically, it is obvious that the optical bandgap energies, E_G, presented in Figure 6.3, are different from those obtained from the values of thermal activation energy of the AC-electrical conduction, E_σ.

It is also worth mentioning that in polymeric complex systems, for example, systems with microdomains dispersed in a phase of other materials, the glassy or semi-crystalline domains can act as physical cross-links and reinforcing filers, whereas the phase determines flexibility. Moreover, the presence of ions into the polymer structure affects significantly its optical properties by a number of factors, including the position and concentration of ionic groups, the compatibility of the polymer chain and the ionic groups, nature of the ion, and the choice of the neutralizing ion [71].

6.4 ORIGIN OF DIELECTRIC RELAXATION IN MODIFIED PSFs

6.4.1 Establishment of Complex Polymer Conformations by Computational Methods

Generally, the following two major polarization mechanisms characteristic to polymeric materials are studied by dielectric spectroscopy:

- Polarization due to charge migration, which gives rise to conductivity.
- Polarization created by orientation of permanent dipoles.

The origin of conductivity in polymer networks is especially due to the intrinsic migrating charges, which can obey a more complex pattern. Unlike the electronic and atomic polarizations, considered instantaneous by dielectric spectroscopy, the permanent dipoles, dipoles orientation, and dipoles polarization results from their alignment in the direction of the applied field, involving cooperative motions of molecular segments with time scale measurable by dielectric spectroscopy. Thus, the time-dependent loss of dipole orientations upon the removal of the electric field is defined by dipole relaxation. In this context, a special interest has been manifested on the fundamental aspects of the dielectric spectroscopy of polymeric materials [72,73] for the elucidation of various molecular motions and relaxation processes, and for enlarging their applicability as electronic interconnected devices, optoelectronic switches, printed board circuitry, and so on.

The derivatives of PSFs possess excellent dielectric properties useful for numerous applications [8,9], such as membranes (hemodialysis, gas separation, etc.), medical accessories (surgical trays, nebulizers, humidifiers, etc.), plumbing (hot-water fittings, manifolds, mixer-tap cartridges, etc.), and in automotives, electrical, electronic, and medical applications, because of their excellent mechanical properties and radiation resistance. Heat stability of PSFs is also quite high, compared to that of other polymeric materials. Because of its excellent electrical properties, PSF is also used as a dielectric element in capacitors.

On the other hand, conformational sampling, necessary to efficiently explore the structure (properties correlation), can be performed by simulation methods using a professional software. It is worth remembering that in relation with the Nobel Prize in chemistry, awarded in 2013 to Kaplus, M., Levitt, M., and Warshel, A. for their activities in the simulation of chemical reactions—*Development of Multiscales for Complex Chemical Systems* [74], special stress has been placed on the new investigations the winners developed on chemical configuration—for elucidating the specific properties of materials by combining quantum and classical mechanics.

Frequently, for understanding the phenomena that determine certain properties and spatial molecular conformations, energy evaluations should be performed. Thus, the HyperChem 8.07 professional program, using the molecular mechanics (MM+) force field approximation method with the Polak-Ribiere algorithm for conjugate gradient, represents a useful computational graphic program that allows rapid structural and geometrical optimizations and molecular display [75,76]. Molecular dynamic is used to calculate the potential, kinetic, and total energy at a temperature over 0K. In addition, the molecular dynamics technique, a powerful method for the evaluation of energy barriers among different stable or metastable conformations, has been proposed in different studies, as it allows a subsequent variation of the geometry. Conformational changes in polymers depend upon their rotation around single bonds. As a consequence of the chemical structure, the torsion angle, Φ, along the linkages between different substructures expresses the main degree of freedom that describes the general shape of polymers. For each of the thus generated conformations, energy must be minimized, whereas the structure can be geometrically optimized with a professional program. In some works [62,63,77–79] on PSF compounds, spatial molecular conformations and energy evaluations were performed with a professional program. Practically, optimized characteristics for adjusting rigidity and flexibility could be achieved by the structural modification of PSFs.

Computational evaluation of some polysulfonic structures, for example, of chelating PSFs containing quaternary and reactive ketone units (KQPSF), and of chelate-modified PSFs with Cu^{2+}-containing quaternary and chelate units (KQPSFCu) (Scheme 6.1) [77,79], showed that the addition of a transient Cu^{2+} cation to the polymer modifies the strength of some bonds among the host polymer atoms. Evaluation of the intensity of certain bonds could demonstrate how the carried metal cation is bound to the structure and is distributed among the polymeric chains. To assess the effect of the metal on the formation of the complex between the carbonyl groups and the free Cu^{2+} cations, the strength of the carbonyl bond can be evaluated.

In addition, the presence of transient metal ions in polysulfonic films affects its properties in two distinct ways: on the one hand, the complex structure between metal cations and electron donor groups of the polymer chains leads to cross-linking formations, decreasing chain mobility and increasing glass transition temperature; on the other hand, the predominant effect is generated by the complexes distributed inside the polymer matrices, which disrupts the uniformity of polymer chains and decrease the glass transition temperature. Therefore, the glass transition temperature is an important factor in interpreting the structure–property relationship, a high value being associated with a high rigidity.

The energies calculated from the computational evaluation energies corresponding to the repeating units (kcal mol^{-1}) of the polymers [e.g., the potential energies at 0K and 300K (E_{pot}^0 and E_{pot}^{300}, respectively), the kinetic energies at 300K ($E_{kinetic}^{300}$), and total energies at 300K (E_{tot}^{300})] detect, on the one hand, the rigidity of structure and, on the other hand, the steric hindrance induced by different structural groups—for example, the SO_2-, which increases the free volume of PSF chain and generates different limited motions, such as phenyl ring oscillations. Therefore, different structural features significantly influence the macromolecular conformation and physicochemical properties of polymers.

6.4.2 AC-Dielectric Measurements at Different Frequency and Temperature Values

The relationships between the structure and the molecular mobility in modified PSFs, which motivate changes in dielectric permittivity, dielectric loss, and conductivity at different frequencies and temperatures, are presented in the literature using dielectric spectroscopy [4,61,62,79]. Generally, dielectric permittivities decrease with increasing frequency and increase with temperature, being influenced by the total polarization arising from dipoles orientation, and also by trapped charge carriers. These aspects are presented as follows:

- In Figure 6.4, for quaternized PSFs with *N*-dimethylethylammonium chloride (PSF-DMEA) or *N*-dimethyloctylammonium chloride pendant groups (PSF-DMOA) [4]
- In Figure 6.5, for phosphorus-modified PSFs with different substitution degrees (PSF-DOPO-1, PSF-DOPO-2) [61] and quaternized PSFs with triphenylphosphonium pendant groups (PSFP) [62]

The interval of variation with frequency at different temperatures becomes narrower for some modified PSFs, such as chelated PSFs with metal ions (Figure 6.6 [79]), as well

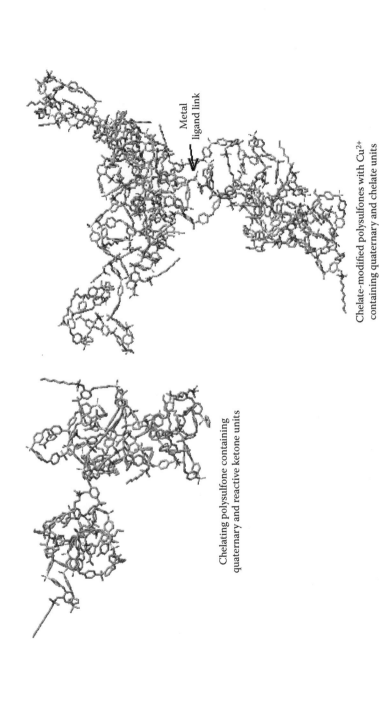

SCHEME 6.1 Conformational structures with minimized energies, considering five repeating units of chelating polysulfone containing quaternary and chelate-modified polysulfones with Cu^{2+} containing quaternary and chelate units. (Data from Albu, R. M. et al., *Polym. Compos.*, 33(4), 573–581, 2012; Albu, R. M., *J. Solid State Electrochem.*, 18(3), 785–794, 2014.)

Chelating polysulfone containing quaternary and reactive ketone units

Chelate-modified polysulfones with Cu^{2+} containing quaternary and chelate units

Metal ligand link

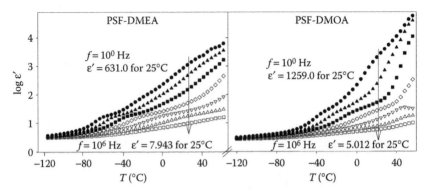

FIGURE 6.4 Logarithmic plot of dielectric permittivity versus temperature at different frequencies, for PSF-DMEA and PSF-DMOA quaternized polysulfones. (Data from Albu, R. M. et al., *High Perform. Polym.*, 23, 85–89, 2011.)

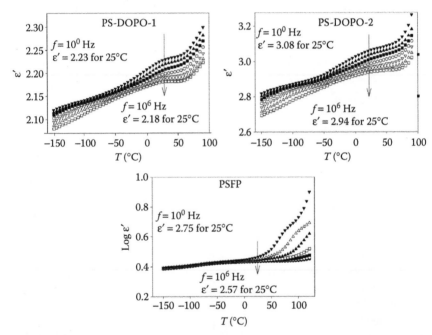

FIGURE 6.5 Dielectric permittivity plot for PS-DOPO-1 and PS-DOPO-2 and logarithmic plot of dielectric permittivity for PSFP, versus temperature at different frequencies. (Data from Ioan, S. et al., *J. Macromol. Sci. Part B Phys.*, 50(8), 1571–1590, 2011; Buruiana, L. I. et al., *Polym. Bull.*, 68, 1641–1661, 2012.)

as for phosphorus-modified PSFs with different substitution degrees (Figure 6.5), whose complex structures induce cumulative effects.

The rapid increase of dielectric permittivity at higher temperatures for the exemplified PSFs was attributed to increased chaotic thermal oscillations of molecules and to the diminishing order degree of dipoles orientation, near the glass transition temperature. In this context, one can assert that dielectric permittivity depends on

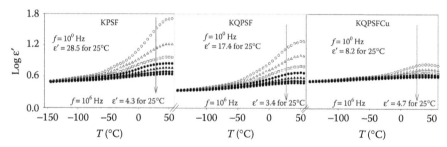

FIGURE 6.6 Logarithmic plot of dielectric permittivity for chelating polysulfone containing ketone units, KPSF, chelating polysulfone containing 60% quaternary and 40% reactive ketone units, KQPSF, and chelate-modified polysulfones containing quaternary and chelate units, KQPSFCu, versus temperature at different frequencies. (Data from Kaplus, M. et al., *Development of Multiscales for Complex Chemical Systems*, The Royal Swedish Academy of Science, Stockholm, Sweden, 2013.)

the complex chemical structures of the modified PSFs. Thus, Figures 6.4 and 6.6 show that, at 25°C, dielectric permittivity takes the following values:

- Between 1259.0 and 5.012, over the same frequency range, for quaternized PSFs with N,N-dimethyloctylamine (PSF-DMOA) pendant groups [4]—outside the reactive ketone units
- Between 28.5 and 4.3, 17.4 and 3.4, and 8.2 and 4.7, over the 10^0–10^6 Hz frequency interval, for chelating PSFs containing ketone units (KPSF), chelating PSFs containing quaternary and reactive ketone units (KQPSF), and chelate-modified PSFs with Cu^{2+}-containing quaternary and chelate units (KQPSFCu) [79]

The high permittivity values are caused by hopping polarization, which represents a migration of electric charges leaving an opposite electric charge behind, as well as by the interfacial polarization induced by the accumulation of free charges at interfaces with different electrical characteristics, such as the electrode–polymer one [80]. On the other hand, the presence of N,N-dimethyloctylamine pendant groups with higher molecular flexibility and mobility determines an increase of electronic conjugation in quaternized PSFs main chain and a higher value of permittivity, comparatively with the more bulky reactive ketone pendant groups from KPSF. In KQPSF, the cumulative effect of both pendant groups reduces permittivity even more. A higher interval of permittivity appears in the 10^0–10^6 Hz range for KPSF, its narrowing being observed for KQPSF (where the reactive ketone side groups alternate with the ammonium quaternary side groups), and especially for KQPSFCu, where retention of copper ions led to the formation of complex structures [79].

6.4.3 INFLUENCE OF FREQUENCY AND TEMPERATURE ON DIELECTRIC LOSS

Structural relaxation phenomena and electrical conduction mechanisms are topics of special theoretical and applicative interest. These phenomena are difficult to describe, considering the complex structure in which the mobile particles diffuse and the effects of the interaction and correlation between different substructures during the transport process. In this context, the α-relaxation process characterizes the structural relaxation and determines the long time behavior of any correlation function, its detection by dielectric spectroscopy being assured by the large accessibility of the frequency domain. At lowest frequencies, the main relaxation process gives rise to a peak characterized by a time constant, τ_α, with a non-Arrhenius temperature dependence, and by the cooperativity of molecular motion—with typical correlation lengths (not exceeding a few nanometers).

While the α-relaxation process is the most discussed relaxation phenomenon related to the physics of glass transition, secondary β- and γ-processes, appear for dielectrically active molecules possessing an internal degree of freedom. The β-process can be observed as a peak in the dielectric spectrum at frequencies higher than those of the α-process, displaying a symmetrical DS peak and being thermally activated—with an activation energy proportional with T_g (with some exceptions), according to the following correlation: $E_\beta = 24T_g$. For several substances, it is reported that, above T_g, the temperature dependence of the time constants for the β-process may differ from the sub-T_g Arrhenius behavior, whereas, above T_g, the dielectric relaxation strength of the β-process strongly decreases with cooling, remaining essentially constant below. In order to explain the molecular origin of the secondary process, Johari and Goldstein introduced the idea of islands of mobility, in which the islands are believed to survive in the glassy state and contain a certain amount of molecules with a considerably higher mobility than that of the environment [81].

Generally, the literature shows that polymer films, characterized by three transition temperatures—α-transition temperature related to the glass transition temperature, and to γ- and β-processes—are initiated by localized motions of atomic groups or molecular segments [63,80]. The local regions containing the smallest group capable of reorientation should produce the γ-relaxation peak, whereas those containing larger groups should produce the β-relaxation peak.

Modified PSF structures can have a cumulative polarization degree, caused by the polar structure of the backbone chains and by the existence of a number of polar side groups. Moreover, these polymers show additional polarity, induced by the polar sulfone linkages from the backbone chain. The small segments easily absorb water from the atmosphere prior to experimental evaluations, thus influencing the dielectric measurements (carried out in nitrogen atmosphere). In addition, for pure PSF films, only two transition temperatures, β and α, are observed:

1. The β-transition appears at approximately 75°C, as a result of the micro-Brownian motion of the main chain segments—due to the flexibility of their molecules.
2. The α-transition appears at 197°C, induced by a rotatory diffusional motion of the molecules from one quasi-stable position to another one, around the skeletal bond, involving large-scale conformational rearrangement of the main chain [9]. In modified PSFs (as illustrated in Figure 6.7 for quaternized PSFs with *N*-dimethylethylammonium chloride and *N*-dimethyloctylammonium chloride pendant groups, and Figure 6.8 for phosphorus-modified PSFs

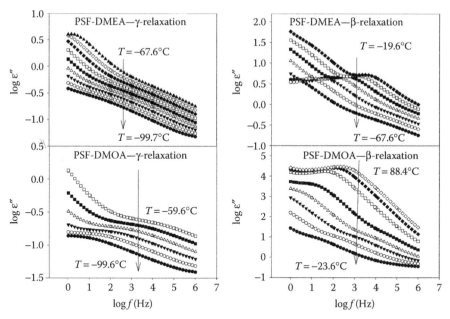

FIGURE 6.7 Dielectric loss versus frequency for PSF-DMEA and PSF-DMOA in the frequency domain of γ- and β-relaxations. (Data from Albu, R. M. et al., *High Perform. Polym.*, 23, 85–89, 2011.)

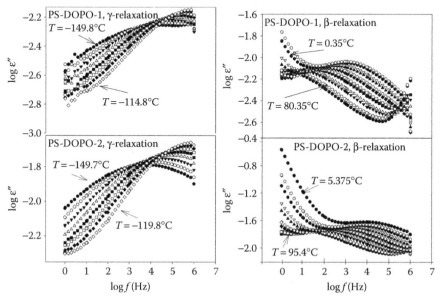

FIGURE 6.8 Dielectric loss versus frequency for PS-DOPO-1 and PS-DOPO-2 in the frequency domain of γ- and β-relaxations. (Data from Ioan, S. et al., *J. Macromol. Sci. Part B Phys.*, 50, 1571–1590, 2011.)

with different substitution degree, respectively), the conformational rearrangement of the main chains is restricted to the introduction of pendant groups in the side chains. In addition, the thermal decomposition temperature of quaternized PSFs does not exceed 170°C–200°C, whereas those of PSFs are around 400°C [82]. In these conditions, no α-dipole relaxation associated to glassy transition occurs, whereas the tri-dimensional variation of dielectric loss, ε'', with frequency and temperature, for the PSFs exemplified in Figures 6.7 and 6.8, reveals only two types of relaxations, γ and β. The measured dielectric loss spectrum includes contributions from dipolar orientation, diffusion of charge carrier and, in some cases, from interfacial polarization [83,84].

The β-relaxation, occurring at higher temperatures for different frequencies, is sometimes difficult to be evidenced, being masked by the conduction of the charged carrier. This statement comes from the literature data [79,85] that specify that dielectric processes are characterized by the superposition of two contributions: a conductivity contribution, which increases both the real, ε', and imaginary part, ε'', of the dielectric function, on decreasing frequency, and a relaxation process exhibiting a maximum in ε'' (which shifts to higher frequency with increasing temperature).

Detailed spectra of dielectric loss versus frequency and temperature and those occurring in the frequency domains of γ- and β-relaxations are plotted in Figures 6.9 through 6.11 for PSFs containing chelating groups, quaternized PSFs containing 60% quaternary and 40% reactive ketone units, and complex structures of chelate-modified PSFs with Cu^{2+}, respectively. A statistical correlation showed that the γ-relaxation temperature is dependent on microstructural characteristics, such as interchain distance and fractional free volume. In this context:

- Chelating PSFs containing ketone units and chelating PSFs containing quaternary and reactive ketone units show no crystallinity, which can be possibly explained by their bulky, nonsymmetrical, and flexible structure. The combined features, responsible for the disturbance of chain packing, are decisive for the amorphous character of these samples.
- In the complex structures of chelate-modified PSFs with Cu^{2+} containing quaternary and chelate units, the noncoplanar orientation of chains and their geometrical constraints induce lower interchain distances and a higher free volume [86], while speeding up segmental motion.

Thus, the experimental data evidenced a γ-transition temperature lower for KQPSFCu, than for KPSF and KQPSF.

6.4.4 Enthalpic and Entropic Contributions of Activation Energy on γ- and β-Relaxation Processes

Considering that the strength and the frequency of relaxation depend on the characteristic properties of dipolar and ionic relaxation, dielectric spectroscopy can also provide some information on the modification of local relaxation [87]. The relaxation

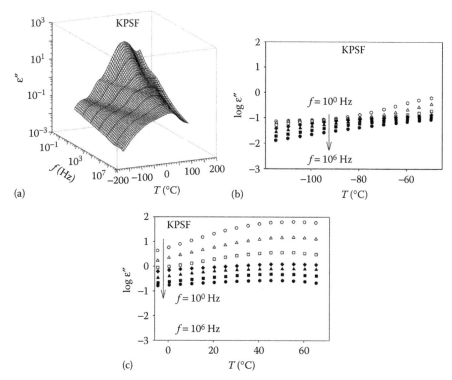

FIGURE 6.9 3D images of dielectric loss versus frequency and temperature (a) and dielectric loss versus temperature of γ-relaxation (b) and β-relaxation (c) domains for chelating polysulfones containing ketone units, KPSF. (Data from Kaplus, M. et al., *Development of Multiscales for Complex Chemical Systems*, The Royal Swedish Academy of Science, Stockholm, Sweden, 2013.)

phenomena described according to HN relationship, Equation 6.34 (see also Equation 6.13) consists of three terms: the first part, on the right side of the equation, describes conductivity, whereas the other two terms refer to the dipole contribution to the $\varepsilon^*(\omega)$ function:

$$\varepsilon^*(\omega) = \varepsilon' - i\varepsilon'' = -i\left(\frac{\sigma_{DC}}{\varepsilon_0\omega}\right)^n + \varepsilon_U + \frac{\varepsilon_R - \varepsilon_U}{\left[1 + (i\omega\tau_{HN})^a\right]^b} \tag{6.34}$$

where:

σ_{DC} is the DC conductivity

ε_0 is the vacuum permittivity

$\Delta\varepsilon = \varepsilon_R - \varepsilon_U$ is the dielectric strength

ε_R and ε_U are the relaxed ($\omega \to 0$) and unrelaxed ($\omega \to \infty$) values, respectively, of the permittivity for each relaxation phenomenon

$\omega = 2\pi f$ is the frequency

τ_{HN} is the relaxation time for each process

a and b are the broadening and skewing parameters, respectively

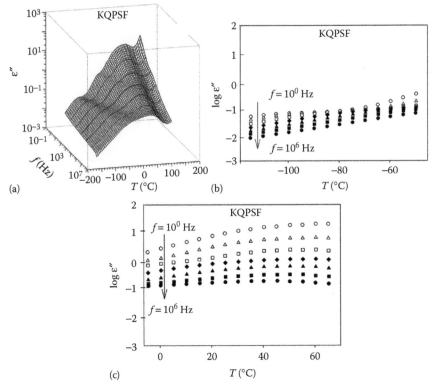

(a)

(b)

(c)

FIGURE 6.10 3D images of dielectric loss versus frequency and temperature (a) and dielectric loss versus temperature of γ-relaxation (b) and β-relaxation (c) domains for chelating polysulfones containing 60% quaternary and 40% reactive ketone units, KQPSF. (Data from Kaplus, M. et al., *Development of Multiscales for Complex Chemical Systems*, The Royal Swedish Academy of Science, Stockholm, Sweden, 2013.)

Thus,

- For $a \ll 1$, the distribution of the relaxation time is broader [88].
- For $b = 1$ or $b < 1$, the dielectric dispersion is either symmetrical or asymmetrical.

Contributions of relaxation and conduction phenomenon are exemplified in Figure 6.12 from the frequency dependence of dielectric loss for chelating PSFs containing ketone units at $-85.15°C$, calculated with Equation 6.34.

Figure 6.12 evidences the deconvolution of the two processes, observed by the fitting technique, which enables the separation of conductivity contributions from the relaxation processes. The circle symbols show the real part of the dielectric loss.

The relaxation time, τ_{max}, associated with the maximum peak of dielectric loss, is derived from the HN relaxation time, τ_{HN}, at each temperature, according to expression:

$$\tau_{max} = \tau_{HN} \left\{ \frac{\sin\left[\pi\, ab/(2+2b)\right]}{\sin\left[\pi\, a/(2+2b)\right]} \right\}^{1/a} \qquad (6.35)$$

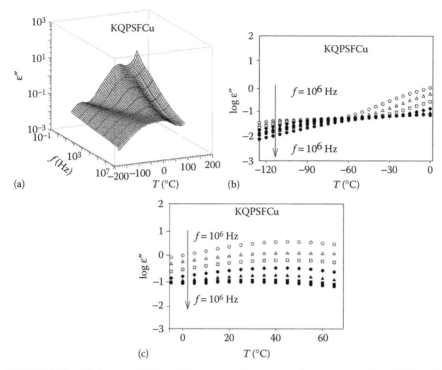

FIGURE 6.11 3D images of dielectric loss versus frequency and temperature (a) and dielectric loss versus temperature of γ-relaxation (b) and β-relaxation (c) domains for chelate-modified polysulfones with Cu^{2+} containing quaternary and chelate units, KQPSFCu. (Data from Kaplus, M. et al., *Development of Multiscales for Complex Chemical Systems*, The Royal Swedish Academy of Science, Stockholm, Sweden, 2013.)

The activation energies for γ- and β-relaxations can be evaluated from the relaxation time for γ- and β-relaxation, τ_{max} (resulting from HN curve fits, correlated with the maximum frequency for dielectric relaxation by the $f_{max} = (2\pi\tau_{max})^{-1}$ dependence) versus the reciprocal temperature (Arrhenius plots), according to Equation 6.36:

$$\tau = \tau_0 \exp\left[\frac{E}{RT}\right] \tag{6.36}$$

where:

E expresses the apparent activation energies

τ_0 is the preexponential factor of the τ_γ relaxation times corresponding to γ- and β-relaxations

Information about the nature of the motions involved in relaxation processes is provided by the preexponential and apparent activation energy parameters. Thus, for the exemplified PSFs (KPSF, KQPSF, and KQPSFCu) [79] and for the

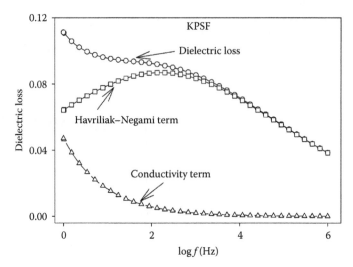

FIGURE 6.12 Dielectric loss versus frequency logarithm for chelating polysulfones containing ketone units, KPSF, at −85.15°C. (Data from Kaplus, M. et al., *Development of Multiscales for Complex Chemical Systems*, The Royal Swedish Academy of Science, Stockholm, Sweden, 2013.)

quaternized PSFs (PSF-DMEA and PSF-DMOA) [4], the following conclusions have been reached:

- The E_γ activation energies have approximately the same low value.
- $\tau_{0\gamma}$ is close to the Debye time, $\tau_D = 10^{-13} \cdot s \ (= 2\pi h/kT$ at room temperature).
- The motions that are associated with γ-relaxation process are considered as localized and noncooperative.
- The intensities of γ-relaxation, $\Delta\varepsilon = \varepsilon_R - \varepsilon_U$, have constant values versus temperature, whereas the chelate-modified PSFs showed lower intensity values. Consequently, the net dipolar moments per volume unity for KPSF and KQPSF are higher than that for KQPSFCu, which means that, for the last sample, polarization is limited mainly by elastic constraints than by thermal agitation [71,88].

In the subglass relaxation domain, the activation energy associated with each relaxation type is related to the relaxation temperature and to its corresponding activation entropy at a frequency of 1 Hz, as expressed by Equation 6.37 [89]:

$$E = RT\left[1 + \ln\left(\frac{kT}{2\pi hf}\right)\right] + T\Delta S \tag{6.37}$$

The first term in this equation expresses the enthalpy contribution of the activation energy with k—Boltzmann constant, h—Planck constant, and T—absolute temperature, whereas the second term, ΔS, represents the entropy contribution of the activation energy of a thermoactivated motion. In this respect, the following observations should be had in view:

- When the activation energy varies linearly with temperature, entropy contribution can be negligible for the limiting low temperature at a given frequency of γ-relaxation, whereas the activation energy is essentially due to an enthalpy contribution.
- β-relaxations are considered to correspond mainly to charge carrier diffusion rather than to dipole-segmental motions. In this context, as already mentioned, the average apparent activation energies for β-relaxations are difficult to separate from the conduction process.

Important phenomena have been explored in different mixtures of PSFs by Saxeba et al. [90]. For example, AC dielectric properties of polyvinylidenefluoride (PVDF)/ PSF blends have been studied to elucidate their molecular motion and relaxation behavior in the frequency range of 100–10000 Hz, at different temperatures (ranging between 30°C and 190°C). The conclusions of these investigations show the following:

- The dielectric permittivity of blends decreased with frequency (due to orientation polarization) and increased with increasing temperature and the PSF content (due to an extended movement of blend's molecular chain at high temperature), a behavior agreeing with the dielectric response of a polar dielectric element.
- The dielectric loss also increased with the increase in temperature and PSF content. The observed characteristics have been consistently explained in terms of dipolar motions and plasticization effect of blends.
- At constant frequency and temperature, the blend establishes a linear relationship between the logarithm of its dielectric constant and different blend ratios.
- The appearance of a peak in the dielectric loss for each concentration suggests the presence of relaxing dipoles in the blend. Increasing of the PSF content determines peak displacement toward higher frequency, which suggests speeding up of the relaxation process.

6.5   AC CONDUCTIVITY

To analyze ionic conductivities by associating a conductivity relaxation time with the ionic process [84], conductivity behavior in the frequency domain is more conveniently interpreted in terms of conductivity relaxation time, τ, using the representation of electrical modulus, $M*$:

$$M* = \frac{1}{\varepsilon *} = M' + iM'' \qquad (6.38)$$

where:

$M' = \dfrac{\varepsilon'}{\varepsilon'^2 + \varepsilon''^2}$ and $M'' = \dfrac{\varepsilon''}{\varepsilon'^2 + \varepsilon''^2}$ represent the real and imaginary parts, respectively

Figures 6.13 and 6.14 illustrate the opportunities of discussing the specific aspects of the interested structures, reflected in conductivity parameters. In this context, graphical representation of M' and M'' versus frequency and temperature for some modified PSFs (Figure 6.13) shows the following:

- At low frequencies, the real part of the modulus approaches zero, indicating that the electrode polarization phenomenon makes a negligible contribution.
- M' represents the ability of the material to store the energy, in the same way as the absence of peak in relation with its dependence on frequency is a consequence of the fact that, in the complex electric modulus ($M*$), M' is equivalent to ε' in complex permittivity ($\varepsilon*$).
- The presence of a peak in the imaginary modulus formalism (M'') at higher frequency suggests ionic conduction in the structure of the studied samples. As temperature increases, peak's maximum shifts to higher frequencies, indicating that the conductivity of the charge carrier has been thermally activated.

The formation of peaks is clearly visible in Figure 6.14 for the imaginary component of the modulus:

- At low frequencies, M'' exhibits low value, which can be caused by a high capacitance value, associated with the electrode polarization effect [91,92] (as a result of the accumulation of charge carriers at the electrode–solid polymer electrolyte interface).
- At high frequencies, well-defined peaks are observed, indicating the relaxation phenomenon of electrical conductivity, dependent on temperature; at higher frequencies, peaks are shifted with increasing temperature, the amplitude remaining almost constant.

For chelate-modified PSFs with Cu^{2+} containing quaternary and chelate units, the peak occurs at temperatures over 100°C, which is not shown in Figure 6.14. In addition, for these samples, electrode polarization is not significant, as in the case of KPSF and KQPSF samples; therefore, M'' does not tend to zero at low frequencies.

The conductivity, $\sigma(f)$, of many materials, particularly of the amorphous ones, is expressed by Equation 6.39 [63,93–95]:

$$\sigma(f) = \sigma_{DC} + Af^n \qquad (6.39)$$

where:
σ_{DC} is the DC conductivity
A is the preexponential factor
n is the fractional exponent, ranging between 0 and 1

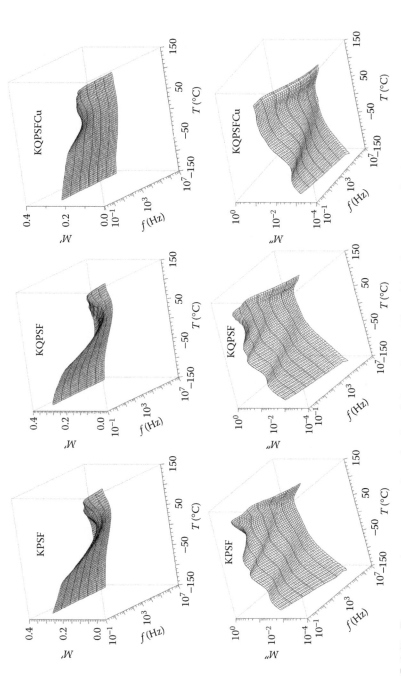

FIGURE 6.13 Frequency and temperature dependencies of the real part, M', and imaginary part, M'', of the dielectric modulus for chelating polysulfones containing ketone units, KPSF, chelating polysulfone containing 60% quaternary and 40% reactive ketone units, KQPSF, and chelate-modified polysulfones with Cu^{2+} containing quaternary and chelate units, KQPSFCu, films.

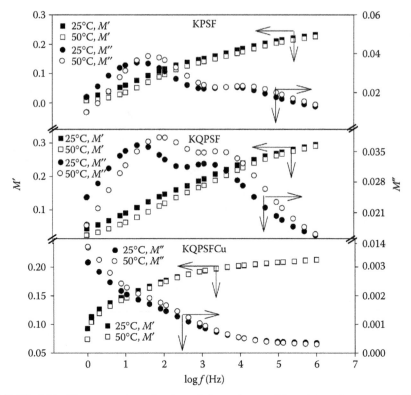

FIGURE 6.14 Frequency dependencies of the real part, M', and imaginary part, M'', of the dielectric modulus for chelating polysulfones containing ketone units, KPSF, chelating polysulfone containing 60% quaternary and 40% reactive ketone units, KQPSF, and chelate-modified polysulfones with Cu^{2+} containing quaternary and chelate units, KQPSFCu, films, at 25°C and 50°C.

The graphical representation of conductivity versus frequency and temperature (Figure 6.15) allows the interpretation and discussion of the parameters from Equation 6.39, as follows:

- Exponent n, calculated from the frequency-dependent conductivity, decreases for all samples with increasing temperature and the frequency domain, being generally < 1.
- Value n, in the region of higher frequency, characterizes electronic conduction via a hopping process [96,97]. The hopping-type conduction manifested as the increase of conductivity at higher frequency takes place at temperatures above the glass transition temperature, through hopping conduction.
- The plateau region of conductivity corresponds to the DC conductivity.
- At high temperatures, AC conductivity is nearly independent on frequency over the low-frequency domain. At these temperatures, the dielectric behavior is less visible, because charge carriers become mobile over large

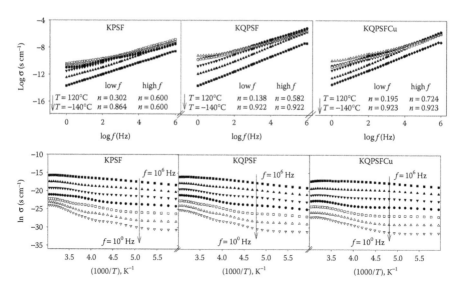

FIGURE 6.15 Electrical conductivity versus frequency and temperature for chelating polysulfones containing ketone units, KPSF, chelating polysulfone containing 60% quaternary and 40% reactive ketone units, KQPSF, and chelate-modified polysulfones with Cu^{2+} containing quaternary and chelate units, KQPSFCu, films.

distances, and a continuous connected network, which permits electric conduction, is formed.

- Deviations from linearity at higher frequencies may be due to the dispersion of charge carriers, produced by dipolar relaxation.

Literature shows that the thermal activation energy of the AC conductivity at different frequency values is evaluated with Equation 6.39 [98,99]:

$$\sigma = \sigma_0 \exp\left(-\frac{E_\sigma}{kT}\right) \tag{6.40}$$

where:
E_σ denotes the thermal activation energy of the electrical conduction
σ_0 is a parameter depending on the polymer nature
$k = 8.617343 \cdot 10^{-5}$ eV K^{-1} is Boltzmann's constant
T represents absolute temperature

The conductivity spectra reported in the literature for PSF complex structures indicate the following [4,61,62,79]:

- The higher slopes obtained from the graphical representation of Equation 6.40 (also Figure 6.15) correspond to the intrinsic electrical conduction.
- The decreasing slopes at lower temperatures indicate a reduction in the impurity concentration of samples [100].

- The activation energy values of the AC conductivity lower than 1 eV can be explained in terms of a band conduction mechanism through a bandgap representation.
- The lower values of activation energy for chelated quaternized PSFs with Cu^{2+} reflect the mobility enhancement of the charge carrier upon complexation.

The optical bandgap energies, E_G, presented in Figure 6.3 are different from those obtained from the values of thermal activation energy of the AC electrical conduction, E_σ. Consequently, electrical conductivity, E_σ, is explained in terms of a band conduction mechanism, through a bandgap representation. On the other hand, considering that light emission in the semiconductor is a photon-creating process, by the annihilation of an electron-hole pair, the gap energy obtained from optical measurements should be higher than the E_G value indicated by conductivity analysis. The values of gap energy evaluated by the Tauc law (E_G) are related to the gap energy values obtained from the conductivity spectrum (E_σ) by $E_G = 2E_a$ equality [70], both processes being attributed to the hopping mechanism characteristic to semiconductor materials. Consequently, the differences observed between optical and electrical gap energy are explained, assuming that the bandgap optical energy of the system is related to the photon energy intensity in the photoluminescence spectra, and that the bandgap electrical energy is an effect of the relaxation process appearing when modifying temperature.

6.6   IMPEDANCE SPECTROSCOPY

Impedance spectroscopy is an AC technique for electrical and interface characterization of materials, based on impedance measurements over a wide frequency range (10^{-6}–10^9 Hz). From these measurements, a direct correlation between the response of a real system and an idealized model circuit composed of electrical components may be established.

Generally, for a system perturbed by a sine-wave input voltage (Equation 6.41), current intensity is also sine wave (Equation 6.42) [101]:

$$v(T) = V_0 \sin \omega t \tag{6.41}$$

$$i(T) = i_0 \sin(\omega T + \phi) \tag{6.42}$$

where:
  Subscript "0" represents the maximum value of voltage and intensity
  ω is the angular frequency
  ϕ is the phase angle

Thus, the admittance function is defined by Equation 6.43 and the impedance functions are defined by Equations 6.44 and 6.45, with the real and imaginary parts expressed by Equations 6.46 and 6.47:

$$Y*(\omega) = \left| Y(\omega)e^{j\phi} \right| \tag{6.43}$$

$$Z^*(\omega) = [Y^*(\omega)]^{-1} \tag{6.44}$$

$$\frac{1}{Z^*(\omega)} = \left(\frac{1}{R}\right) + (j\omega C) \tag{6.45}$$

where:

Resistance R is the dissipative component of the dielectric response

Capacitance C is the storage component of the material

$$Z_{real} = \left\{ \frac{R}{\left[1+(\omega RC)^2\right]} \right\} \tag{6.46}$$

$$Z_{img} = \left\{ \frac{-\omega R^2 C}{\left[1+(\omega RC)^2\right]} \right\} \tag{6.47}$$

In the Nyquist plot, $-Z_{img}$ is represented versus Z_{real}, where, for a parallel (RC) circuit, $Z^*(\omega)$ is represented by a semicircle, which:

- Intercepts the Z_{real}-axis at R_∞ and R_0 for $\omega \to \infty$ and $\omega \to 0$, respectively
- Records a maximum at $0.5(R_0 - R_\infty)$, occurring at a frequency where $\omega RC = 1$, RC being the τ relaxation time

In the Bode plot, $-Z_{img}$ represented versus frequency allows the evaluation of the frequency interval associated with each relaxation process.

For heterogeneous systems composed of several subsystems with different dielectric properties, different semicircles exist, associated with different relaxation processes; therefore, impedance is expressed by Equation 6.48:

$$Q(\omega)^* = Y_0(j\omega)^{-n} \tag{6.48}$$

where:

Admittance $Y_0 = R_0\tau_0^{-n}$ is a real parameter $(0 \le n \le 1)$

Thus, the distribution of the relaxation times and the resulting plot appears as a depressed semicircle, which requires the interpretation of system inhomogeneities through the following:

- A nonideal capacitor or a constant phase element. In these situations, an equivalent capacitance $C^{eq} = (RY_0)^{1/n}/R$ can be considered.
- A plane capacitor for the dense active sublayer of composite membranes is expressed by Equation 6.49:

$$C = \varepsilon_0\varepsilon_r S/\Delta x_m \tag{6.49}$$

where:

ε_0 and ε_r represent the permittivity of vacuum and the relative dielectric constant, respectively

S and Δx_m represent membrane surface and thickness, respectively

The impedance plots provide information about the different sublayers of heterogeneous systems, such as those formed by membrane/electrolyte solutions.

Performances of PSF membranes for different applications involve the evaluation of the changes observed in their electrical resistance, through impedance spectroscopy. Benavente et al. [101] described the changes in the electrical resistance of composite membranes having asymmetric sulfonated PSF membranes as support layer. The skin layer of membranes contains different ratios of polyethylene glycol in the casting solution, while lignosulfonate was used for manufacturing membranes. Measurements were carried out on membranes in contact with NaCl solutions at different concentrations. The thus determined electrical resistance and equivalent capacitance values show a clear decrease in the membrane electrical resistance, as a result of both PSF sulfonation and increased concentration of the modifying substances, although a concentration limit was established for both polyethylene glycol and lignosulfonate, whereas the dielectric constant value (hydrated state) clearly increased.

In the same context, the electrical properties of dense membranes based on three samples of sulfonated PSFs of different sulfonation degrees were characterized spectroscopically, by their inherent viscosity and water absorption [102]. Electrical characterization of membranes was carried out on dense membranes in contact with NaCl solutions, by impedance spectroscopy measurements using equivalent circuits as models. Literature shows that sulfonation process affects the membrane electrical characteristics by modifying concentration, reducing membrane resistance, and changing the type of circuit associated with the membrane—which can be related to the increase of the amount of electrolyte taken over by the membrane when the sulfonation degree increases. The electrical and electrochemical properties of sulfonated poly(ether ether sulfone) membranes with different sulfonation degrees (0%, 5%, and 10%) were determined in another investigation, by measuring the electrical resistance and concentration potential with the membranes in contact with HCl solutions of different concentrations [103]. Impedance spectroscopy used to determine membrane resistance using equivalent circuits as models led to the conclusion, that the sulfonation affects the electrical characteristics of the membranes.

In addition, the transport properties of polymer blend membranes of sulfonated and nonsulfonated PSFs (for direct methanol fuel cell applications) with various morphologies, induced by different drying conditions, were measured and analyzed on the basis of the absorbed water molecules [104]. AC-impedance spectroscopy used to measure proton conductivity allowed the design of a liquid permeability instrument to measure methanol permeability.

It should be noted that the cross-linking of sulfonated aromatic polymers is one of the ways used to reduce swelling at high proton conductivity. For this reason, Furtado Filho and Gomez [105] performed the radiation-induced cross-linking on a sulfonated PSF membrane, with doses ranging from 2.5 to 25.0 kGy (dose rate: 45 Gy min^{-1}), using gamma rays from a ^{60}Co source. The pristine sulfonated PSFs were obtained by a mild sulfonation of bisphenol-A-PSF with trimethylsilyl chlorosulfonate as a sulfonating agent. The proton conductivity of membranes, determined by electrical impedance spectroscopy techniques, showed that the mechanical, chemical, and thermal stability values of the membrane improved after irradiation, and that the degree of sulfonation and proton conductivity tended to decrease with increasing the total irradiation dose.

6.7   GENERAL REMARKS

An understanding of the charge transport mechanism in composite materials is important from both fundamental and technological viewpoints. Studies on the dielectric properties of some new systems are interesting for possible applications. Some described aspects concerning the charge transport and dipolar relaxations phenomena in a series of complex structures of modified PSFs can be investigated by broadband dielectric spectroscopy. A general observation is found that dielectric permittivity decreases with increasing frequency and increases with increasing temperature, being influenced by the total polarization arising from dipoles orientation and also by trapped charge carriers. The interval of variation with frequency at different temperatures becomes narrower for complex PSF structures—which can induce some cumulative effects. The γ- and β-relaxation effects observed in dielectric loss spectra are related to chain motions: γ-relaxation corresponds to the isolated motions occurring without cooperative contributions at low temperature, their main activation energy having an enthalpic character, symmetrical in the frequency domain, with the skewing parameter $b = 1$. The γ-transition temperature can be lower due to the steric hindrance effect induced by the different groups, which increases the free volume and facilitates different limited motions of polymer segments, comparatively with those of some simple structures. The entropy contribution, $T\Delta S$, for the β-process is not negligible, having a greater influence on the activation energy for more flexible polymers, and being characterized by a specific cooperation between the intramolecular and intermolecular contributions, in correlation with the chemical structure of samples. In some complex structures, for the β-process, which corresponds mainly to charge carrier diffusion than to dipole-segmental motions, the average apparent activation energies were difficult to separate from the conduction process. Thus, the dielectric processes occurring in the β-relaxation domain are characterized by the superposition of conductivity contribution with the relaxation process. Therefore, decoupling between conductivity and structural relaxation is possible only in the temperature range of γ-dielectric relaxation. On the other hand, as in the case of γ-transition, in the β-relaxation domain, a narrow distribution of dielectric loss versus temperature appears for complex PSF structures, involving a steady-state constant polarization produced by a field.

Stress should be laid on the fact that modification in the AC conductivity with temperature and frequency is dependent on the structural parameters of polymers. Representation of the electrical modulus shows the presence of a peak in the imaginary modulus formalism at higher frequency, suggesting that ionic conduction is predominant in the analyzed structure. The maximum peak shifts to higher frequencies as temperature increases, revealing that the conductivity of the charge carrier is thermally activated; at lower frequencies, the real and imaginary parts of the modulus approach zero, indicating a negligible contribution of the electrode polarization phenomenon. At the same time, it evidences that the values of thermal activation energy of electrical conduction, below 1, indicate a model of modified PSFs representation based on energy bandgap, and reflect an enhanced mobility of the charge carrier upon complexation structures.

In conclusion, this chapter summarizes the main aspects that correlate the structure of polysulfonic compounds with the phenomena occurring under the action of electrical fields at different frequencies and different temperatures. The examples provided allow the elucidation of the origin of the dielectric response and conductivity type in some functionalized PSFs. All discussed properties recommend these compounds (with typical behavior of semiconductor materials) as potential candidates for various applications in electrotechnical domains.

On the other hand, special interest is being manifested for the development of micro and nanotechnologies that contribute to creating miniaturized devices applied in medical fields [25,26,106]. In this respect, PSF materials, involving organic–inorganic composite materials with different mechanical and electrical properties [18,107] as well, offer exceptional opportunities to create unique properties in the bioindustry.

REFERENCES

1. Nagese, Y., Naruse, A., and Matsui, K., Chemical modification of polysulphone: 1. Synthesis of polysulphone/polydimethylsiloxane graft copolymer. *Polymer*, 30(10), 1931–1937, 1989.
2. Nagese, Y., Naruse, A., and Matsui, K., Chemical modification of polysulphone: 2. Gas and liquid permeability of polysulphone/polydimethylsiloxane graft copolymer membranes. *Polymer*, 31(1), 121–125, 1990.
3. Filimon, A., Avram, E., and Ioan, S., Influence of mixed solvents and of temperature on the solution properties of quaternized polysulfones. *J. Macromol. Sci. Part B Phys.*, 46(3), 503–520, 2007.
4. Albu, R. M., Avram, E., Musteata, V. E., Homocianu, M., and Ioan, S., Opto-electrical properties of some quaternized polysulfones. *High Perform. Polym.*, 23(1), 85–89, 2011.
5. Petreus, O., Avram, E., and Serbezeanu, D., Synthesis and characterization of phosphorus-containing polysulfone. *Polym. Eng. Sci.*, 50(1), 48–56, 2010.
6. Sheldon, J., The fine-structure of ultrafiltration membranes. I. Clean membranes. *J. Membr. Sci.*, 62(1), 75–86, 1991.
7. Summers, G. J., Ndawuni, M. P., and Summers, C. A., Dipyridyl functionalized polysulfones for membrane production. *J. Membrane Sci.*, 226(1,2), 21–33, 2003.
8. Cha, D. I., Kim, K. W., Chu, G. H., Kim, H. Y., Lee, K. H., and Bhattarai, N., Mechanical behaviors and characterization of electrospun polysulfone/polyurethane blend nonwovens. *Macromol. Res.*, 14(3), 331–337, 2006.
9. Saxena, P., Gaur, M. S., Shukla, P., and Khare, P. K., Relaxation investigation in polysulfone: Thermally stimulated discharge current and dielectric spectroscopy. *J. Electrostatics*, 66(11–12), 584–588, 2008.
10. Ioan, S., Filimon, A., and Avram, E., Influence of the degree of substitution on the solution properties of chloromethylated polysulfone. *J. Appl. Polym. Sci.*, 101(1), 524–531, 2006.
11. Ioan, S., Filimon, A., and Avram, E., Conformational and visometric behavior of quaternized polysulfone in dilute solution. *Polym. Eng. Sci.*, 46(7), 827–836, 2006.
12. Filimon, A., Albu, R. M., Avram, E., and Ioan, S., Effect of alkyl side chain on the conformational properties of polysulfones with quaternary groups. *J. Macromol. Sci. Part B Phys.*, 49(1), 207–217, 2010.

13. Guan, R., Zou, H., Lu, D., Gong, C., and Liu, Y., Polyethersulfone sulfonated by chlorosulfonic acid and its membrane characteristics. *Eur. Polym. J.*, 41(7), 1554–1560, 2005.

14. Yu, H., Huang, Y., Ying, H., and Xiao, C., Preparation and characterization of a quaternary ammonium derivative of konjac glucomannan. *Carbohydr. Polym.*, 69(1), 29–40, 2007.

15. Filimon, A., Avram, E., Dunca, S., Stoica, I., and Ioan, S., Surface properties and antibacterial activity of quaternized polysulfones. *J. Appl. Polym. Sci.*, 112(3), 1808–1816, 2009.

16. Idris, A. and Zain, N. M., Effect of heat treatment on the performance and structural details of polyethersulfone ultrafiltration membranes. *J. Technol.*, 44(F), 27–40, 2006.

17. Kochkodan, V., Tsarenko, S., Potapchenko, N., Kosinova, V., and Goncharuk, V., Adhesion of microorganisms to polymer membranes: A photobactericidal effect of surface treatment with TiO_2. *Desalination*, 220(1–3), 380–385, 2008.

18. Lukowska, E., Wojciechowski, C., and Chwojnowski, A., Dudzinski, K., Sabalinska, S., Ciechanowska, A., and Czapiewska, G., Preparation of sulfonated polysulfone membrane for enzymes immobilization. *Biocyber. Biomed. Eng.*, 32(2), 77–86, 2012.

19. Möckel, D., Staude, E., and Guiver, M. D., Static protein adsorption, ultrafiltration behavior and cleanability of hydrophilized polysulfone membranes. *J. Membr. Sci.*, 158(1/2), 63–75, 1999.

20. Genova-Dimitrova, P., Baradie, B., Foscallo, D., Poinsignon, C., and Sanchez, J. Y., Ionomeric membranes for proton exchange membrane fuel cell (PEMFC): Sulfonated polysulfone associated with phosphatoantimonic acid. *J. Membr. Sci.*, 185(1), 59–71, 2001.

21. Matsumoto, Y., Sudoh, M., and Suzuki, Y., Preparation of composite UF membranes of sulfonated polysulfone coated on ceramics. *J. Membr. Sci.*, 158(1/2), 55–62, 1999.

22. Zschocke, P. and Quellmalz, D., Novel ion exchange membranes based on an aromatic polyethersulfone. *J. Membr. Sci.*, 22(2/3), 325–332, 1985.

23. Rucka, M., Poźniak, G., Turkiewicz, B., and Trochimczuk, W., Ultrafiltration membranes from polysulfone/aminated polysulfone blends with proteolytic activity. *Enzyme Microb. Technol.*, 18(7), 477–481, 1996.

24. Nayak, L., Khastgir, D., and Chaki, T. K., Influence of carbon nanofibers reinforcement on thermal and electrical behavior of polysulfone nanocomposites, *Polym. Eng. Sci.*, 52(11), 2424–2434, 2012.

25. Bojorge Ramírez, N., Salgado, A. M., and Valdman, B., The evolution and developments of immunosensors for health and environmental monitoring: Problems and perspectives. *Braz. J. Chem. Eng.*, 26(2), 227–249, 2009.

26. Ordóñez, S. S. and Fàbregas, E., New antibodies immobilization system into a graphite-polysulfone membrane for amperometric immunosensors. *Biosens. Bioelectron.*, 22(6), 965–972, 2007.

27. Gainaru, C., Hecksher, T., Olsen, N. B., Böhmer, R., and Dyre, J. C., Shear and dielectric responses of propylene carbonate, tripropylene glycol, and a mixture of two secondary amides. *J. Chem. Phys.*, 137(6), 064508, 2012.

28. Bottchear, J. F. and Bordewijk, P., *Theory of Electric Polarization*, Vol. 2, second edition, Elsevier Science, Amsterdam, the Netherlands, 1992.

29. Havriliak, S. and Negami S., A complex plane analysis of α-dispersions in some polymer systems. *J. Polym. Sci. Part C Polym. Symposia*, 14(1), 99–117, 1966.

30. Cole, K. S. and Cole, R. H., Dispersion and absorption in dielectrics I. Alternating current characteristics. *J. Chem. Phys.*, 9(4), 341–351, 1941.

31. Davidson, D. W. and Cole, R. H., Dielectric relaxation in glycerol, propylene glycol, and n-propanol. *J. Chem. Phys.*, 19(12), 1484–1490, 1951.

32. Jonscher, A. K., *Universal Relaxation Law*. Chelsea Dielectric Press, London, UK, 1996.
33. Dasari, M. P., Sambasiva Rao, K., Murali Krishna, P., and Gopala Krishna, G., Barium strontium bismuth niobate layered perovskites: Dielectric, impedance and electrical modulus characteristics. *Acta Phys. Pol. A*, 119(3), 387–394, 2011.
34. Dyre, J. C. and Schrøder, T. B., Universality of AC-conduction in disordered solids. *Rev. Mod. Phys.*, 72(3), 873–892, 2000.
35. Cole, R. H., Dielectric polarization and relaxation, Molecular Liquids. *NATO ASI Series C*, 135, 59–110, 1984.
36. Khamzin, A. A., Nigmatullin, R, R., Popov, I. I., and Murzaliev, B. A., Microscopic model of dielectric α-relaxation in disordered media. *Fract. Calc. Appl. Anal.*, 16(1), 158–170, 2013.
37. Bottchear, J. F., *Theory of Electric Polarization*, Vol. 2, second edition, Elsevier Science, Amsterdam, the Netherlands, 1993.
38. Barthel, J., Buchner, R., and Wurm, B., The dynamics of liquid formamide, *N*-methylformamide, *N*,*N*-dimethylformamide, and *N*,*N*-dimethylacetamide. A dielectric relaxation study. *J. Mol. Liq.*, 98–99, 51–69, 2002.
39. Zhang, X. X., Liang, M., Hunger, J., Buchner, R., and Maroncelli, M., Dielectric relaxation and solvation dynamics in a prototypical ionic liquid + dipolar protic liquid mixture: 1-butyl-3-methylimidazolium tetrafluoroborate + water. *J. Phys. Chem. B.*, 117(49), 15356–15368, 2013.
40. Brand, R., Lunkenheimer, P., and Loidl, A., Relaxation dynamic in plastic crystals. *J. Chem. Phys.*, 116(23), 10386–10401, 2002.
41. Thomas, G., Fox, T.G., and Flory, P. J., The glass temperature and related properties of polystyrene. Influence of molecular weight. *J. Polym. Sci. Part A Polym. Chem.*, 14(75), 315–319, 1954.
42. Turnbull, D. and Cohen, M. H., Free-volume model of the amorphous glass transition. *J. Chem. Phys.*, 34(1), 120–125, 1961.
43. Stevenson, D. J. and Wolynes, P. G., A universal origin for secondary relaxations in supercooled liquids and structural glasses. *Nat. Phys.*, 6(1), 62–68, 2010.
44. Goedhart, D. J., Specific refractive index of segmented polyurethanes. *Proceedings of International GPC Seminar*. Monaco, Vol. 12, p. 2, 1969.
45. van Krevelen, D. W., *Properties of Polymers*. Elsevier, Amsterdam, the Netherlands, 1972.
46. Groh, W. and Zimmermann, A., What is the refractive index of an organic polymer? *Macromolecules*, 24(25), 6660–6663, 1991.
47. Huglin, M. B. In *Polymers Handbook*, J. Brandrup, Immergut E.H. Eds., New York, 1989, third Edition, 409–484.
48. Lorenz, L. V., Ueber die Refractionsconstante. *Wied. Ann. Phys.*, 11, 70–103, 1880.
49. Lorentz, H. A., Ueber die Beziehung zwischen der Fortpflanzungeschwindigkeit des Lightes und der Körperdichte. *Wied. Ann. Phys.*, 9, 641–665, 1880.
50. Gladstone, J. H. and Dale, T. P., On the influence of temperature on the refraction of light. *Phil. Trans. R. Soc. Lond.*, 148, 887–894, 1858.
51. Schultz, G., Wehrstedt, C., and Gnauck, R., Zur Bestimmung und Berechnung des Brechungsinkrements von Polyurethanen in Abhängigkeit von ihrer Struktur. *Plaste u Kautsch*, 32(4), 153–155, 1985.
52. Neumann, G. and Becker, M. Über die Schrumpfung bei harten Polyurethangießharzen. *Plaste u Kautsch*, 23, 26–31, 1976.
53. Ioan, S,. Filimon, A., and Avram, E., Influence of degree of substitution on the optical properties of chloromethylated polysulfone. *J. Macromol. Sci. Part B Phys.*, 44(1), 129–135, 2005.
54. Seferis, J. C., Refractive index of polymers. In *Polymers Handbook*, Brandrup, J., Immergut, E. H., Grulke E. A. Eds., Wiley, Toronto, Ontario, Canada, 1999, Chapter VI, 581.

55. Kelly, K. L., Coronado, E., Zhao, L. L., and Schatz, G. C., The optical properties of metal nanoparticles: The influence of size, shape, and dielectric environment. *J. Phys. Chem. B*, 107(3), 668–677, 2003.

56. Gaur, M. S., Singh, P. K., Suruchi, K., and Chauhan, R. S., Structural and thermal properties of polysulfone-ZnO nanocomposites. *J. Therm. Anal. Calorim.*, 111 (1), 743–751, 2013.

57. Salzano de Luna, M., Galizia, M., Wojnarowicz, J., Rosa, R., Lojkowski, W., Leonelli, C., Acierno, D., and Filippone, G., Dispersing hydrophilic nanoparticles in hydrophobic polymers: HDPE/ZnO nanocomposites by a novel template-based approach. *eXPRESS Polym. Lett.*, 8(5), 362–372, 2014.

58. Caseri, W., Nanocomposites of polymers and metals or semiconductors: Historical background and optical properties. *Macromol. Rapid Commun.*, 21(11), 705–722, 2000.

59. Ogieglo, W., Wormeester, H., Wessling, M., and Benes, N. E., Spectroscopic ellipsometry analysis of a thin film composite membrane consisting of polysulfone on a porous α-alumina support. *ACS Appl. Mater. Interfaces*, 4(2), 935–943, 2012.

60. Arshak, K. and Korostynska, O., Advanced materials and techniques for radiation dosimetry. Artech House Publishers, Boston, MA, pp. 91–114, 2006, ISBN: 158053340X.

61. Ioan, S., Buruiana, L. I., Avram, E., Petreus, O., and Musteata, V. E., Optical, dielectric and conduction properties of new phosphorus-modified polysulfones. *J. Macromol. Sci. Part B Phys.*, 50(8), 1571–1590, 2011.

62. Buruiana, L. I., Avram, E., Popa, A., Musteata, V. E., and Ioan, S., Electrical conductivity and optical properties of a new quaternized polysulfone. *Polym. Bull.*, 68(6), 1641–1661, 2012.

63. Ioan, S., Hulubei, C., Popovici, D., and Musteata, V. E., Origin of dielectric response and conductivity of some alicyclic polyimides. *Polym. Eng. Sci.*, 53(7), 1430–1447, 2013.

64. Tauc, J. and Menth, A., States in the gap. *J. Non-Cryst. Solids*, 8–10, 569–585, 1972.

65. Jarząbek, B., Weszka, J., Burian, A., and Pocztowski, G., Optical-properties of amorphous thin-films of the Zn-P system. *Thin Solid Films*, 279(1/2), 204–208, 1996.

66. Jarząbek, B., Schab-Balcerzak, E., Chamenko, T., Sek, D., Cisowski, J., and Volozhin, A., Optical properties of new aliphatic-aromatic co-polyimides. *J. Non-Cryst. Solids*, 299–302(Part 2), 1057–1061, 2002.

67. Moss, T. S., Burell, G. T., and Ellis, B., *Semiconductor Opto-Electronics*. Wiley, New York, 1973.

68. Kazmerski, L. L., *Polycrystalline and Amorphous Thin Films and Devices*, Academic Press, New York, 1998.

69. Jarząbek, B., Weszka, J., Domański, M., Jurusik, J., and Cisowski, J., Optical studies of aromatic polyazomethine thin films. *J. Non-Cryst. Solids*, 354(10/11), 856–862, 2008.

70. Meier, M., *Organic Semiconductors*. Verlag Chemie, Weinheim, Germany, 1974.

71. Georgoussis, G., Kanapitsas, A., Pissis, P., Savelyev, Yu. V., Veselov, V. Ya., and Privalko, E. G., Structure-property relationships in segmented polyurethanes with metal chelats in the main chain. *Eur. Polym. J.*, 36(6), 1113–1126, 2000.

72. Parka, S. J., Choa, K. S., and Kimb, S. H., A study on dielectric characteristics of fluorinated polyimide thin film. *J. Colloid Interface Sci.*, 272(2), 384–390, 2004.

73. Kripotoua, S., Pissisa, P., Bershteinb, V. A., Syselc, P., and Hobzovac, R., Dielectric studies of molecular mobility in hybrid polyimide–poly(dimethylsiloxane) networks. *Polymer*, 44(12), 2781–2984, 2003.

74. Kaplus, M., Levitt, M., and Warshel, A., Scientific background on the Nobel Prize in Chemistry from 2013. *Development of Multiscales for Complex Chemical Systems*, The Royal Swedish Academy of Science, Stockholm, Sweden, October 2013.

75. Bawden, D., Computerized chemical structure-handling techniques in structure-activity studies and molecular property prediction. *J. Chem. Inf. Comput.*, 23(1), 14–22, 1983.

76. HyperChem™, HyperChem 8.07, HyperChem Professional Program, Hypercube, Gainesville, FL, 2001.

77. Albu, R. M., Avram, E., Stoica, I., and Ioan, S., Polysulfones with chelating groups for heavy metals retention. *Polym. Compos.*, 33(4), 573–581, 2012.
78. Li, M., Liu, X. Y., Qin, Q., and Gu Y., Molecular dynamics simulation on glass transition temperature of isomeric polyimide. *eXPRESS Polym. Lett.*, 3(10), 665–675, 2009.
79. Albu, R. M., Avram, E., Musteata, V. E., and Ioan, S., Dielectric relaxation and AC conductivity of modified polysulfones with chelating groups. *J. Solid State Electrochem.*, 18(3), 785–794, 2014.
80. Montes, H., Mazeau, K., and Cavaille, J. Y., Secondary mechanical relaxations in amorphous cellulose. *Macromolecules*, 30(22), 6977–6984, 1997.
81. Vogel, M., Tschirwitz, C., Schneider, G., Koplin, C., Medick, P., and Rőssler, E., A ^{2}H NMR and dielectric spectroscopy study of the slow β-process in organic glass formers. *J Non-Cryst. Solids*, 307–310, 326–335, 2002.
82. Rudnik, E. and Dobkowski, Z., Investigations and molecular modeling of some thermophysical properties of polysulfones. *J. Therm. Anal. Calorim.*, 45(5), 1153–1158, 1995.
83. Kao, K. C. *Dielectric Phenomena in Solids*. Elsevier Academic Press, San Diego, CA, p. 75, 2004.
84. Pradhan, K. D., Choudhary. R. N. P., and Samantaray, B. K., Studies of dielectric relaxation and AC conductivity behavior of plasticized polymer nanocomposite electrolytes. *Int. J. Electrochem. Sci.*, 3(5), 597–608, 2008.
85. Havriliak, S. and Havriliak, S. J., *Dielectric and Mechanical Relaxation in Materials*. Hanser Publishers, Cincinnati, OH, 1997.
86. Bas, C., Tamagna, C, Pascal, T., and Alberola, D., On the dynamic mechanical behavior of polyimides based on aromatic and alicyclic dianhydrides. *Polym. Eng. Sci.*, 43, 344–355, 2003.
87. Comer, A. C., Kalika, D. S., Rowe, B. W., Freeman, B. D., and Paul, D. R., Dynamic relaxation characteristics of matrimid polyimide. *Polymer*, 5(3), 891–897, 2009.
88. Tsuwi, J., Pospiech, D., Jehnichen, D., Häußler, L., and Kremer, F. Molecular dynamics in semifluorinated-side-chain polysulfone studied by broadband dielectric spectroscopy. *J. Appl. Polym. Sci.*, 105(1), 201–207, 2007.
89. Starkweather, H. W., Aspects of simple, non-cooperative relaxations. *Polymer*, 32(13), 2443–2448, 1991.
90. Saxena, P., Gaur, M. S., Khare, P. K., and Tiwari, R. K., Dielectric relaxation in polyvinylidenefluoride polysulfone blends. *J. Electostatics*, 69(3), 214–219, 2011.
91. Aziz, S. B., Abidin, Z. H. Z., and Arof, A. K., Influence of silver ion reduction on electrical modulus parameters of solid polymer electrolyte based on chitosansilver triflate electrolyte membrane. *eXPRESS Polym. Lett.*, 4(5), 300–310, 2010.
92. Khazaka, R., Locatelli, M. L., Diaham, S., Bidan, P., Dupuy, L., and Grosset, G., Broadband dielectric spectroscopy of BPDA/ODA polyimide films. *J. Phys. D Appl. Phys.*, 46(6) 065501 (7pp.), 2013.
93. Yakuphanoglu, F., Aydogdu, Y., Schatzschneider, U., and Rentschler, E., DC and AC conductivity and dielectric properties of the metal-radical compound: Aqua[bis(2-dimethylaminomethyl-4-NIT-phenolato)]copper(II) *Solid State Commun* 128(2/3), 63–67, 2003.
94. Damaceanu, M. D., Rusu, R. D., Musteata, V. E., and Bruma, M., Insulating polyimide films containing n-type perylenediimide moieties. *Polym. Int.*, 61(10), 1582–1591, 2012.
95. Chisca, S., Musteata, V. E., Sava, I., and Bruma, M., Dielectric behavior of some aromatic polyimide films. *Eur. Polym. J.*, 47(5), 1186–1197, 2011.
96. Kuczkowski, A. and Zielinski, R., The AC conductivity of the polyvinylcarbazole-tetracyanoquinodimethane (PVK:TCNQ) CT complex. *J. Phys. D Appl. Phys.* 15, 1765–1768, 1982.
97. Clarke, P. J., Ray, A. K., Tsibouklis, J., and Werninck, A. R., Dielectric loss in novel disubstituted polydiacetylenes. *J. Mater. Sci. Mater. Electron.*, 2(1), 18–20, 1991.

98. Muruganand, S., Narayandass, S. K., Mangalaraj, D., and Vijayanm, T. M., Dielectric and conduction properties of pure polyimide films. *Polym. Int.*, 50(10), 1089–1094, 2001.

99. Banik, I., One way to explain the Meyer-Neldel Rule. *Chalcogenide Lett.*, 6(12), 629–633, 2009.

100. Smith, R., *Semiconductors*. Cambridge University Press, London, 1980.

101. Benavente, J., Zhang, X., and Garcia Valls, R., Modification of polysulfone membranes with polyethylene glycol and lignosulfate: Electrical characterization by impedance spectroscopy measurements. *J. Colloid Interface Sci.*, 285(1), 273–280, 2005.

102. Benavente, J., Garcia, J. M., Riley, R., and Lozano, A. E., Sulfonated poly(ether ether sulfones): Characterization and study of dielectrical properties by impedance spectroscopy. *J. Membr. Sci.*, 175(1), 43–52, 2000.

103. Benavente, J., Cañas, A., Ariza, M. J., Lozano, A. E., and de Abajo, J., Electrochemical parameters of sulfonated poly(ether ether sulfone) membranes in HCl solutions determined by impedance spectroscopy and membrane potential measurements. *Solid State Ionics*, 145(1–4), 53–60, 2001.

104. Kim, D. H. and Kim, S. C., Transport properties of polymer blend membranes of sulfonated and nonsulfonated polysulfones for direct methanol fuel cell application. *Macromol. Res.*, 16(5), 457–466, 2008.

105. Furtado Filho, A. A. M. and Gomes, A., de S., Crosslinked sulfonated polysulfone-based polymer electrolyte membranes induced by gamma ray irradiation. *Int. J. Polym. Mat. Polym. Biomater.*, 59(6), 429–437, 2010.

106. Ciobanu, M., Marin, L., Cozan, V., and Bruma, M., Aromatic polysulfones used in sensor applications. *Rev. Adv. Mater. Sci.*, 22(1/2), 89–96, 2009.

107. Zhang, J., Fei, G., Liang, Y., Zhang, Y., and Zhao, J., Influence of silica content in sulfonated polysulfone/phosphotungstic acid hybrid membranes on properties for fuel cell application. *e-Polymers*, (102), 1–10, 2010, ISSN: 1618-7229.

7 Functionalized Polysulfone–Metal Complexes

Raluca Marinica Albu

CONTENTS

7.1 INTRODUCTION

In recent years, polymer–metal complexes have attracted interest in many scientific and technological fields, such as bioinorganic industry [1], wastewater treatment [2], pollution control [3], hydrometallurgy [4], preconcentration [5], anionic polyelectrolyte hydrogels [6], and cation-exchange resins [7]. They are an important class of new materials due to the coupling of the chemical, optical, and electronic properties of the metal moiety to those of the polymer. Originating whether from either natural or synthetic sources, the polymeric materials that possess the ability to create complexes with different metal ions have attracted a great deal of attention recently and are commonly considered as a new frontier in material systems [8–10]. The incorporation of metals into a nonmetallic matrix component is a key step in the functional behavior of many industrially important applications such as heterogeneous catalysts and ion exchange resins. In all of these cases, on the other hand, the properties of metal-containing surfaces are influenced by the binding of the metal atoms to the surrounding matrix and the chemical state of the metal centers, such as the type of complexation and the possibility for charge transfer. In addition, the possibilities of obtaining polymer–metal complexes and their relation to the chemical structure can be intensively investigated even in bulk samples. Normally, metals do not bind to polymers. Binding of metals to polymers used in industrial applications is a complex phenomenon, which requires changes in different places, such as at the adhesive interface or within a thicker interphase layer. To create these possibilities, it is necessary to obtain bond formation at the interface by the functionalization of the polymer or the polymer surface through various techniques for surface treatment. Functionalized polymers are highly versatile and complex, providing new opportunities in an excellent area of research. A functionalized polymer contains a desired functional group that is able to perform a chemical transformation. Hence, by varying the polymer chain and the nature of the ligand and the metal ion, it is possible to prepare polymer complexes having different uses. A polymer–metal complex is composed of a synthetic polymer and metal ions, the latter being bound to the polymer ligand by a coordinate bond. A polymer ligand contains anchoring sites such as nitrogen, oxygen, and sulfur obtained either by polymerization of a monomer possessing the coordinating site or by a chemical reaction between a polymer and a low-molecular-weight compound with coordinating ability. The metal atoms attached to the polymer backbone exhibit a characteristic catalytic behavior, distinctly different from their low-molecular-weight analogues. Indeed, many synthetic polymer complexes have been found to possess high catalytic activity, in addition to semiconductivity, heat resistance, and biomedical potentials.

The chemical activity of the polymer support depends greatly on structural factors and the chemical nature of the functional group. Polymer-supported ligands are found to be efficient complexing agents and their high selectivity enables the removal and analysis of traces of heavy metal ions from polluted environments.

Polymer–metal complexes are used in various fields and their main applications are in organic synthesis such as catalysts, environmental remediation agents, as well as in hydrometallurgy, sensing, and biomedical fields [11]. Heavy metal ions are toxic to all the living organisms of both land and sea. Therefore, metal ion removal studies have been carried out to develop optimum conditions using different processes/polymers as supports for base ligands and various functional groups (carbonyl, carboxyl, amino, amido, sulfonate, phosphate, etc.) present on the surface or inside the polymeric support. Also, different binding mechanisms such as ion exchange, physical adsorption, chemisorption, complexation, and microprecipitation that may occur in metal-binding processes by an adsorbent have been in the research focus [12].

Metal–polymer composites are attractive for many applications, especially in microelectronics [13]. Generally, the interaction between metals and polymers is very weak, but it can be increased if the polymer surface is modified before metal deposition. For this reason, some physical and chemical modification techniques are necessary to intensify metal adhesion [14]. Due to the unique properties of the metal, its nanoparticles are preferred in a variety of potential applications in the field of electronics, sensor materials [15,16], medical diagnostics [17], Raman spectroscopy [18], biological imaging [19], and biosensors [20]. In this context, reports indicate that the fabrication of structurally continuous gold films below 15–20 nm is generally difficult to achieve on commonly used optical surfaces—including amorphous and crystalline materials (such as glass, native silicon oxide, Si_3N_4, TiO_2, and certain transparent polymers) [21]. Deposition of metal films onto a polymeric support is recommended due to their high conductivity, large surface, and low temperature processing; the use of gold is especially attractive due to its chemical stability and high atomic mass (electromigration resistance).

Aromatic polysulfones [Udel polysulfones, poly(ether sulfone)s, and poly(phenyl sulfones)] are a family of amorphous thermoplastics, characterized by unique high-performance properties as engineering materials: excellent thermal stability, high strength, low creep, good electrical characteristics, transparency, and good resistance to many solvents and chemicals. The aromatic structural elements and sulfone groups from the structural unit are responsible for the resistance to heat and oxidation, whereas the ether and isopropylidene groups contribute to some chain flexibility [22]. Therefore, polysulfones (PSFs) and their derivatives have been used in the manufacture of medical equipment (e.g., surgical trays, nebulizers, and dialysis components), devices (e.g., coffeemakers, humidifiers, and microwave ovens), automobile parts (e.g., steering column lockswitches, relay insulators, and pistons), and electronic equipment (e.g., television components and capacitor film) [23–26]. Due to their excellent electrical properties, PSFs have a wide application in the field of sensors (such as humidity sensors, gas sensors, biosensors, immobilization of enzyme, enzyme membrane reactor), providing information about the physical, chemical, and biological environments. Consequently, the introduction of functional groups into the PSF backbone, as well as the metal deposition on these polymers, extends the range of potential applications of these high-performance materials through the specific properties obtained and thus provides a wider scope [22,27].

7.2 FUNCTIONALIZED PSFs FOR SPECIAL APPLICATIONS

PSFs possess many properties required in various fields of materials science, biology, and polymer science, which underlies their numerous applications. However, these materials also have some limitations related to stress cracking with certain solvents, poor tracking resistance, and weathering properties; therefore, a chemical modification is necessary for overcoming this inconvenience by obtaining new specific properties. PSFs functionalized with different groups, such as halides, acids, alcohols, alkyls, amines, phenyls, and polymerizable groups, have been the subject of intense research interest due to their improved properties and versatility. PSFs can be chemically modified by a number of techniques: one of them is to bond the desired functional groups (such as carboxylic, fluorine, and methyl chloride) to the aromatic ring, or by sulfonation, nitration, and lithiation to the main chain through chemical reaction. Another approach is to form difunctional PSF oligomers by the incorporation of functional groups into their aromatic groups and use in the formation of graft polymers or PSF-based networks [28].

The chemical modification of PSFs, especially the chloromethylation [29–31] and quaternization reactions [32], is a subject of considerable scientific interest from both theoretical and practical viewpoints, considering their area of application. Quaternization with tertiary amines of the PSF backbone represents a useful way to change some properties of the material, such as solubility [33–36] and hydrophilicity (which is of special interest for biomedical applications) [37–39], allowing higher water permeability and better separation [26,40,41].

In addition, the modification of polymers through the introduction of chelating units into the modified PSF structures allows new potential applications, such as surface coatings on metals and glasses, adhesives, high-temperature lubricants, electrical insulators, semiconductors, and applications for reducing heavy metal pollution in ecosystems [42]. As generally known, heavy metal contamination occurs in the aqueous waste effluents of many industries, such as metal-plating facilities, fertilizer industry, mining operations, and tanneries. Various techniques, such as precipitation, extraction, membrane filtration, ion exchange, adsorption, and neutralization [43,44], to remove heavy metals from wastewater have been reported. Heavy metals are not biodegradable and tend to accumulate in living organisms, causing various diseases and disorders [45]. In this context, copper removal by polymers possessing complex groups would be of great importance in environmental applications [46–48]. The presence of transient metal ions in polysulfonic films affects different properties in two distinct ways [48,49]: on the one hand, the complex structure between metal cations and the electron donor groups of the polymer chains leads to cross-link formation, decreasing chain mobility, and enhancing the glass transition temperature; on the other hand, the main effect is generated by the complexes distributed in polymer matrices, which disrupts the uniformity of the polymer chains and decreases the glass transition temperature. For all these reasons, the PSF–metal chelates present interest especially for environmental applications [46,47,50].

7.3   DEPOSITION OF METAL NANOPARTICLES AND NANO-LAYERS ON MODIFIED PSFs

7.3.1   Deposition Mechanisms

Metals and metal–polymer interfaces have played an important role in many materials applications, in microelectronics, device packaging, and protective coatings. Reactions at the metal–polymer interface or adhesion can determine whether a device will work or fail. The growth and morphology of a metal thin film deposited on a polymer should be determined as a function of the metal adsorption energy, particle diameter, and metal layer thickness.

Metallized polymer films have considerable technological importance for a wide range of applications, from food packaging to biosensors [51]. Thus, thin-film metallized polymeric substrates are used, for example, in gas-barrier applications, composite and photoconductive materials, cryogenics engineering, and protective coatings [52,53]. Most synthetic polymers used as commercial materials have a low surface energy and, as a result, these materials have a low adhesion to metal coatings. Therefore, many studies have been focusing on the adhesion phenomena, properties at the metal–polymer interface, as well as the control of the microstructure and thermal stability, with the aim to prevent degradation and improve adhesion.

The realization and reproducibility of metal adhesion on polymer substrates is an important industrial and scientific problem [54]. The interaction between a metal and a polymer strongly depends on the type of the metal and on the functional groups present in the polymer. The techniques most commonly used to improve the adhesion of polymers to metals are as follows:

- Oxidation of polymer substrate surfaces [55]
- Chemical modification of the interfacial polymer chains with polar groups, such as hydroxyl, carbonyl, and carboxylic acid moieties
- Plasma treatment of the metallic surfaces [56]

The mechanisms of formation of the interfacial region—where metal atoms come into contact with the film surface—can be classified as follows:

- Mechanical—interlocking
- Chemical—bonding
- Diffusion—dispersion forces
- Combinations of these types, depending upon substrate morphology, contamination on the surface, chemical interactions, the energy available during interface formation, and the nucleation behavior of the deposited metal

PSFs have received a great attention as regards such applications, due to their thermal and chemical stabilities, excellent electrical properties, and the ease of processing into coatings and films.

In the case of metallizing PSF films, the most important aspects of adhesion arise from mechanical and chemical bonding at the interface. The mechanical interface is characterized by an interlocking of the depositing metal with the rough surface of the substrate [57]. The strength of this interface will depend upon the mechanical properties of the materials being brought together: metal and film. According to Scheme 7.1, the chemical bonding depends upon the formation of chelates of the polymer oxygen atoms with the metal atoms [58].

Chemical bonding can be

- Covalent, by exchange of electrons between atoms
- Ionic, by interaction between ionic crystals (loss of electrons)
- Metallic, classified as covalent, with much greater mobility of electrons (this bonding does not occur on the surface, but rather in building metal layers)

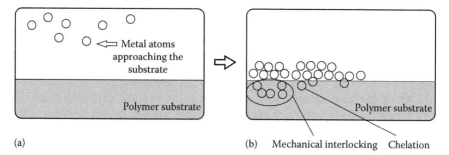

(a)   (b) Mechanical interlocking Chelation

SCHEME 7.1 Diagram of mechanical interlocking phenomenon of appearing at the metal–polymer substrate interface: (a) interface—incoming metal atoms and the film surface and (b) chelation—when the metal reacts with the polymer.

The interaction of the polymer chain with the incoming metal atom can result in a chelation reaction with the oxygen atoms, and in chain breaking and reaction with the end groups formed. Generally, as the metal atoms strike the surface, they lose energy to the surface and condense on the polymeric substrate. During the condensation process, the atoms have some degree of mobility on the surface—determined by their kinetic energy, strength and the type of interaction between the metal atoms, clusters of metal atoms, and the substrate surface.

The metal atoms/clusters will grow to form a continuous metallic film. The atom density and growth mode determine the effective interfacial contact area and the development of voids in the interfacial regions. Atom density and metallic crystal orientation formed during the deposition can be affected by the environment, contamination, surface inclusions, and deposition techniques. Moreover, to the effective contact area, the growth mode of the metallic film will determine the defect morphology in the interface region and the amount of diffusion and reaction between depositing atoms and the polymeric substrate.

All of these contribute to the mechanical adhesion of the metal film being formed to the functionalized PSF substrate and to the barrier properties of the final metallized film. Therefore, the adhesion of the metal and the barrier properties of quaternized PSFs are related to the following:

- The PSF film surface
- The interaction of the metal with the surface
- The way the metal builds a structure beyond the surface
- The thickness of the metal deposited

Chemical bonds on the PSF surfaces, such as carbonyl, hydroxyl, and ketone groups, also influence the adhesion of the metal to the PSF film.

7.3.2 Metal Film Deposition on Modified PSFs

Metals such as gold constitute important materials for numerous applications in optics, electronics, photonics, plasmonics, biosensing, and chemical catalysis, as they possess a number of favorable electrical, optical, physical, and chemical properties [59]. The realization of continuous gold films is, generally, difficult to achieve on usually used amorphous and crystalline materials, and certain transparent polymers. For a range of crystalline substrates, including sapphire, mica, silicon, NaCl, KCl, and LiF, epitaxial single-crystal gold islands or sheets can be formed. However, these substrates and the required deposition methods are, in most cases, incompatible with the fabrication of multilayer devices, as they typically require special conditions such as *in situ* cleaving, high-temperature substrate surface reconstruction, elevated deposition temperatures, seeding layers of different chemical species, and template stripping. On the other hand, the dynamics of gold film formation on the surface of certain polymers can be different from that on inorganic substrates. The possibility of fabricating and patterning high-mass-density, low-roughness gold films has interesting implications for electronics, optics, photonics, biosensing, and surface chemistry. The high structural quality of the thin metal films, combined with the large effective-index variations that can be introduced through very small metal thickness modulation, translates into a high degree of control over device structure and required properties.

It has been established that the adhesion strength between quaternized PSF surfaces (PSF-DMEA and PSF-DMOA, containing different tertiary amines—*N,N*-dimethylethylamine or *N,N*-dimethyloctylamine) and gold nanoparticles can be modified by plasma treatment and by different physical and chemical conditions [26,60]. It is generally known that there are two major functions of the plasma surface treatment: (1) removal of impurities and (2) the activation of surface [54,55,61]. Such changes may generate several kinds of reactions, such as breakage of the covalent bonds along the chain, cross-linking, grafting, interactions of surface free radicals, alterations of the existing functional groups, and the incorporation of chemical groups originating in the plasma. Considering this, after the plasma treatment, the PSF surfaces undergo several changes in their chemical functionality, surface morphology, wettability, and bondability. The adhesion and morphology of untreated PSFs [atomic force microscopy (AFM) images from Figure 7.1] and of those treated through gold sputtering for different time periods, can be investigated by AFM (Figures 7.2 through 7.6, Table 7.1) [62,63]. Thus, the mean adhesion force values between the cantilever and the studied surfaces can be correlated with the quaternized

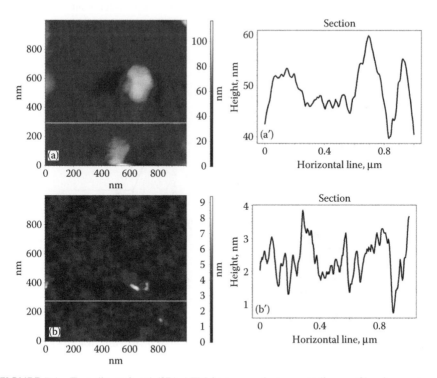

FIGURE 7.1 Two-dimensional (2D) AFM images and corresponding profiles for: quaternized polysulfone films with *N,N*-dimethylethylamine (PSF-DMEA)—(a) and (a'), respectively; quaternized polysulfone films with *N,N*-dimethyloctylamine (PSF-DMOA)—(b) and (b'), respectively.

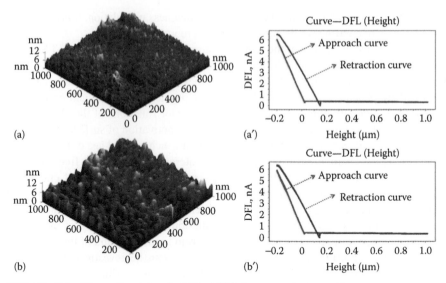

FIGURE 7.2 Three-dimensional (3D) AFM image and force–distance spectroscopy DFL (height) performed on: PSF-DMEA$_{p0}$ + Au$_{t11}$ film—(a) and (a'), respectively; PSF-DMOA$_{p0}$ + Au$_{t11}$ film—(b) and (b'), respectively. Subscript "p0" refers to untreated plasma film, and subscript "t11" refers to 11 min gold sputtering time.

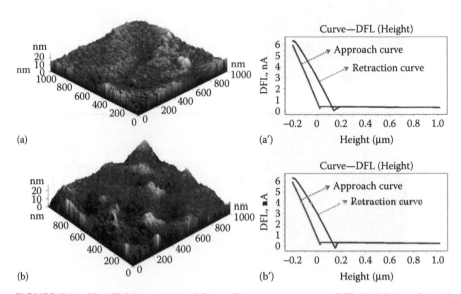

FIGURE 7.3 3D AFM image (a) and force–distance spectroscopy DFL (height) performed on: PSF-DMEA$_{p10}$ + Au$_{t6}$ film—(a) and (a'), respectively; PSF-DMEA$_{p10}$ + Au$_{t11}$ film—(b) and (b'), respectively. Subscript "p10" refers to 10 min of plasma treatment, and subscripts "t6" and "t11" refer to 6 and 11 min gold sputtering time, respectively.

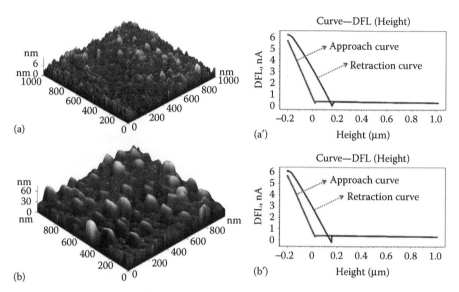

FIGURE 7.4 3D AFM images and force–distance spectroscopy DFL (height) performed on: PSF-DMOA$_{p10}$ + Au$_{t6}$ film—(a) and (a′), respectively; PSF-DMOA$_{p10}$ + Au$_{t11}$ film—(b) and (b′), respectively. Subscript "p10" refers to 10 min of plasma treatment, and subscripts "t6" and "t11" refer to 6 and 11 min gold sputtering time, respectively.

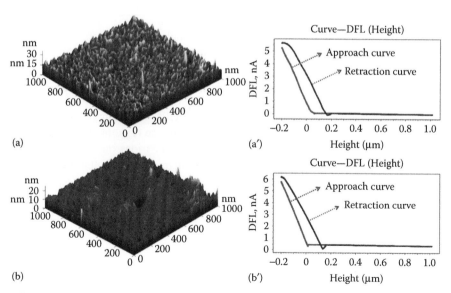

FIGURE 7.5 3D AFM images and force–distance spectroscopy DFL (height) performed on: PSF-PSF-DMEA$_{p20}$ + Au$_{t6}$ film—(a) and (a′), respectively; PSF-DMEA$_{p20}$ + Au$_{t11}$ film—(b) and (b′), respectively. Subscript "p20" refers to 20 min of plasma treatment, and subscripts "t6" and "t11" refer to 6 and 11 min gold sputtering time, respectively.

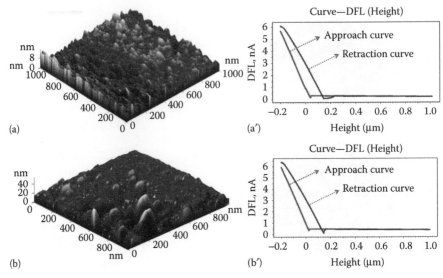

FIGURE 7.6 3D AFM image and force–distance spectroscopy DFL (height) performed on: PSF-PSF-DMOA$_{p20}$ + Au$_{t6}$ film—(a) and (a′), respectively; PSF-DMOA$_{p20}$ + Au$_{t11}$ film—(b) and (b′), respectively. Subscript "p20" refers to 20 min of plasma treatment, and subscripts "t6" and "t11" refer to 6 and 11 min gold sputtering time, respectively.

TABLE 7.1

Average Height (H_a, nm) and Root Mean Square Roughness (S_q, nm) Parameters, DFL Spectroscopy Measurements for Five Force-Distance Curves [Mean Adhesion Force (F_{adh}, nN)], and Average Grain Diameter (nm)

Sample	Surface Roughness Parameters		F_{adh}	Average Grain Diameter
	H_a	S_q		
PSF-DMEA	49.18	11.44	–	–
PSF-DMEA$_{p0}$ + Au$_{t11}$	5.59	1.42	32.4 ± 1.8	34.00 ± 3.2
PSF-DMEA$_{p10}$ + Au$_{t6}$	14.22	2.36	27.3 ± 1.0	51.50 ± 13.0
PSF-DMEA$_{p10}$ + Au$_{t11}$	12.17	3.40	39.7 ± 3.9	23.50 ± 3.6
PSF-DMEA$_{p20}$ + Au$_{t6}$	14.66	2.82	19.9 ± 2.4	46.67 ± 13.0
PSF-DMEA$_{p20}$ + Au$_{t11}$	10.62	2.04	27.9 ± 0.9	28.33 ± 7.4
PSF-DMOA	2.36	0.68	–	–
PSF-DMOA$_{p0}$ + Au$_{t11}$	8.57	1.71	32.2 ± 4.8	68.33 ± 4.1
PSF-DMOA$_{p10}$ + Au$_{t6}$	4.97	1.26	32.01 ± 1.8	72.67 ± 7.0
PSF-DMOA$_{p10}$ + Au$_{t11}$	34.30	10.34	43.3 ± 7.3	111.00 ± 11.3
PSF-DMOA$_{p20}$ + Au$_{t6}$	7.45	1.96	24.1 ± 1.1	39.00 ± 9.1
PSF-DMOA$_{p20}$ + Au$_{t11}$	19.27	6.64	32.4 ± 2.3	133.17 ± 9.8

PSF structures, modification of hydrophobicity after the plasma treatment, and gold deposition time on polymer surfaces (Table 7.1).

The AFM analysis permits to observe the hydrophobic characteristics of PSF-DMEA and PSF-DMOA PSFs, where the amount of polar components (γ_p) is lower than that of the disperse components (γ_d): $\gamma_p = 5.9$, $\gamma_d = 43.7$, for PSF-DMEA, and $\gamma_p = 5.1$, $\gamma_d = 40.9$ for PSF-DMOA. The hydrophobic character is offered by the ethyl radical from the N-dimethylethylammonium chloride pendant group and by the octyl radical from the N-dimethyloctylammonium chloride pendant group. After the plasma treatment of the corresponding films, the surface tension changes by modifications in the interaction between the high-energy particles and the polymer surface, so that the amount of polar components of the surface tension increases significantly for both the samples presented. According to the literature data, these modifications correspond to increases in wettability and adhesion [64,65].

On the other hand, the surface roughness parameters—listed in Table 7.1—are higher for the PSF-DMEA film than for the PSF-DMOA film. In addition, Table 7.1 shows that plasma treatment increases the surface roughness and, consequently, adhesion and gold sputtering time of the polymer surfaces.

The increasing number of studies devoted to new materials and their impact on the new technologies, including those associated with nanotechnology, emphasize the importance of intermolecular and surface forces in micro and nanosystems. Some experimental methods, such as the AFM, accurately measure these forces in air, vacuum, and solution, providing information on local material properties, such as elasticity, hardness, and adhesion [66].

AFM studies on the adhesion between the cantilever and the polymer surface modified by plasma treatment and metal deposition allow the assessment of the degree of adhesion between the polymer and the surface layer deposited [67]. The adhesion forces between the surface of the PSF samples surface and the silicon cantilever in the AFM technique allow the assessment of the interface properties, investigated by force–distance spectroscopy DFL (height) (Equation 7.1). Figures 7.2b through 7.6b illustrate the values of the mean adhesion force between the cantilever and the studied surfaces of quaternized PSFs [60], measured by AFM investigation. These data can be correlated with the structures, the modification of hydrophobicity after the plasma treatment, and metal (gold) deposition on polymer surfaces.

In contact mode, the adhesion forces have a significant effect on the cantilever during its withdrawal from the sample, causing its deflection before it interrupts the contact with the surface. The z-scanner length being reduced, the DFL (normal deflection distribution of the cantilever) first falls below its value, observed well away from the surface and then abruptly reaches the free-state value, thus forming a specific dip. The adhesion force can be calculated as a linear function of probe displacement relatively to the sample surface along the Z-axis, according to Hooke's law, expressed by Equation 7.1 as follows:

$$F = -k \cdot \Delta x \qquad (7.1)$$

where:

k is cantilever stiffness

Δx is deflection of the cantilever comparatively with PSF film surface [68–70]

Cantilever's normal spring constant, k, of 1.97 Nm^{-1} was determined by Sader's method, using data on the resonance peak of 93 kHz and the planar dimensions of the cantilever [69,70].

Because the silica surface of the cantilever is cleaned and dried and is hydrophobic, it can be estimated that the interaction between the cantilever and a hydrophobic substrate is greater than that between a hydrophobic substrate and a hydrophilic one [71].

7.3.3   Self-Assembly of Metal Particles on Polymeric Films

The self-assembly of metal particles generates a great interest as a powerful method of fabrication of macroscopic surfaces with well-defined and controllable nanostructures [72,73]. The interest in nanoscale materials stems from the fact that their properties (optical, electrical, mechanical, chemical, etc.) are a function of their size, composition, and structural order. Effective strategies to build tailored nanomaterials reliably and predictably are required in order to meet the ever-increasing demands (e.g., structural and compositional complexity) placed on material synthesis and performance by nanotechnology. Metallic colloids exhibit behaviors between those of single atoms and bulk materials. Controlling the particle diameter, aggregation degree, and coverage of metallic colloids on polymeric substrates allows obtaining materials with interesting optical and electrical properties [74], surface plasmon resonance substrates—where optical surface plasmon resonance spectroscopy is a powerful tool for *in situ* real-time characterization of solid–liquid interface [75], substrates for surface-enhanced Raman spectroscopy [75], catalytic surfaces [76], and the production of metal patterns in both microscale and nanoscale metallic structures [77].

Electrical conductivities close to that of bulk metal have been achieved by one of the following:

- Self-assembly of colloidal metal particles using linker molecules between gold particles.
- Increasing the metal coverage via a reduction process.

The interest in making conductive films on flexible polymer surfaces is motivated by the idea of making electronic or optical devices on mechanically flexible materials. Methods such as sputtering or vacuum deposition of metals have been presented in the literature [78]. Also, conductive gold films were successfully assembled on flexible polymer substrates, where the surface of the polymers is modified. Supriya and Claus reported that this method led to the formation of a shiny gold layer on the surface with a surface resistance of about 1 Ω/sq [72].

Nano-grained (10–100 nm grain size) and ultrafine-grained (up to 500 nm in size) polycrystalline metals and alloys based on 3d elements (Co, Ni, and Fe) have been researched, owing to the novel properties they present. Fellah et al. [79] emphasize that such novel properties appear to be promising for several magnetic, optical, and structural applications. It is now well established that the factors behind these properties are the morphology and size of the crystallites, along with the intercrystallite interactions that occur in bulk nanostructured materials. In this context, a literature review reveals two types of techniques that have been adopted to process these materials [80]:

- In the first category, ultrafine structured or nanostructured materials are obtained from the bulk material using a structural disintegration process, based on severe plastic deformation methods, such as high-energy ball milling, equal channel angular pressing [80], high pressure torsion [81], surface mechanical attrition treatment [82], and dynamic severe plastic deformation [83].
- The second category includes a one-step processing method, such as electro-deposition, which, in most cases, leads to porosity-free samples [84], and a two-step processing approach, in which the nanoparticle synthesis is followed by consolidation.

The main methods used to synthesize these nanoparticles are physical, electrochemical, and seldom chemical-based processing—despite its numerous advantages, such as sol-gel, forced hydrolysis, and reduction in a liquid medium.

7.3.4 ELASTOPLASTIC PROPERTIES OF METAL LAYER/PSF COMPLEXES

In the light of the above examples, the new trends in nano-, micro-, and macroelectronic domains require materials with portability and flexibility characteristics, thus flexible polymeric materials are ideal candidates for this area. The elastoplastic behavior of thin metallic films with grain sizes in the nanometric range can differ significantly to the mechanical behavior of coarse grain materials [85–87]. The substrate may play an important role on the mechanical properties of the film, suggesting that those properties depend on the substrate employed and on the microstructure. Generally, it has been found that the mechanical properties of thin metallic/polymeric films depend on the deposition technique, amount of residual stresses, film microtexture and grain size. Thus, a commercial PSF material used in substrate production has excellent thermal properties, resisting to the temperatures achieved during the thermal deposition of film. Also, the thin gold films (50–300 nm) deposited over flexible PSF substrate and their mechanical properties have been studied by tensile testing and by mathematical modeling [88]. Figure 7.7 illustrates the stress–strain curve (tensile response) of the PSF substrate, where a linear elastic region at low attained strain, followed by a plastic region at a large deformation, is observed. According to Figure 7.7, the average deviation values of strength, σ_{max}, ultimate strain, ε_{ult}, and elastic modulus, E, are 16.9 MPa, 27.6%, and 735 MPa, respectively. The elastic modulus is obtained from the initial slope of the curve.

In the case of different film thickness of the gold layer deposited onto the PSF support, the mechanical response of Au/PSF is presented in Figure 7.8, leading to the following observations:

- An increase in resistance occurs compared to the polysulfonic substrate, for values remarks.
- The ultimate strain values of the Au/PSF complex are strongly reduced with respect to that of the substrate and decrease with thickness.
- The flexibility of the polysulfonic substrate provides increased film ductility in the gold/polysufone system [89,90].

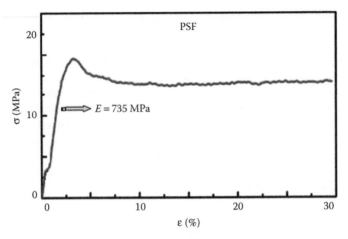

FIGURE 7.7   Tensile stress–strain curves for the PSF substrate.

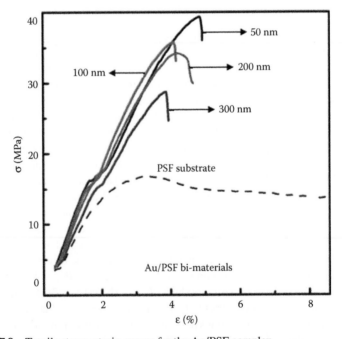

FIGURE 7.8   Tensile stress–strain curves for the Au/PSF complex.

The mechanical properties of gold films are dependent on the polymeric substrate. Therefore, it is necessary to know the specimen geometry in order to record the stress–strain curves of the substrate, applying Equations 7.2 and 7.3 (if $t_s \gg t_f$) [88], and to determine the elastic modulus of the Au film. The mechanical properties of the film will be determined as the difference between the curves of the substrate and those of the bi-material.

$$E_f = \left(\frac{t_s}{t_f}\right) \cdot \left(E_{bim} - E_s\right) \tag{7.2}$$

where:

E_f and E_s are elastic modulus of film and substrate, respectively
E_{bim} is total elastic modulus of Au/PSF bi-material
t_s and t_f are thickness of the film and substrate, respectively

$$\sigma_f = \left(\frac{t_s}{t_f}\right) \cdot \left(\sigma_{bim} - \sigma_s\right) \tag{7.3}$$

where:

σ_f and σ_s are the stresses of the film and substrate, respectively
σ_{bim} is the total stress applied to the Au/PSF bi-material

Because the plastic zone of the Au film deposited over PSF substrates is very limited, the offset method [91] was used to determine its yield strength. In this method, described by Aviles et al. [88,92], a strain offset is fixed and a straight line parallel to the initial slope of the $\sigma - \varepsilon$ curve is drawn starting from the offset point. It can be observed that the values of the yield strength and strain determined in this manner are very close to the maximum stress (strength) and ultimate strain, given the reduced extension of the plastic zone.

The data on the elastic modulus of the film and the yield strength *versus* film thickness film listed in Figure 7.9 and Table 7.2 indicate that (a) with the increase in the layer gold from 50 to 300 nm, the elastic modulus of the film decreases from 520 to 100 GPa, respectively; (b) the minimum value of the elastic modulus corresponding

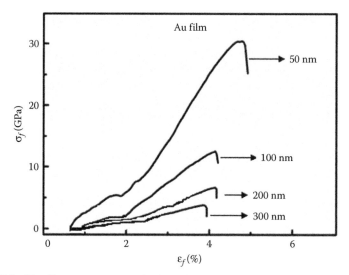

FIGURE 7.9 Tensile stress versus strain dependence for Au films extracted from the difference between Au/PSF and PSF (substrate), according to Equation 7.3.

TABLE 7.2

Variation of Elastic Modulus (E_f), and Offset Yield Strength (σ_y) with Film Thickness (t_f), and Grain Size Determined by AFM (d_f)

t_f, nm	d_f, nm	E_f, GPa	σ_y, GPa
50	83	520	30.2
100	113	360	8.8
200	127	190	7.5
300	133	100	3.9
Bulk value	–	77	0.2

to a thickness of 300 nm is close to that of gold in bulk geometry (77 GPa) [92]; (c) the film microstructure and confinement effects, as well as the deposition method, influence the dependence of the film's Young's modulus on the film thickness, making it nonlinear [88]; and (d) the mean yield strength values of 30.2 GPa predicted for 50 nm thick films, and of 3.85 GPa for 300 nm thick films are substantially higher than the bulk value of 205 MPa reported in other works [92,93].

The correlation between the film microstructure and its yield strength was determined by the means of AFM, which imaged every different surface of Au/PSF bi-materials. The morphological analysis evidences grain formations, whose dimensions differ from a film to another (Table 7.2). It has been observed that the grain size, d_f, is the largest for the thickest film. Also, the average grain size increases from 83 to 133 nm when film thickness increases from 50 to 300 nm. In the end, in case of thin films, there appear confinement effects, which could affect the yield strength of the film, modifying the elastic response of the material.

In summary, it may be stated that the yield strength and elastic modulus of films depend on the film thickness. The elastoplastic behavior of thin films is strongly influenced by factors such as deposition type, substrate type, thermal history, grain size, thickness confinement, and microstructural parameters. It would be important to determine the individual contribution of each factor by more extensive investigation in specific scientific and technological areas.

7.4 PSF COMPOSITES

7.4.1 Formation of Metal Nanoparticles in PSF Matrices

A number of methods of incorporating metal nanoparticles in polymer matrices have been reported. Thus, the metal nanoparticles can be synthesized *ex situ*, being then added to the polymer solution [94]. The organosol is prepared by adding salt-containing metal to a reducing agent and heating the solution under intense stirring conditions. Finally, the organosol is added to the casting mixtures containing solvent, polymer, and porogen. Other approaches involve *in situ* reduction of an ionic metal by the addition of solvent to the membrane casting mixture [95]. In this case, the salt-containing metal is first dissolved in the solvent at room temperature to minimize metal reduction. The polymer solution is subjected to intense stirring under heating; once the casting mixture becomes homogeneous, the salt solution is added to it to initiate the reduction of metal ions, with the concomitant formation of metal nanoparticles.

Literature data confirm that the microstructural changes induced by nanoparticle incorporation can be controlled for obtaining membranes with desirable properties. On the other hand, the formation of the polymer matrix and the nanoparticles include the chemical reduction of metal ions by a component of the membrane casting solution [96]. Porous nanocomposite membranes are dependent on essential variables such as:

- Nanoparticles dimension - relative to the characteristic size of matrix pores,
- The affinity of the filler material for the components of the casting mixture.

Different studies describe the formation of PSF membranes [97–101] by adding different particles (Ag—[102–104], Al_2O_3—[105,106], ZrO_2—[97,107], TiO_2—[101,108], SiO_2—[98,99,109,110]) to the casting solution.

Many studies have been conducted to increase the hydrophilic properties of the PSF membrane with excellent separation performance, good thermal and chemical resistances, and adaptability to the harsh wastewater environments by different methods:

- Blending PSFs with hydrophilic nanoparticles, such as SiO_2, ZrO_2, and TiO_2.
- Grafting with hydrophilic polymers, monomers or functional groups (in this case, a phase-inversion process takes place, where a polymer is transformed from a liquid state to a solid state).
- Coating with hydrophilic polymers.

Blending involves dissolving or dispersing the metal nanoparticles in a suitable solvent (N,N'-dimethylacetamide or N-methyl-2-pyrrolidone).

On the other hand, the process of solidification by phase inversion (involving different techniques, such as solvent evaporation, thermal precipitation, and immersion precipitation) is initiated by the transition from one liquid state into two liquids (liquid–liquid demixing). At a certain stage during demixing, the high polymer-concentration phase will solidify, so that a solid matrix is formed. Richards et al. [111] point out that some commercially available membranes are prepared using immersion precipitation, where a solution of the polymer and the solvent is cast on a suitable support and immersed in a coagulation bath containing a nonsolvent. Precipitation occurs because of the exchange of solvent (organic solvent such as methanol) and nonsolvent (water) and eventually the polymer is observed to precipitate. The obtained membrane structure results from a combination of mass transfer and phase separation. Also, various metal nanoparticles are used in wastewater treatment membrane technology with varying degrees of success, and metal nanocomposite membranes are applied to remediate membrane fouling due to organic matter and biofouling.

7.4.2 PSF WITH CHELATING GROUPS FOR HEAVY METALS RETENTION

It is well known that in recent years a rapid expansion in the industrial activities has generated an increase in the complexity of toxic effluents of chemical industries and mining. Some industrial processes produce variable amounts of dissolved toxic metals, which constitute a serious pollution problem because they cannot be degraded or destroyed and can affect human health by bioaccumulation. Many metals, such as copper (Cu), mercury (Hg), lead (Pb), chromium (Cr), and manganese (Mn), are known to be harmful to the majority of living organisms and the environment [112]. Moreover, the aquatic flora and fauna are affected by this pollution. Using polluted waters as irrigation sources is not recommended because the heavy metals accumulate in the soil and in some plants. Animals that consume these plants carry the accumulated heavy metals further in milk and meat products that we humans consume. For this reason, various techniques have been developed for removing and recovering these metallic species accumulated in the soil and water [113]. Conventional technologies for the purification of contaminated soil consist of washing with strong acids or caustics, which might lead to secondary pollution and large deposits of sludge that sometimes reach waste deposits. Traditional methods of cleaning wastewater include through precipitation with chemical agents, adsorption onto activated carbon, ion-exchange resins, and membrane filtration processes. All these methods are quite satisfactory in terms of removing pollutants, but they produce solid residues containing toxic compounds and their final disposal is generally done by land filling, with high costs and with the probability of groundwater contamination [114]. Membrane separation methods are quite effective, but cannot be used as potential solutions to remediate broad areas because of the high costs associated with their implementation [115]. The utilization of polymeric materials originating from both natural and synthetic sources and having the ability to form complexes with heavy metals is also very common [116].

Recently, the use of chelating polymers for the remediation of water and soil has attracted much attention. By incorporating into the polymeric side chains or backbone chelating groups, chelate-forming polymers are obtained, which can form complexes with heavy metals. The metal ion is connected to a ligand of the functional groups from the polymer matrix by a coordinate bond forming a polymer–metal complex. Hence, new PSFs functionalized with chelating groups have been realized for the retention of heavy metals from aqueous media [48]. As known, copper, which is a widely used material, may affect biological species if used excessively. Its harmfulness has been a motivating factor for an increasing number of research works devoted to copper. In this regard, chelate-modified PSF (KQPSFCu – Scheme 7.2) were obtained starting from chloromethylated polysulfone (CMPSF), which was initially partially functionalized with methyl 3-pyridyl ketone (3-MPK) for attaining a molar degree of modified PSF (KPSF – Scheme 7.2) of 0.4. Second, N,N-dimethyloctylamine (DMOA) was added to react with the remaining chloromethylene groups, which led to a quaternized molar degree of 0.6. The final product of the reaction, containing quaternary and reactive ketone groups (KQPSF – Scheme 7.2) in the side chain (Scheme 7.2), was used to analyze the capacity of retaining heavy metals—copper (Cu^{2+}) cations—from an aqueous $CuCl_2 \cdot 2H_2O$ solution, at different molarity, temperature, and time [48].

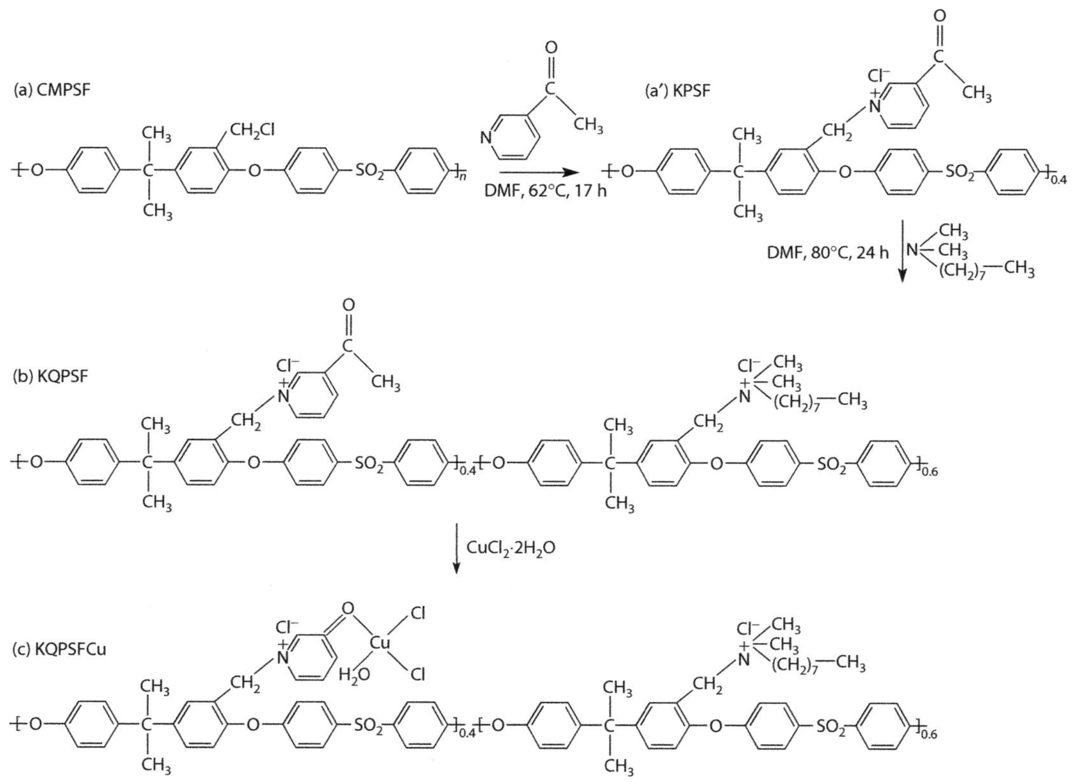

SCHEME 7.2 The general structure of chloromethylated polysulfone (a—CMPSF), chelating polysulfone containing ketone units (a'—KPSF), chelating polysulfone containing quaternary and reactive ketone units (b—KQPSF), and chelate-modified polysulfones containing quaternary and reactive ketone units (c—KQPSFCu) formed from the complexation of KQPSF with copper ions.

Techniques, such as attenuated total reflection-Fourier transform infrared (ATR-FTIR) spectroscopy, AFM, environmental scanning electron microscopy (ESEM), and differential scanning calorimetry (DSC), have been used to study the copper ions retention ability of films immersed in aqueous solution and of the formed KQPSFCu compounds. The addition of transient Cu^{2+} cations to the chelated polymers changes the strength of some bonds between the basic polymer atoms. ATR-FTIR spectroscopy has helped to evaluate the intensity of some bonds, demonstrating how the carried metal cation binds to the membrane structure and is distributed among the polymeric chains, as seen in Figure 7.10. In this case, the strength of the carbonyl bond is evaluated to assess the effect of the metal on the complex formed between the carbonyl groups and the free Cu^{2+} cations. The identified bond is considered a characteristic of metal–ligand links [117].

Also, the band frequency at 1705 cm^{-1} corresponding to $\tilde{v}$ (—C = O) vibrations in KQPSF depends on the physical parameters of each aqueous solution (such as temperature, molarity, time of immersion). As a result, when the —C = O groups participate in the formation of Cu^{2+}–KQPSF linkages, the peaks for the stretching vibrations (in the KQPSFCu sample spectra) are shifted in the direction of lower wave number or lower frequency, comparatively with the reference peak (KQPSF). This proves the increased number of complexes formed and also that the concentration

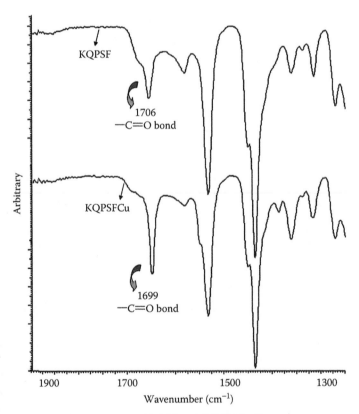

FIGURE 7.10   ATR-FTIR spectra of KQPSF and KQPSFCu films.

of the free carbonyl bonds decreases by metal addition. Therefore, the distribution
of the carried metal is larger and more suitable. ATR spectra of the KQPSF and
KQPSFCu demonstrate that the wave number corresponding to carbonyl groups
vibrations depends on temperature, immersion time, and molarity of the $CuCl_2 \cdot 2H_2O$
aqueous solutions.

It can be remarked that the increase in temperature and time of KQPSF immer-
sions in $CuCl_2 \cdot 2H2O$ aqueous solutions favors the binding of Cu^{2+} ions. When the
temperature and molarity of the $CuCl_2 \cdot 2H_2O$ aqueous solution exceed a certain
threshold, the film structure is disrupted, and the salt becomes aggregated on the
polymer chains, which affects the uniformity of the chains. Later, a powerful interaction occurs on one side of the active layer, whereas no interaction appears on the
other side. The irregularities observed in the sample spectra are due to the heterogeneous distribution of the coordination interactions [49,118]. The shift of the peak to
a lower frequency shows that the carbonyl bond is weakened. Thus, changes in the $\tilde{v}$
(C = O) frequency are correlated with the decrease in the stretching force constant
of the C = O bond, as a consequence of oxygen atoms coordination with the metal
ion. As complexation with copper is higher, ketone absorption moves toward lower
values of the $-C = O$ frequency vibration, due to the decrease in the stretching force
constant, K, according to the proportionality expressed by Equation 7.4:

$$\tilde{v} = \frac{1}{2\pi c} \cdot \sqrt{\frac{K}{\mu}} \tag{7.4}$$

where:
  $\tilde{v}$ is the wave number (cm^{-1})
  $c = 300 \cdot 10^{10}\,cm/s$ is the speed of light in vacuum
  K is the stretching force constant (N/m)
  $\mu = M_C \cdot M_O / M_C + M_O$ is the reduced mass (kg)

With increasing time and molarity, the retention of copper by complexation increases
up to certain limit values when equilibrium is attained (Table 7.3). The exception
observed in Table 7.3 regarding the shift in wave number, as a function of temperature, would refer to the conditions of obtaining the KQPSFCu films resulted from the
immersion of KQPSF in a $CuCl_2 \cdot 2H_2O$ aqueous solution. An explanation might be
the excess of chlorine anions among the polymer chains, which prevents complexation between cations and the carbonyl groups.

The initiation of wrinkling and deformation of the polymer matrix is the result
of the electrostatic interactions between Cu^{2+} ions and the ketone groups from the
KQPSF sample, the metal ions distributed among the polymer chains and the complex formations. In time, these contribute to a decrease in the smoothness of the film
surface. The changes in the wavenumber of the analyzed bands are definitely associated with alterations at the macromolecular level, which are illustrated by the AFM
images from Figure 7.11. The bright and dark regions in the AFM images represent
the highest points (or peaks) and valleys (or membrane pores), respectively [119].
Average roughness, root-mean-square roughness, and average surface peak height

TABLE 7.3

Wavenumber of ATR-FTIR Spectra, $\bar{v}$, and Surface Roughness Parameters[a]

Sample	KQPSF	T, °C for KQPSFCu, 48 h and 1.5 M			t, hour for KQPSFCu, 20°C and 1.5 M			M, for KQPSFCu, 20°C and 48 h		
	20	20	40	60	8	24	48	0.5	1.5	3
$\bar{v}$, cm^{-1}	1706	1699	1704	1704	1705	1700	1699	1706	1699	1699
S_a, nm	2.1	41	9	15	16	16	41	24	41	0.8
S_q, nm	3.3	59	14	23	22	27	59	39	59	1
S_z, nm	22.2	288	72	140	135	220	288	205	288	259

Note: [a] Parameters include average roughness, S_a; root mean square roughness, S_q; average surface peak height, S_z, for KQPSF at 20°C; and for KQPSFCu—obtained by KQPSF immersion in CuCl$_2$·2H$_2$O aqueous solution at different time, t; temperature, T; and molarity values, M.

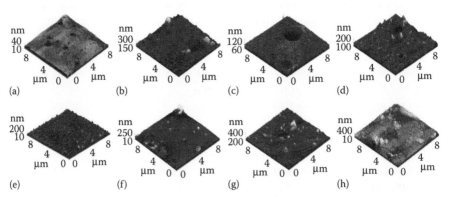

FIGURE 7.11   3D AFM images with $10 \times 10 \mu m^2$ scanned areas of KQPSF (a) and KQPSFCu films obtained by immersion in CuCl$_2$·2H$_2$O aqueous solution under different conditions: (b) 20°C, 48 h, 1.5 M; (c) 40°C, 48 h, 1.5 M; (d) 60°C, 48 h, 1.5 M; (e) 20°C, 8 h, 1.5 M; (f) 20°C, 24 h, 1.5 M; (g) 20°C, 48 h, 0.5 M; (h) 20°C, 48 h, 3.0 M.

are listed in Table 7.3. The modification of wave number of the metal–ligand links involved the appearance of the higher and lower surface roughness values of the compounds, as noted in the AFM images. Also, the retention of metal ions by KQPSF is higher when surface roughness increases. In addition, the differences in surface height between the KQPSF and KQPSFCu films are explained by the occurrence of complex and cross-linked structures.

The results of FTIR and AFM analyses are in good agreement with those obtained by the EDX-SEM spectrometry. The quantitative results of copper after KQPSF immersion in the CuCl$_2$·2H$_2$O aqueous solution extracted from Representative EDX elemental analyses (Figure 7.12) indicate that Cu^{2+} retention is higher for chelate-modified PSF obtained at a temperature of 60°C, time of 48 h, and a molarity of 1.5 M. Due to the complex combinations of copper with the 3-MPK ligand,

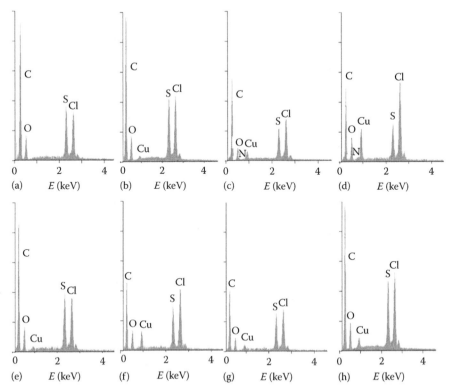

FIGURE 7.12 ESEM profile and analytical results for KQPSF and KQPSFCu films obtained at different temperatures, time, and molarity values. (a) KQPSF film obtained and KQPSFCu films obtained under different conditions: (b) 20°C, 48 h, 1.5 M; (c) 40°C, 48 h, 1.5 M; (d) 60°C, 48 h, 1.5 M; (e) 20°C, 8 h, 1.5 M; (f) 20°C, 24 h, 1.5 M; (g) 20°C, 48 h, 0.5 M; (h) 20°C, 48 h, 3 M.

formations appear, which generate multiple coordinative links among the elements of the different structural units [120].

It is known that generally the presence of transient metal ions in polymeric films affects glass transition temperature (T_g) in two distinct ways [49]. Complex formation between metal cations and the electron donor groups of the polymer chains leads to cross-linking formations, which decreases chain mobility and increases T_g. On the other hand, the formation of distributed complexes in polymer matrices disrupts the uniformity of polymer chains, which decreases both polymer crystallinity and T_g. Moreover, according to DSC studies, the glass transition temperatures of PSF-DMOA and KQPSF are 139.8°C and 174.6°C, respectively (Figure 7.13). In this case, the addition of Cu^{2+} decreases T_g, from 174.6°C for KQPSF, to approximately 165.4°C for KQPSFCu—resulted from KQPSF immersion in a $CuCl_2 \cdot 2H_2O$ aqueous solution, at temperatures of 20°C and 40°C.

This outcome leads to the conclusion that complex formation has a higher effect in disturbing the structural order of the polymer than cross-linking, lowering the value of T_g. In the cases of the KQPSFCu obtained at a higher temperature (60°C),

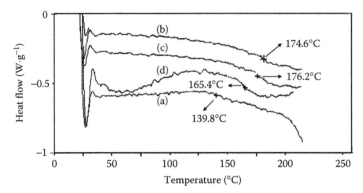

FIGURE 7.13 DSC curves for: (a) PSF-DMOA; (b) KQPSF; (c) KQPSFCu—obtained at temperatures of 20°C and 40°C, time of 48 h and molarity of 1.5 M; (d) KQPSFCu—obtained at temperature of 60°C, time of 48 h and molarity of 1.5 M.

cross-linking formation has a strong effect, slightly increasing the T_g value (176.2°C). Correlating these results with EDX analysis evidences a copper retention value of 9.31 wt%, much higher than that of other KQPSFCu samples. Moreover, a higher percentage of copper ions generates more cross-linking formation. From the results obtained, it may conclude that PSFs functionalized with chelating groups possess specific properties, which make them suitable for wastewater purification.

7.5 GENERAL REMARKS

Functionalized PSF–metal complexes are an important class of new materials due to coupling of the chemical, optical, and electronic properties of the metal moiety to those of the polymer. This chapter offers a broad, interdisciplinary view of the synthesis, characterization, and application of functionalized PSF–metal compounds, demonstrating their importance in different fields, such as technology, biomedicine, and environmental remediation. Thus, the aspects presented in this chapter comprise the special applications of functionalized PSFs, deposition mechanisms of metal nanoparticles and nano-layers on modified PSFs, self-assembly of metal particles on polymeric films, elastoplastic properties of metal layer/PSF complexes, and PSF composites characterized by the formation of metal nanoparticles in PSF matrices or chelating groups in PSFs for heavy metal retention.

Finally, this chapter offers an accessible overview to students, industrial researchers, pharmaceutical innovators, medical and public health personnel, environmental scientists and engineers, and anyone interested in this interdisciplinary field.

REFERENCES

1. Lazaro, N., Sevilla, A. L., Morales, S., and Marques, A. M., Heavy metal biosorption by gellan gum gel beads. *WaterRes.*, 37(21), 2118–2126, 2003.
2. Rhazi, M., Desbrieres, J., Tolaimate, A., Rinaudo, M., Vottero, P., Alagui, A., and El Meray, M., Influence of the nature of the metal ions on the complexation with chitosan. Application to the treatment of liquid waste. *Eur. Polym. J.*, 38(8), 1523–1530, 2002.

3. Rhazi, M., Desbrieres, J., Tolaimate, A., Rinaudo, M., Vottero, P., and Alagui A., Contribution to the study of the complexation of copper by chitosan and oligomers. *Polymer*, 43(4), 1267–1276, 2002.

4. Vinod, V. T. P., Sashidhar, R. B., and Černík, M., Morphology and metal binding characteristics of a natural polymer-kondagogu (*Cochlospermum gossypium*) gum. *Molecules*, 18(7), 8264–8274, 2013.

5. Utgikar, V., Chen, B. Y., Tabak, H. H., Bishop, D. F., and Govind, R., Treatment of acid mine drainage. I: Equilibrium biosorption of zinc and copper on non-viable activated sludge. *Int. Biodeterior. Biodegrad.*, 46(1), 19–28, 2000.

6. Fenger, I. and Le Drian, C., Reusable polymer-supported palladium catalysts: An alternative to tetrakis(triphenylphine) palladium in the suzuki cross-coupling reaction. *Tetrahedron Lett.* 39(24), 4287–4290, 1998.

7. Mizuta, T., Onishi, M., and Miyoshi, K., Photolytic ring-opening polymerization of phosphorous-bridged [1] ferrocenophane coordinating to an organometallic fragment. *Organometallics*, 19(24), 5005–5009, 2000.

8. Orazzhanova, L. K., Yashkarova, H. G., Issue, L. A., and Kudaibergenov, S. E., Binary and ternary polymer-strontium complexes and the capture of radioactive strontium-90 from the polluted soil of the semipalatinsk nuclear test site. *J. Appl. Polym. Sci.*, 87(5), 759–764, 2003.

9. Varvara, S., Muresane, L., Popescu, I. C., and Maurin, G., Copper electrodeposition from sulfate electrolytes in the presence of hydroxyethylated-2-butyne-1, 4-diol. *Hydrometallurgy*, 75(1–4), 147–156, 2004.

10. Ro, K. W., Chang, W. J., Kim, H., Koo, Y. M., and Hahn, J. H., Capilary electrochromatography and preconcentration of neutral compounds on poly(dimethylsiloxane) microchips. *Electrophoresis*, 24(18), 3253–3259, 2003.

11. Varghese, S., Lele, A. K., Sirnivas, D., and Mashellear, R. A., Role of hydrophobicity on structure of polymer-metal complexes. *J. Phys. Chem. B*, 105(23), 5368–5373, 2001.

12. Ahmed, M., Malik, M. A., Pervez, S., and Raffiq, M., Effect of porosity on sulfonation of macroporous styrene-divinylbenzene beads. *Eur. Polym. J.*, 40(8), 1609–1613, 2004.

13. Li, Z., Friedrich, A., and Taubert A., Gold microcrystal synthesis via reduction of $HAuCl_4$ by cellulose in the ionic liquid 1-butyl-3-methyl imidazolium chloride. *J. Mater. Chem.* 18(9), 1008–1014, 2008.

14. Švorčík, V., Kotál, V., Slepicka, P., Bláhová, O., and Šutta, P., Gold coating of polyethylene modified by argon plasma discharge. *Polym. Eng. Sci.* 46(9), 1326–1332, 2006.

15. Haruta, M., Gold as a novel catalyst in the 21st century: Preparation, working mechanism and applications. *Gold Bull.*, 37(1/2), 27–36, 2004.

16. Goia, D. V., Preparation and formation mechanisms of uniform metallic particles in homogeneous solutions. *J. Mater. Chem.*, 14(4), 451–458, 2004.

17. Cheng, M. M. C., Cuda, G., Bunimovich, Y. L., Heath, J. R., Mirkin, C. A., Nijdam, A., Terracciano, J. R., Thundat, T., Ferrari, M., Nanotechnologies for biomolecular detection and medical. *Curr. Opin. Chem. Biol.*, 10, 11–19, 2006.

18. Hering, K., Cialla, D., Ackermann, K., Dörfer, T., Möller, R., Mattheis, R., Fritzsche, W., Rösch, P., and Popp, J., SERS: A versatile tool in chemical and biochemical diagnostics. *Anal. Bioanal. Chem.*, 390(1), 113–124, 2008.

19. Hainfeld, J. F., Slatkin, D. N., and Smilowitz, H. M., The use of gold nanoparticles to enhance radiotherapy in mice. *Phys. Med. Biol.* 49(18), N309–N315, 2004.

20. Sinha, A. K., Seelan, S., Tsubota, S., and Haruta, M., Catalysis by gold nanoparticles: Epoxidation of propene. *Top. Catal.* 29(3/4), 95–102, 2004.

21. Leosson, K., Ingason, A. S., Agnarsson, B., Kossoy, A., Olafsson, S., and Gather, M. C., Ultra-thin gold films on transparent polymers. *Nanophotonics*, 2(1), 3–11, 2013.

22. Ciobanu, M., Marin, L., Cozan, V., and Bruma, M., Aromatic polysulfone used in sensor applications, *Rev. Adv. Mater. Sci.*, 22(1/2), 89–96, 2009.

23. Voicu, S. I., Pandele M. A., Vasile E., Rughinis, R., Crica, L., Pilan L., Ionita, M., The impact of sonication time through polysulfone-graphene oxide composite films properties. *Dig. J. Nanomater. Bios.*, 8(4), 1389–1394, 2013.

24. Cha, D. I., Kim, K. W., Chu, G. H., Kim, H. Y., Lee, K. H., and Bhattarai, N., Mechanical behaviors and characterization of electrospun polysulfone/polyurethane blend nonwovens. *Macromol. Res.*, 14(3), 331–337, 2006.

25. Saxena, P., Gaur, M. S., Shukla, P., and Khare, P. K., Relaxation investigation in polysulfone: Thermally stimulated discharge current and dielectric spectroscopy. *J. Electrostat.*, 66(11), 584–588, 2008.

26. Albu, R. M., Avram, E., Musteata, V. E., Homocianu, M., and Ioan, S., Opto-electrical properties of some quaternized polysulfones. *High. Perform. Polym.*, 23(1), 85–96, 2011.

27. Albu, R. M., Macromolecular assemblies in solution. PhD Thesis, "Petru Poni" Institute of Macromolecular Chemistry, Romanian Academy, Iasi, Romania, Supervisor Ioan, S., 2012.

28. Ersoz, M., Gugul, I. H., Cimen, A., Leylek, B., and Yildiz, S., The sorption of metals on the polysulfone cation exchange membranes. *Turk. J. Chem.* 25(1), 39–48, 2001.

29. Väisänen, P., and Nyström, M., Comparison of polysulfone membranes and polysulfone films. *Acta Polytech. Scand.*, 247, 25–34, 1997.

30. Higuchi, A., Shirano, K., Harashima, M., Yoon, B. O., Hara, M., Hattori, M., and Imamura, K., Chemically modified polysulfone hollow fibers with vinylpyrrolidone having improved blood compatibility. *Biomaterials*, 23(13), 2659–2666, 2002.

31. Tomaszewska, M., Jarosiewicz, A., and Karakulski, K., Physical and chemical characteristics of polymer coatings in CRF formulation. *Desalination*, 146(1), 319–323, 2002.

32. Ydens, I., Moins, S., Degée, P., and Dubois, P., Solution properties of well-defined 2-(dimethylamino)ethyl methacrylate-based (co)polymers: A viscometric approach. *Eur. Polym. J.*, 41(7), 1502–1509, 2005.

33. Ioan, S., Filimon, A., and Avram, E., Influence of the degree of substitution on the solution properties of chloromethylated polysulfone. *J. Appl. Polym. Sci.*, 101(1), 524–531, 2006.

34. Ioan, S., Filimon, A., and Avram, E., Conformational and viscometric behavior of quaternized polysulfone in dilute solution. *Polym. Eng. Sci.*, 46(7), 827–836, 2006.

35. Filimon, A., Avram, E., and Ioan, S., Influence of mixed solvents and temperature on the solution properties of quaternized polysulfones. *J. Macromol. Sci. Part B Phys.*, 46(3), 503–520, 2007.

36. Filimon, A., Albu, R. M., Avram, E., and Ioan, S., Effect of alkyl side chain on the conformational properties of polysulfones with quaternary groups. *J. Macromol. Sci. Part B Phys.*, 49(1), 207–217, 2010.

37. Guan, R., Zou, H., Lu, D., Gong, C., and Liu, Y., Polyethersulfone sulfonated by chlorosulfonic acid and its membrane characteristics. *Eur. Polym. J.*, 41(7), 1554–1560, 2005.

38. Yu, H., Huang, Y., Ying, H., and Xiao, C., Preparation and characterization of a quaternary ammonium derivative of konjac glucomannan. *Carbohydr. Polym.*, 69(1), 29–40, 2007.

39. Filimon, A., Avram, E., Dunca, S., Stoica, I., and Ioan, S., Surface properties and antibacterial activity of quaternized polysulfones. *J. Appl. Polym. Sci.*, 112(3), 1808–1816, 2009.

40. Idris, A., and Zain, N. M., Effect of heat treatment on the performance and structural details of polyethersulfone ultrafiltration membranes. *J. Teknol.*, 44(1), 27–40, 2006.

41. Kochkodan, V., Tsarenko, S., Potapchenko, N., Kosinova, V., and Goncharuk, V., Adhesion of microorganisms to polymer membranes: A photobactericidal effect of surface treatment with TiO_2. *Desalination*, 220(1–3), 380–385, 2008.

42. Cozan, V., Butuc, E., Avram, E., and Airinei, A., Pendant functional group copolyether sulfones: III. Modified copolyether sulfones with bisphenolic copper chelate. *Appl. Organomet. Chem.*, 17(5), 282–286, 2003.

43. Rivas, B. L., Pooley, S. A., Maturana, H. A., and Villegas, S., Metal ions uptake of acrylamide derivatives resins. *Macromol. Chem. Phys.*, 202(3), 443–447, 2001.

44. George, B., Pillai, V. N. R., and Mathew, B. J., Effect of the nature of the crosslinking agent on the metal-ion complexation characteristics of 4 mol% DVB- and NNMBA-crosslinked polyacrylamide-supported glycines. *J. Appl. Polym. Sci.*, 74(14), 3432–3444, 1999.

45. Song, L., Wang, J., Zheng, Q., and Zhang, Z., Characterization of Cu(II) ion adsorption behavior of the polyacrylic acid-polyvinylidene fluoride blended polymer. *Tsinghua Sci. Technol.*, 13(2), 249–256, 2008.

46. Li, W., Zhao, H., Teasdale, P. R., John, R., and Zhang, S., Synthesis and characterization of a polyacrylamide-polyacrylic acid copolymer hydrogel for environmental analysis of Cu and Cd. *React. Funct. Polym.*, 52(1), 31–41, 2002.

47. Pizarro, G. D. C., Marambio, O. G., Jeria-Orell, M., and Huerta, M. R., Preparation, characterization, and thermal properties of hydrophilic polymers: *p*-chlorophenylmaleimides with hydroxyethyl methacrylate and β-methylitaconate. *Polym. Int.*, 56(1), 93–103, 2007.

48. Albu, R. M., Avram, E., Stoica, I., and Ioan, S., Polysulfones with chelating groups for heavy metals retention. *Polym. Compos.*, 33(4), 573–581, 2012.

49. Esmaeili, M., Madaeni, S. S., and Barzin, J., The dependence of morphology of solid polymer electrolyte membranes on transient salt type: Effect of cation type. *Polym. Int.*, 59(7), 1006–1013, 2010.

50. Albu, R. M., Avram, E., Musteata, V. E., and Ioan, S., Dielectric relaxation and AC-conductivity of modified polysulfones with chelating groups. *J. Solid State Electrochem.*, 18(3), 785–794, 2014.

51. Siegel, J., and Kotál, V., Preparation of thin metal layers on polymers. *Acta Polytech.*, 47(1), 9–11, 2007.

52. Tian, W. J., Zhang, H. Y., and Shen, J. C., Some properties of interfaces between metals and polymers. *Surf. Rev. Lett.*, 4(4), 703–708, 1997.

53. Birgerson, J., Fahlman, M., Bröms, P., and Salaneck W. R., Conjugated polymer surfaces and interfaces: A mini-review and some new results. *Synth. Met.*, 80(2), 125–130, 1996.

54. Rånby, B., Surface modification and lamination of polymers by photografting. *Int. J. Adhes. Adhes.*, 19(5), 337–343, 1999.

55. Siau, S., Vervaet, A., Schacht, E., Degrande, S., Callewaert, K., and van Calster, A., Chemical modification of buildup epoxy surfaces for altering the adhesion of electrochemically deposited copper. *J. Electrochem. Soc.*, 152(9), d136–d150, 2005.

56. Liston, E. M., Martinu L., and Wertheimer, M.R., Plasma surface modification of polymers for improved adhesion: A critical review. *J. Adhesion Sci. Technol.*, 7(10), 1091–1127, 1993.

57. Jem-Kun Chen, J. K., and Chang, C. J., Fabrications and applications of stimulus-responsive polymer films and patterns on surfaces: A review. *Materials*, 7(2), 805–875, 2014.

58. Culbertson, E. C., Metal adhesion to PET film. *PLACE Conference*, September 16-20, St. Louis, MO, 2007. http://www.tappi.org/content/events/07place/papers/culbertson.pdf.

59. Daniel, M. C., and Astruc, D., Gold nanoparticles: Assembly, supramolecular chemistry, quantum-size-related properties, and applications toward biology, catalysis, and nanotechnology. *Chem. Rev.*, 104, 293–346, 2004.

60. Albu, R. M., Stoica, I., Avram, E., Ioanid, E. G., and Ioan, S., Gold layers on untreated and plasma-treated substrates of quaternized polysulfones. *J. Solid State Electrochem.*, 18(10), 2803–2813, 2014.

61. Sanchis, M. R., Calvo, O., Fenollar, O., Garcia, D., and Balart, R., Characterization of the surface changes and the aging effects of low-pressure nitrogen plasma treatment in a polyurethane film. *Polym. Test.*, 27(1), 75–83, 2008.

62. Albu, R. M., Avram, E., Stoica, I., Ioanid, E. G., Popovici, D., and Ioan, S., Surface properties and compatibility with blood of new quaternized polysulfones. *J. Biomat. Nanobiotechnol.*, 2(2), 114–124, 2011.

63. Ioan, S., Albu, R. M., Avram, E., Stoica, I., and Ioanid, E. G., Surface characterization of quaternized polysulfone films and biocompatibility studies. *J. Appl. Polym. Sci.*, 121(1), 127–137, 2011.

64. Gadre, K. S., and Alford, T. L., Contact angle measurements for adhesion energy evaluation of silver and copper films on parylene-*n* and SiO$_2$ substrates. *J. Appl. Phys.*, 93(2), 919–923, 2003.

65. Lee, J. H., Hwang, K. S., Kim, T. S., Seong, J. W., Yoon, K. H., and Ahn, S., Effect of oxygen plasma treatment on adhesion improvement of Au deposited on Pa-c substrates, *J. Korean Phys. Soc.*, 44(5), 1177–1181, 2004.

66. Leite, F. L., Bueno, C. C., Da Róz, A. L., Ziemath, E. C., and Oliveira, O. N., Theoretical models for surface forces and adhesion and their measurement using atomic force microscopy. *Int. J. Mol. Sci.*, 13(10), 12773–12856, 2012.

67. Schirmeisen, A., Weiner, D., and Fuchs, H., Measurements of metal–polymer adhesion properties with dynamic force spectroscopy. *Surface Sci.*, 545(3) 155–162, 2003.

68. Yeager, J. D. and Bahr, D. F., Microstructural characterization of thin gold films on a polyimide substrate. *Thin Solid Films*, 518(21), 5896–5900, 2010.

69. Sader, J. E., Chon, J. W. M., and Mulvaney, P., Calibration of rectangular atomic force microscope cantilevers. *Rev. Sci. Instrum.*, 70(10), 3967–3969, 1999.

70. Sader, E., Pacifico, J., Green, C. P., and Mulvaney, P., General scaling law for stiffness measurement of small bodies with applications to the atomic force microscope. *J. Appl. Phys.*, 97(12), 124903–124909, 2005.

71. Noy, A., Vezenov, D. V., and Lieber, C. M., Chemical force microscopy. *Annu. Rev. Mater. Sci.*, 27, 381–421, 1997.

72. Supriya, L. and Claus, R. O., Solution-based assembly of conductive gold film on flexible polymer substrates. *Langmuir*, 20(20), 8870–8876, 2004.

73. Caruso, F., Nanoengineering of particle surfaces. *Adv. Mater.*, 13(1), 1122, 2001.

74. Schmitt, J., Mächtle, P., Eck, D., Möhwald, H., and Helm, C. A., Preparation and optical properties of colloidal gold monolayers. *Langmuir*, 15(9), 3256–3266, 1999.

75. Jin, Y., Kang, X., Song, Y., Zhang, B., Cheng, G., and Dong, S., Controlled nucleation and growth of surface-confined gold nanoparticles on a (3-aminopropyl)trimethoxysilane modified glass slide: A strategy for SPR substrates. *Anal. Chem.*, 73(13), 2843–2849, 2001.

76. Grabar, K. C., Freeman, R. G., Hommer, M. B., and Natan, M. J., Preparation and characterization of Au colloid monolayers. *Anal. Chem.*, 67(4), 735–743, 1995.

77. Doron, A., Katz, E., and Willner, I., Organization of Au colloids as monolayer films onto ITO glass surfaces: Application of the metal colloid films as base interfaces to construct redox-active monolayers. *Langmuir*, 11(4), 1313–1317, 1995.

78. Hidber, P. C., Helbig, W., Kim, E., and Whitesides, G. M., Microcontact printing of palladium colloids: Micron-scale patterning by electroless deposition of copper. *Langmuir*, 12(5), 1375–1380, 1996.

79. Fellah, F., Schoenstein, F., Dakhlaoui-Omrani, A., Chérif, S. M., Dirras, G., and Jouini, N., Nanostructured cobalt powders synthesised by polyol process and consolidated by spark plasma sintering: Microstructure and mechanical properties. *Mater. Character.*, 69, 1–8, 2012.

80. Langdon, T. G., The principle of grain refinement in equal-channel angular pressing. *Mater. Sci. Eng. Part A*, 462(1/2), 3–11, 2007.

81. Wetscher, F., Vorhauer, A., and Pippan, R., Strain hardening during high pressure torsion deformation. *Mater. Sci. Eng. Part A*, 410–411, 213–216, 2005.

82. Wu, X., Tao, N., Hong, Y., Liu, G., Xu, B., Lu, J., and Lu, K., Strain-induced grain refinement of cobalt during surface mechanical attrition treatment. *Acta Mater.*, 53(3), 681–691, 2005.

83. Abdul-Latif, A., Dirras, G. F., Ramtani, S., and Hocini A., A new concept for producing ultrafine grained metallic structures via an intermediate strain rate: Experiments and modeling. *Int. J. Mech. Sci.*, 51(11/12), 797–806, 2009.

84. Erb, U., Electrodeposited nanocrystals: Synthesis, properties and industrial applications. *Nanostruct. Mater.*, 6(5–8), 533–538, 1995.

85. Rajagopalan, J., Han, J. H., and Saif, M. T. A., Plastic deformation recovery in free-standing nanocrystalline aluminum and gold thin films. *Science*, 315(5820), 1831–1834, 2007.

86. Meyers, M. A., Mishra, A., and Benson, D. J., Mechanical properties of nanostructured materials. *Prog. Mater. Sci.*, 51(4), 427–556, 2006.

87. Greer, J. R., Oliver, W. C., and Nix, W. D., Size dependence of mechanical properties of gold at the micronscale in the absence of strain gradients. *Acta. Mater.*, 53(6), 1821–1830, 2005.

88. Aviles, F., Llanes, L., and Oliva, A. I., Elasto-plastic properties of gold thin films deposited onto polymeric substrates. *J. Mater. Sci.*, 44(10), 2590–2598, 2009.

89. Xiang, Y., Li, T., Suo Z., and Vlassak, J. J., High ductility of a metal film adherent on a polymer substrate. *Appl. Phys. Lett.*, 87(16), 161910–161913, 2005.

90. Li, T. and Suo, Z., Deformability of thin metal films on elastomer substrates. *Int. J. Solids Struct.*, 43(7/8), 2351–2363, 2006.

91. Niu, R. M., Liu, G., Wang, C., Zhang, G., Ding X. D., and Sun, J., Thickness dependent critical strain in submicron Cu films adherent to polymer substrate. *Appl. Phys. Lett.*, 90(16), 161907, 2007.

92. Avilés, F., Oliva, A.I., and May-Pat, A., Determination of elastic modulus in a bimaterial through a one dimensional laminated model. *J. Mater. Eng. Perform.*, 17(4), 482–488, 2008.

93. Cao, Y., Allameh, S., Nankivil, D., Sethiaraj, S., Otiti, T., and Soboyejo, W., Nanoindentation measurements of the mechanical properties of polycrystalline Au and Ag thin films on silicon substrates: Effects of grain size and film thickness. *Mater. Sci. Eng., Part A*, 427(1/2), 232–240, 2006.

94. Pastoriza-Santos, I. and Liz-Marzan, L.M., Formation and stabilization of silver nanoparticles through reduction by *N,N*-dimethylformamide. *Langmuir*, 15(4), 948–951, 1999.

95. Taurozzia, J. S., Arul, H., Bosak, V. Z., Burban, A. F., Voice, T. C., Bruening, M. L., and Tarabara, V. V., Effect of filler incorporation route on the properties of polysulfone-silver nanocomposite membranes of different porosities. *J. Membr. Sci.*, 325(1), 58–68, 2008.

96. Meyer, D. E. and Bhattacharyya, D., Impact of membrane immobilization on particle formation and trichloroethylene dechlorination for bimetallic Fe/Ni nanoparticles in cellulose acetate membranes. *J. Phys. Chem. B*, 111(25) 7142–7154, 2007.

97. Genne, I., Kuypers, S., and Leysen, R., Effect of the addition of ZrO_2 to polysulfone based UF membranes. *J. Membr. Sci.*, 113(2) 343–350, 1996.

98. Aerts, P., Genne, I., Kuypers, S., Leysen, R., Vankelecom, I. F. J., and Jacobs, P. A., Polysulfone-aerosil composite membranes. Part 2. The influence of the addition of aerosil on the skin characteristics and membrane properties. *J. Membr. Sci.*, 178(1/2), 1–11, 2000.

99. Aerts, P., VanHoof, E., Leysen, R., Vankelecom, I. F. J., and Jacobs, P. A., Polysulfone–aerosil composite membranes. Part 1. The influence of the addition of aerosil on the formation process and membrane morphology. *J. Membr. Sci.* 176(1) 63–73, 2000.

100. Monticelli, O., Bottino, A., Scandale, I., Capannelli, G., and Russo S., Preparation and properties of polysulfone–clay composite membranes. *J. Appl. Polym. Sci.* 103(6), 3637–3644, 2007.

101. Yang, Y., Zhang, H., Wang, P., Zheng, Q., and Li, J., The influence of nano-sized TiO_2 fillers on the morphologies and properties of PSF UF membrane. *J. Membr. Sci.*, 288(1/2), 231–238, 2007.

102. Yu, D. G., Teng, M. Y., Chou, W. L., and Yang, M. C., Characterization and inhibitory effect of antibacterial PAN-based hollow fiber loaded with silver nitrate. *J. Membr. Sci.* 225(1/2), 115–123. 2003.

103. Son, W. K., Youk, J. H., Lee, T. S., and Park, W. H., Preparation of antimicrobial ultrafine cellulose acetate fibers with silver nanoparticles. *Macromol. Rapid Commun.*, 25(18), 1632–1637, 2004.

104. Chou, W. L., Yu, D. G., and Yang, M. C., The preparation and characterization of silver loading cellulose acetate hollow fiber membrane for water treatment. *Polym. Advan. Technol.*, 16(8), 600–607, 2005.

105. Wara, N. M., Francis, L. F., and Velamakanni, B. V., Addition of alumina to cellulose acetate membranes. *J. Membr. Sci.*, 104(1/2), 43–49, 1995.

106. Yan, L., Li, Y. S., Xiang, C. B., and Xianda S., Effect of nano-sized Al_2O_3-particle addition on PVDF ultrafiltration membrane performance. *J. Membr. Sci.*, 276(1/2), 162–167, 2006.

107. Bottino, A., Capannelli, G., and Comite, A., Preparation and characterization of novel porous PVDF–ZrO_2 composite membranes. *Desalination*, 146(1–3), 35–40, 2002.

108. Li, J. B., Zhu, J. W., and Zheng, M. S., Morphologies and properties of poly(phthalazinone ether sulfone ketone) matrix ultrafiltration membranes with entrapped TiO2 nanoparticles. *J. Appl. Polym. Sci.*, 103(6), 3623–3629, 2006.

109. Bottino, A., Capannelli, G., D'Asti, V., and Piaggio, P., Preparation and properties of novel organic–inorganic porous membranes. *Separ. Purif. Technol.*, 22–23, 269–275, 2001.

110. He, X., Shi, Q., Zhou, X., Wan, C., and Jiang, C., In situ composite of nano SiO_2-P(VDFHFP) porous polymer electrolytes for Li-ion batteries. *Electrochim. Acta*, 51(6), 1069–1075, 2005.

111. Richards, H. L., Baker, P. G. L., and Iwuoha, E., Metal nanoparticle modified polysulfone membranes for use in wastewater treatment: A critical review. *J. Surf. Eng. Mater. Adv. Techn.*, 2(3A), 183–193, 2012.

112. Landaburu-Aguirre, J., García, V., Pongrácz, E., and Keiski, R., Applicability of membrane technologies for the removal of heavy metals. *Desalination*, 200(1–3), 272–273, 2006.

113. Araneda, C., Fonseca, C., Sapag, J., Basualto, C., Yazdani-Pedram, M., Kondo, K., Kamio, E., and Valenzuela, F., Removal of metal ions from aqueous solutions by sorption onto microcapsules prepared by copolymerization of ethylene glycol dimethacrylate with styrene. *Sep. Purif. Technol.*, 63(3), 517–523, 2008.

114. Mocioi, M., Albu, A. M., Mateescu, C., Voicu, G., Rusen, E., Marculescu, B., and Mutihac, L., New polymeric structures designed for the removal of Cu(II) ions from aqueous solutions. *J. Appl. Polym. Sci.*, 103(3), 1397–1405, 2007.

115. Lebrun, L., Vallée, F., Alexandre, B., and Nguyen, Q., Preparation of chelating membranes to remove metal cations from aqueous solutions. *Desalination*, 207(1–3), 9–23, 2007.

116. Vasiliu, S., Racovita, S., Neagu, V., Popa, M., and Desbrieres, J., Polymer-metal complexes based on gellan, *Polimery*, 55(11/12), 839–845, 2010.

117. An, B., Fu, Z., Xiong, Z., Zhao, D., and Sengupta A. K., Synthesis and characterization of a new class of polymeric ligand exchangers for selective removal of arsenate from drinking water. *React. Funct. Polym.*, 70(8), 497–507, 2010.

118. Kim, J. H., Min, B. R., Kim, C. K., Won, J., and Kang, Y. S., New insights into the coordination mode of silver ions dissolved in poly(2-ethyl-2-oxazoline) and its relation to facilitated olefin transport. *Macromolecules*, 35(13), 5250–5255, 2002.

119. Rahimpour, A., Madaeni, S. S., Shockravi, A., Ghorbani, S., Preparation and characterization of hydrophile nano-porous polyethersulfone membranes using synthesized poly(sulfoxide-amide) as additive in the casting solution. *J. Membr. Sci.*, 334, 64–73, 2009.
120. Breeze, S. R., Wang, S., Greedan, J. E., and Raju, N. P., Copper and bismuth complexes containing dipyridyl gem-diolato ligands: BiIII2[2-PY)2CO(OH]2(O2CCF3)4(THF)2,CUII-[(2-PY)2CO(OH)]2(HO2CCH3)2 and CUII4[(2-PY)2CO(OH)]2(O2CCH3)6(H2O)2, a ferromagnetically coupled tetranuclear copper(II) chain. *Inorg. Chem.*, 35(24), 6944–6951, 1996.

8 Biocompatibility of Polysulfone Compounds

Silvia Ioan and Luminta-Ioana Buruiana

CONTENTS

8.1 INTRODUCTION

Different materials, including polysulfones, polyurethanes, polyamides, silicone rubber, and polysaccharides, are used in biomedical domains, as implant materials, tissue engineering scaffolds, blood-contacting devices, and disposable clinical apparatus [1–4]. To establish blood-compatible polymeric compounds, bio-reactions and bio-responses involving the adhesion of blood components, platelet adhesion, plasma protein phase, and coagulation process activation must be known [5,6]. Adverse reactions of cellular response caused by polymeric materials are major subjects in the fundamental research of biomedical polymers. Thus, in order to obtain the desired properties of biomedical applications, studies concerning a delicate control of interactions between blood and surface of the polymer compound should be performed [7]. Generally, blood is a fluid consisting of red blood cells ($4.2–6.2·10^6/mm^3$, 99.9%), white blood cells, or leukocytes, ($5–9·10^3/mm^3$, <0.1%), platelets ($250–400·10^3/mm^3$, <0.1%), and a intracellular liquid substance (plasma) consisting of a water solution with protein and salts. Blood fixes oxygen in the lungs and transports it to the tissues and cells of the whole body; in the intestine, it also takes the nutrients resulting from digestion and intestinal absorption, transporting them for use in the tissues and organs. The unnecessary substances resulting from the cellular assimilation and nonassimilation are carried by the blood to the bodies responsible for transformation and elimination. Blood (which constitutes about 8% of the total body weight of the human organism, with a volume around 5 liters, in adults) has also the role of transporting the hormones produced by the endocrine glands. White blood cells play the important role of defending the body against microbes, destroying them by phagocytosis (potting and digestion) or immunological (antibodies) processes. Outside the body, the blood coagulates, due to the transformation of fibrinogen—a protein occurring in solution in plasma—into fibrin, under the action of various coagulation factors present in the plasma and platelets. Plasma without fibrinogen becomes a serum. On the other hand, plasma proteins in the body of 7% (albumin—58%, globulins—38%, and fibrinogen—4%) have multiple roles in establishing and carrying water or other substances in protecting the body against infection (immunological function by γ-globulin, antibodies) to achieve coagulation and hemostasis with the fibrinogen and coagulation factors existing in the plasma, and to meet different enzymatic activities. Besides proteins, some mineral salts (Na^+, K^+, Ca^{2+}, Mg^{2+}, Cl^-, HCO_3^-, HPO_4^{2-}, SO_4^{2-}), organic nutrients (lipids, carbohydrates, amino acids), and organic wastes (urea, uric acid, creatine, bilirubin), which contribute to the preservation of the biological constants of blood and fluids in maintaining tissue reactivity, may also be found in the plasma. Each of these blood components has a specific role that should not be disrupted by the presence of foreign materials.

A considerable attention has been devoted in the scientific literature to the investigation of new applications of polysulfones in biomedical fields. Chain rigidity and toughness derived from the relatively inflexible and immobile phenyl and SO_2 groups, and from the connecting ether oxygen, as well as their intrinsic hydrophobic nature precludes their use in the some applications that require a hydrophilic character. Therefore, the chemical modification of polysulfones, especially by the chloromethylation reaction, is a subject of considerable interest from both theoretical and practical viewpoints, including obtaining precursors for functional membranes, coatings, ion exchange resins, ion exchange fibers, and selectively permeable membranes [8–10]. Functionalized polymers, chloromethylated and quaternized polysulfones, and block copolymers able to form nanostructures, including nanospheres, nanofibers, nanochannels, as well as blends between polysulfone or modified polysulfones, and other synthetic polymers have evidenced several interesting properties useful in biomedical applications. Furthermore, the addition of functional groups to the polysulfone can enhance some properties of the material, such as hydrophilicity (of special interest for biomedical applications) [11], antimicrobial action [12], solubility characteristics [13,14], allowing higher water permeability, and better separation [15,16]. In addition, the functional groups are an intrinsic requirement for affinity, ion exchange, and other specialty membranes [17]. From these reasons, this chapter will present some recent applications of polysulfone compounds.

8.2 BIOCOMPATIBLE HEMODIALYSIS MEMBRANES

The literature shows that the interactions between blood and the hemodialysis membrane from cellulosic materials include complement activation, direct activation of cellular components, and the initiation of the coagulation cascade [18]. Studies have established that synthetic polysulfone membranes can minimize the effect of complement activation and improve the biocompatibility of synthetic versus cellulosic membranes [19]. However, Jams and Post [18] draw attention on the scarce knowledge concerning different biocompatibilities of membranes made from the same type of polysulfones by different manufacturers, for example, Fresenius Medical Care Optiflux polysulfone membrane (F-160) or Asahi REXEED 25S polysulfone membrane (AR-25S). The thrombogenicity difference between AR-25S and other polysulfone membranes is generated by the chemical nature of the internal membrane surface, consisting of polysulfone/polyvinylpirrolidone copolymers. Also, it is observed that differences in the membrane composition may be responsible for these findings. Literature shows that thrombogenicity and protein absorption of these membranes decrease with the formation of a few nanometers-thick hydrogel layer [20].

Therefore, in the hemodialysis process (defined as a widely used treatment for kidney failure), biocompatibility represents a sum of specific interactions between blood and the artificial materials of the hemodialysis circuit, and can be evaluated by the *inflammatory response* degree [21]. Generally, artificial materials from synthetic polymers are grouped by their hydrophobic and hydrophilic characteristics. The hydrophobic membranes (such as those obtained from polysulfone, polymethylmethacrylate, and polyacrylonitrile) are apolar, have a low energy of interaction with water, adsorb proteins, are more porous, and have high ultrafiltration coefficients. Among other materials, polysulfone-based membranes show outstanding oxidative, thermal, and hydrolytic stability; good mechanical and film-forming characteristics; and permeability for low-molecular-weight proteins, being widely acknowledged as providing an optimal biocompatibility in terms of solute removal and complement activation [22].

Although polysulfone is extensively used as a membrane material, its hydrophobic nature does not recommend it for blood-contacting applications [23]. Adsorption of serum proteins onto polysulfone hemodialysis membranes can cause serious or life-threatening complications, due to the activation of the complement alternative pathways [C1] and [C3] (a group of blood proteins that mediate the specific antibody response). Anticoagulants are often administered during dialysis treatments to avoid clot formation. Protein deposition on membranes during dialysis additionally reduces throughput and results in modified rejection characteristics. In this context, different researchers created hydrophilic polysulfone membrane surfaces using a variety of methods summarized by Park et al. [23]:

- Hydrophilic polymer coatings deposited onto polysulfone surfaces.
- Hydrophilic layers graft-polymerized onto polysulfone membranes using radical reactions generated with low-temperature plasma.
- Ultraviolet or gamma radiation.
- Chemical reaction of hydrophilic components onto the membrane surface or bulk polysulfone, using, for example, radiation techniques to graft polymerize hydrophilic monomers such as 2-hydroxy-ethyl methacrylate, acrylic acid, and methacrylic acid onto polysulfone membrane surfaces. The resulting membranes showed increased flux and higher bovine serum albumin (BSA) retention than unmodified polysulfone membranes.
- Chemically grafted sulfonyl and hydroxyl end-terminated groups onto polysulfone membrane surfaces and obtaining of reduced protein adsorption.
- Chemical modification of bulk polysulfone using lithiation chemistry, by the incorporation of hydrophilic components, such as carboxylated and hydroxylated derivatives.

Amphiphilic graft copolymers with polysulfone backbones and poly(ethylene glycol) side chain [synthesized reaction of an alkoxide formed from poly(ethylene glycol) and a base (sodium hydride) with chloromethylated polysulfone] become hydrophilic materials, even if water insoluble, which makes them suitable as potential biomaterial coatings. Their films exhibit high resistance to protein adsorption and cell attachment. When used as an additive in polysulfone membranes prepared by immersion precipitation, the graft copolymer preferentially segregates to the membrane surface, delivering enhanced wettability, porosity, and protein resistance compared to unmodified polysulfone membranes [23].

The surface properties of these membranes render them desirable candidates for hemodialysis.

8.3 BIOCOMPATIBILITY IN THE MEDICAL DEVICE INDUSTRY OF POLYSULFONE COMPOUNDS

As in the case of other polymeric compounds, the utilization of different polysulfones for medical devices must ensure biocompatibility, which includes the ability of a material to act without causing negative effects on the immunological basic functions of the body. Generally, biomaterials and cell surfaces coming into contact with the tissue and blood are analyzed especially in terms of their biocompatibility. These materials are used in therapeutic medicine as implants (e.g., heart valves and stents), extracorporeal circuits (e.g., in hemodialysis or cardiopulmonary bypass surgery), bioengineered devices (e.g., pumps or drug delivery vehicles), soft and hard tissue implants, whole organ transplants, and cell therapies. As they can sometimes negatively affect clinical outcomes by activating defense systems—such as the complement, contact, and coagulation cascades, and contribute to anaphylactoid reactions, ischemia-reperfusion injury, thromboinflammation, and immune responses that negatively affect the clinical outcome—several studies develop methods for maintaining the anticipated functions, thus avoiding adverse effects [24]. The literature presents different evaluations, such as thermal and mechanical tests, implants, intracutaneous and systemic injection, for establishing the biocompatibility [25]. Most of the biocompatible plastics having undergone stringent tests before they can be used as medical devices include the following medical classes of polymers:

- *Polyvinyl chloride*—for blood bags and blood tubing
- *Polycarbonate*—for medical instruments and containers with glass-like transparency, check valves, and tubing connectors
- *Polyetherimide*—for reusable and sterilizable applications, or as surgical skin staplers
- *Polypropylene*—heart valve structures
- *Polysulfone*—for surgical and medical devices, clamps, artificial heart components, and heart valves
- *Polyethersulfone*—for single and multilumen tubing and catheters
- *Polyurethane*—breathable wound dressings
- *Polytetrafluoroethylene*—for catheter linings, single and multilumen tubing, synthetic blood vessels, endoscopes, surgical sutures, reconstructive surgery, and soft tissue regeneration patches

- *Polyethylene*—surgical cables, artificial tendons and orthopedic sutures, and tubing
- *Polycarbonate*—medical instruments and containers with glass-like transparency, check valves, and tubing connectors
- *Polyetheretherketone*—dentistry products and rigid tubing

Recently, Solvay Specialty Polymers, part of Belgian Chemical and Plastics Manufacturer Solvay, has presented two medical applications for its sulfone polymer technology—an implantable drug infusion system made of polysulfone resin, and a highly durable nonimplantable impeller for blowers and fans made of polyphenylsulfone resin [26]. Thus, an implantable catheter port made from polysulfone resin has been developed. The resin was selected for its biocompatibility and dimensional stability, and was used to improve a previous all-titanium model of the port. This new port system, the Plastics Low Profile model, is said to be versatile and highly reliable for the delivery of drugs, antibiotics, and nutrient-therapy solutions. The system is lightweight and cost effective, and features a low-profile polysulfone housing suitable for all patients. The catheter port is a multipiece assembly consisting of an injection-molded housing, a ring component, and a titanium inner chamber.

On the other hand, high-performance thermoplastics, replacing competitive materials such as modified polyphenylene ethers, and offering improved stress crack performance, were presented by Solvay Specialty Polymers. Modified polyphenylene ether is a *super-tough thermoplastic* with high heat resistance, hydrolytic stability, and chemical resistance. It can withstand over 1000 cycles of steam sterilization without significant loss of properties; it is inherently flame retardant and resistant to bases and other chemicals.

In the context of modern techniques, the literature presents new effective methods in image analysis, covering segmentation, registration, and visualization and focuses on the key theories, algorithms, and applications that have emerged from recent progress recorded in computer vision, imaging, and computational biomedical science. Recently, Farag elaborated on a solid overview of the field—signals, systems, image formation and modality, stochastic models, computational geometry, level set methods, and tools and computer-aided design models—for biomedical image analysis [27]. On the other hand, Slevin presented some nanotechnologies for new medical therapies, more rapid and sensitive diagnosis instruments for normal and diseased tissues [28]. Chapters 9 and 10 include nanobiological approaches to imaging, diagnosis, and the treatment of disease using targeted monoclonal antibodies, the medical use of nanomaterials, nanoelectronic biosensors, and possible future applications of molecular nanotechnology for cell repair. Generally, studies in the field are conducted with respect to the requirements of the modern scientific context, to obtain superior medical solutions and convenient costs. From these materials, researchers developed a number of medical devices that are now largely used as heart valve prostheses, left ventricular assist devices, pacemakers, vascular grafts, stents, artificial kidney, hip and knee prostheses, dental implants, intraocular lenses, and breast implants [29,30]. Thus, short carbon fiber–reinforced composites can replace some of the metal alloys used in orthopedic implants. In particular, polysulfone and polyetheretherketone have been considered as the matrix material for carbon fiber–reinforced composite implant materials. To determine the *in vitro* biocompatibility between a carbon fiber composite of polyetheretherketone and a carbon fiber–reinforced polysulfone composite, ASTM standards F813 and F619 were employed for direct contact cell culture evaluation and extraction [31]. The cell cultures were evaluated qualitatively by microscopy and quantitatively by enzyme assay, to determine cytotoxicity.

The most important property of biomedical devices is represented by their biocompatibility, to avoid different side effects, such as formation of clot or thrombus composed of various blood elements, shedding or nucleation of emboli, destruction of circulating blood components, or activation of the complement system, and other immunologic pathways [30].

The first step in the detection of toxic materials or materials that do not react with blood or coagulant factors is to obtain information on the possible modification of the physicochemical properties of polymer surfaces [32]. Surface modification of the polymers present in a polysulfone hollow-fiber hemodialyzer by covalent binding of heparin or endothelial cell surface heparin sulfate, while observation of flow characteristics and platelet adhesion, shows that endothelial cell surface heparin sulfate represents a promising method for improving membrane properties and for generating biocompatibility characteristics similar to those of natural blood vessels [33]. Polysulfone hollow-fiber membranes have been widely used in blood purification, in spite of their low biocompatibility. To improve biocompatibility, the polysulfone/d-α -tocopheryl polyethylene glycol 1000 succinate composite hollow-fiber membranes and 2-methacryloyloxyethyl phosphorylcholine-coated polysulfone hollow-fiber membranes have been prepared, with good results. The effects of these implanted membrane materials on liver, kidney, and so on have been studied by hematology, serum biochemistry, and peritoneal fluid cytology. Tissue and immunological responses to hollow-fiber membranes have been evaluated using histopathological observations and immunohistochemistry [34].

On the other hand, the modification of polysulfone/poly(vinylidene fluoride) surface properties by oxygen plasma treatment and dopamine coating on these two polymers for acquiring a better biocompatibility was realized [35]. All modification steps were verified by electron spectroscopy for chemical analysis, contact angle, atomic force, and scanning electron microscopy measurements. The effects of surface modifications on protein adsorption and cell attachments have been tested with BSA and L-929 mouse fibroblasts. Thus, biocompatibility was promoted to twofold and fourfold on both hydrophobic polysulfone and poly(vinylidene fluoride), by applying oxygen plasma treatments, whereas simple immobilization of polymers in dopamine solution lead to a hydrophilic surface coating with increased stability and biocompatibility.

Several studies have reported the surface modification of polysulfone and polysulfone membranes with potential use in biomedical fields through chemical methods—wet chemical reaction, photochemical method, plasma treatment, and so on—or physical methods—blending, coating, physical adsorption, and so on [36]. Polysulfone membranes are widely employed in advanced separation technology and biomedical fields as artificial organs and medical devices used for blood purification—hemodialysis, hemodiafiltration, hemofiltration, plasmapheresis, and plasma collection. From these studies arise the idea that, in contact with blood, proteins will rapidly adsorb onto the surface of the membrane and also that the adsorbed protein layer may lead to further undesirable results, such as platelet adhesion, aggregation, and coagulation. As a consequence, the blood compatibility of the membrane is not adequate, and injections of anticoagulants are needed during its clinical application. Therefore, it is necessary to modify the membrane surface to improve blood compatibility. One of the materials that can be used in these modifications is serum albumin—a protein of highest concentration in the plasma of prime importance in maintaining the osmotic pressure of blood, which can be regarded as a naturally occurring and highly specific functional biopolymer, to be used as a polymeric material. To reduce deposition of the protein from the modified membrane, grafting of acrylic acid onto the polysulfone and polyethersulfone membrane (through heterogeneous photoinitiated grafting polymerization), followed by BSA immobilization on their surface, were realized. Similar methods were adopted to investigate the adsorptive and covalent binding of a variety of proteins and peptides to poly(D,L-lactide) grafted with poly(acrylic acid). Liu et al. [36] show that it is difficult to modify the internal surface of hollow-fiber membranes, because the diameter of the fiber is very small, hardly permitting modification through UV radiation. In addition, the photochemical method may have some adverse effect on the molecular structure of the membrane. Replacing the photochemical treatment by blending the polyethersulfone with the copolymer of acrylic acid and N-vinylpyrrolidone, followed by the immobilization of BSA onto the surface, leads to obtaining membranes with a good biocompatibility.

Thus, it can be concluded that BSA immobilized onto the polysulfone membrane surface plays an important role in improving blood compatibility. Cell-culture results demonstrated that BSA immobilized onto the membrane surface promoted endothelial cell adhesion and proliferation, leading to the production of biomaterials with potential use in blood-contacting apparatuses and many other artificial organs.

Biocompatibility of any material involves the study of different phases, both the receptor tissue and the implant, at macroscopic and microscopic levels [37]:

- Macroscopic analysis provides important information regarding the healing process, which, even it involving a number of inflammatory phenomena, was free of complications for polyslfone and ultra-high-molecular-weight polyethylene materials. The findings about a good-quality healing and an adequate interaction of the implant, without presence of local hyperemia, are early clues of material toleration by the receptor tissue.
- Microscopic evaluation, on the other hand, gives the cellular and receptor tissue response as a whole, so that immunologic and metabolic systems can participate and express their influence when facing substances released by implant degradation. Both testing material and control must be implanted as particles and rods. Particles aim to increase contact surface and facilitate implant integration, sensitizing the inflammatory response and toxic effects. Comparative analysis of the cellular population in both acute and evolution stages, as well as quantitative and qualitative features associated to cellular necrosis and vessel neoformation, are important to characterize implant compatibility.

Another aspect studied over the years has been directed toward obtaining dialyzer membranes, with maximum potential to retain toxins. Hörl [38] and Mansoor [39] discuss the different advantages and disadvantages of synthetic membranes and the possible optimization techniques for toxin removal through these membranes.

Besides defining the biocompatibility of hemodialysis membranes in the context of traditional membranes or upcoming trends, the activation of the terminal pathway of complement during hemodialysis, indices of complement activation allied with the hemodialysis membranes, and/or adsorption of dialysis membranes as an index of biocompatibility should be studied. These investigations stipulate that the synthetic membranes, including polysulfone, can be structurally symmetrical and asymmetrical and have a minimum wall thickness of 20 μm. To avoid too much protein adsorption on blood-contact membranes, the introduction of different hydrophilic agents was necessary. In this context, alterations of the blood elements, when they come into contact with the hemodialysis membranes having limited therapy, generated a series of investigations for obtaining membranes with specific destinations, such as the membranes with leverage materials and implanted devices.

Polysulfone is often indicated in medical equipment such as blood dialysis membranes and in targeted drug delivery applications using the microrobot [40–42]. Polysulfone capillary fibers used for intraocular drug delivery have been modified using a suspension coating of silver, gold, or calcium carbonate ($CaCO_3$) nanoparticles, which were subsequently removed selectively, resulting in a network of nanometer-sized pores in the polysulfone. These nanoporous membranes ensure and enhance the adsorption of drug and the release of, for example, Rhodamine B (Rh-B—a model drug) from porous polysulfone coatings [43].

Permeability and biocompatibility of synthetic membranes can be established only by knowing the clinical correlations. The concept of biocompatibility also refers to any harmful effects induced by the contact of blood with the dialysis membrane, as well as to anaphylactoid reactions, which are related more frequently to contaminated dialysate or leachable chemicals than to the sustained activation of the contact phase of coagulation in patients treated with angiotensin-converting enzyme inhibitors. A highlight of the roles played by the absorptive properties of dialysis membranes in determining biocompatibility, including the heparin-binding property, was presented in numerous works [43].

Biocompatibility estimation must take into account the phenomena of coagulation cascade and the activation of the blood platelets [44]. Contact of blood with foreign material surfaces may be accompanied by the following:

- Blood coagulation and platelet activation.
- Activation of thrombin initiated during the coagulation process.
- The strongest activator of the blood platelets (which provokes platelet shape change, release of fibrinogen, platelet factor 4, and β-thromboglobulin, and stimulates platelet aggregation). Activated platelets, on the other hand, provide the following:
  - A procoagulant surface for the formation of the prothrombin complex
  - Stimulate the release of procoagulant and proinflammatory molecules

Blood coagulation is promoted particularly on negatively charged biomaterial (hydrophilic) surfaces. In this context, autoactivation of Factor XII, activation of further components of the contact phase or intrinsic coagulation systems (such as pre-kallikrein to kallikrein), and more of Factor XII in a positive feedback loop occur, which finally leads to the generation of thrombin. Although the contact system is activated on the hydrophilic surfaces with a high density of negative charges, platelet adhesion and activation are promoted by hydrophobic materials.

The literature shows that a polysulfone film with immobilized heparin considerably enhances the selective adsorption of the level of low-density lipoprotein (LDL) from protein mixtures [45,46]. In addition to and compared to plain polysulfone, adsorbed LDL could be easily desorbed from the polysulfone-heparin surface with NaCl or urea solutions, respectively. Therefore, it was suggested to apply a heparin-modified polysulfone membrane for simultaneous application in hemodialysis and LDL aphaeresis therapy. It is also shown that the treatment of end-stage renal disease patients with membranes that continuously remove LDL during the hemodialysis session would not only reduce expenses, but probably will provide more safety and comfort for the patients. Surface-induced blood coagulation and fouling of membranes by irreversible protein adsorption with significant loss of performance are serious obstacles for the application of membranes in hemodialysis [47].

Recently, biocompatible polysulfone membranes with double porosity level were realized and characterized for applications in liver tissue engineering [48]. To acquire a double porosity level, these membranes were designed with surface macroporosity emerging in macrochambers—accessible to hepatic cell colonization, and with microporosity—to ensure gas and molecule transfers between macrochambers and supernatant, as well as potential immune barriers. Obtained membranes are biocompatible and offer a three-dimensional (3D) environment that can be colonized by hepatocytes, leading to a potentially high cell density. Therefore, these membranes with double porosity offer an inner 3D environment adequate to cell proliferation, thus forming a liver tissue.

The assessment of biocompatibility in systems consisting of a host, permiselective membrane, and a biological material encapsulated within may be standardized for biological material immunoisolation purposes. The procedures for the evaluation of membrane nontoxicity against the biological material, post implantation membrane physical and chemical stability, and biomaterial ability to perform with the host are standardized for biological material immunoisolation purposes. According to Granicka et al. [48], the following three types of membranes should be considered:

1. Membrane nontoxicity against the encapsulated biological materials, which may be evaluated with different cell lines. Thus, in the case of biomaterials for direct contact with blood, blood compatibility is established by testing the hemolytic action, coagulative and fibrinolytic parameters, and blood viscosity, whereas their cytocompatibility—the urinary catheters being evaluated using human urothelial cells, for urinary reconstructions—may be evaluated using human bladder smooth muscle, and their cytotoxicity for oxygenators is established on the human lung WI-38 cell line.
2. Post implantation membrane physical and chemical stability—which can be established using the diffusive transport and Fourier transform infrared

evaluation. Diffusive permeability was appreciated using a thermodynamic description of diffusive mass transport over a homogenous membrane (Fick's law) and a two-compartment model.

3. Biomaterial ability to perform with the host, by analyzing the cell structures surrounding the membrane.

Descriptions of membrane types and the more commonly used dialyzers technologies are presented by Clarck and Gao [49]. Hollow-fiber dimensions, surface area, porosity, and water permeability are important characteristics determining membrane performances.

A hollow fiber can be represented by a cylinder in which the central region is removed, forming the blood compartment with dimensions dictated by the operating conditions of hemodialysis (approximately 180–220 μm in diameter and 20–24 cm long). The blood flow rate along the length of a cylinder, Q_B, is correlated with axial pressure drop, ΔP, blood viscosity, fiber length, L, and hollow fiber radius, r, using Equations 8.1 or 8.2:

$$Q_B = \frac{\Delta P}{(8\mu L / \pi r^4)} \tag{8.1}$$

or

$$Q_B = \frac{\Delta P}{R} \tag{8.2}$$

where:

$R = 8\mu L/\pi r^4$ is the resistance to blood flow

These relations show that a small decrease in the inner diameter of the hollow fiber and increase in fiber length and hematocrit (μ) are associated with an increase in flow resistance, which in turn results in an increase of axial pressure drop at a constant blood flow rate.

The inner annular surface of a hollow fiber, depending on fiber length, L, inner diameter, $2r$, and the overall number (which generally takes values in the range of 7000–14000), represents the theoretically maximal area available for blood contact in the dialyzer. The surface area (A), defined as the cylindrical surface, is given by Equation 8.3:

$$A_{fiber} = 2\pi r L \tag{8.3}$$

Finally, the straight cylindrical pore model is used to estimate pore parameters. The rate of ultrafiltrate flow is directly related to r^4—at constant transmembrane pressure. Also, the dimensions and number of pores influence water permittivity. In this context, Seito exemplified the following dialyzer membranes with advanced level of performance [50]: cellulose triacetate (hollow fiber, Nipro), polysulfone (hollow fiber, Asahi Kasei Kuraray Medical), polyethersulfone (hollow fiber, Nipro

Membrana), polymethylmethacrylate (hollow fiber, Toray), polyester polymer alloy (hollow fiber, Toray), ethylene vinyl alcohol copolymer (hollow fiber, Asahi Kasei Kuraray Medical), and polyacrylonitrile (hollow fiber laminated, Gambro). The criteria for these high-performance membranes include excellent biocompatibility, effective clearance of target solutes, larger pore size than that of conventional hemodialysis membranes, for promoting the removal of protein-bound uremic toxins, and middle-to-large molecular-weight solutes.

8.4 INTERACTION OF BLOOD COMPONENTS WITH POLYSULFONE SURFACES

The medical devices that come into contact with blood must be biocompatible, without inducing adverse reactions—such as the formation of clot or thrombus composed of various blood elements. Modification of biosurfaces and pharmaceutical intervention are strategies that produced many successful examples, but rejection phenomena, local and systemic inflammation, and the thrombosis of biosurface can induce complications, remain major clinical problems. It becomes progressively evident that the complexities of the underlying processes require a multidisciplinary approach between basic sciences—such as immunology, cell biology, materials sciences, and drug discovery—and clinical specialties in adjacent fields for advancing to enhanced treatment options [24].

Thrombotic and thromboembolic effects, and the risks associated with the necessary anticoagulant therapy remain a serious concern with some medical devices. In addition, blood represents about 8% of the total human body weight, including water (more then 90%), proteins (albumin, globulins, fibrinogen), different types of cells (platelets, white and red cells), ions, and different organic nutrients—lipids and carbohydrates. These components are involved in the transport of gases, nutrients, waste products, processed molecules, and regulatory molecules, and, also, in pH regulation and osmosis, maintenance of body temperature, protection against foreign substances (complement system), and clot formation, for preventing bleeding after injury (coagulation cascade) [30]. Thrombus formation and all related pathologies occur by cascade coagulation, and the inflammation surrounding the implant is associated with the activation of the complement system.

In view of a direct contact of the biomaterial with blood, a clear understanding of their interactions is a prerequisite. The material interacts instantaneously with blood constituents, which is critical in determining their potential side effects on the circulatory system and, eventually, on the whole organism [51,52]. Second, the interactions with blood can affect the *in vivo* pharmacokinetic behavior of polymers and their ability to leave the blood compartment and enter other tissues. Blood has important physiological functions and a complex composition, being divided into two compartments: plasma—which contains proteins, lipids, and salts—and specific cells, including red blood cells, white blood cells, and platelets. Cells adhesion occurs at a later stage and is mediated by the proteins initially adsorbed on the surface. Platelets, among the other cells present in blood, play the most important role in blood–material interactions. Thus:

- Adhesion is related to protein adsorption.
- Interaction of platelets with the adsorbed fibrinogen or γ-globulin has been attributed to the formation of a complex between glycosyltransferases located in the platelet membrane and incomplete heterosaccharides in the protein layer;
- Fibrinogen, fibronectin, and γ-globulin precoating causes an increase of platelet adhesion. Generally, the literature states that polyurethane, polyethylene oxide, silicone rubber, and polytetrafluoroethylene most often appear as passive materials to platelets, whereas polystyrene, polyvinylchloride, polyethylene, and polymethylmethacrylate are recognized to be reactive to platelets.

The artificial surfaces interact with the blood platelets, initially causing platelet adherence and aggregation. In contact with the circulating blood, this interaction is believed to lead to thrombosis and thromboembolism, and to the removal of platelets from the circulation [53,54].

Traditional methods for improving blood compatibility of implants were focused on the minimization of blood interaction with materials; however, it is nowadays believed that the biomaterial surface should interact with the biological material to elicit the appropriate biological response [55]. The hemocompatible devices are generally obtained by the treatment of materials with chemicals or by their bioactive coatings.

The surface characteristics of biomaterials, such as chemical properties, hydrophilicity/hydrophobicity surface, roughness, and flexibility may affect the cell-surface interactions, protein adsorption, behavior of cells adhesion and proliferation, and the host response, too. Therefore, cellular adhesion has a direct bearing on the thrombogenicity and immuogenicity of a specific material, predicting its blood compatibility and deciding the long-term use for a blood-contacting material application [54,56]. This property is described from different perspectives. Interfacial fibrin polymerization and fibrillation kinetics contribution by nanoscale roughness and fibrinogen-fibrin cleavage in solution [57,58], influence of nanopore size on platelet adhesion and activation [59], *in vitro* reaction of endothelial cells to polymer demixed nanotopography [60], platelet shape modification and cytoskeletal reorganization on polyurethaneureas [61] are only a few issues mentioned in the literature.

Generally, the biocompatible properties of polysulfones are intensely discussed as two categories of applications: blood-contacting devices—hemodialysis, hemodiafiltration, and hemofiltration membranes—and cell- or tissue-contacting devices—bioreactors (made of hollow-fiber membranes), nerve generation through polysulfone semipermeable hollow membrane, etc. [62].

Some studies present the correlation between the characteristics of functionalized polysulfones, as well as of their complex structures, and the red blood cells, platelets, sanguine plasma proteins, and finally the adhesion/cohesion of blood components and plasma proteins [32,63–66]. In the cited literature, one of the aspects refers to the determination of surface polymer properties. Static contact angles measurements of different test liquids on surface polymer films using the Lifshitz-van der Waals/acid-base method (LW/AB) (Equations 8.4 through 8.6) are considered in the evaluation of total surface tension parameter, with their disperse and polar contributions [67–72]:

$$1 + \cos\theta = \frac{2}{\gamma_{lv}} \left(\sqrt{\gamma_{sv}^{LW} \gamma_{lv}^{LW}} + \sqrt{\gamma_{sv}^{+} \gamma_{lv}^{-}} + \sqrt{\gamma_{sv}^{-} \gamma_{lv}^{+}} \right) \qquad (8.4)$$

$$\gamma_{sv}^{AB} = 2\sqrt{\gamma_{sv}^{+} \gamma_{sv}^{-}} \qquad (8.5)$$

$$\gamma_{sv}^{LW/AB} = \gamma_{sv}^{LW} + \gamma_{sv}^{AB} \qquad (8.6)$$

where:

superscripts LW/AB, AB, and LW refer to the total surface tension, polar component (calculated from the electron-donor, γ_{sv}^{-}, and electron-acceptor, γ_{sv}^{+}, interactions, according to Equation 8.4), and disperse component, respectively

The effect of the chemical structure on the surface and interfacial properties (evaluated by Equations 8.7 through 8.9) can evidence hydrophobicity or hydrophilicity—characterized by a surface free energy (ΔG_w) higher or lower than −113 mJ m^{-2}, respectively [32,67], and, on the other hand, attraction or rejection between the two surfaces, s, immersed in water or in other liquid, as a function of the obtained negative or positive values of the interfacial free energy, respectively (Equation 8.7):

$$\Delta G_w = -\gamma_{lv} \left(1 + \cos\theta_{water} \right) \qquad (8.7)$$

$$\Delta G_{sls} = -2\gamma_{sl} \qquad (8.8)$$

$$\gamma_{sl} = \left(\sqrt{\gamma_{lv}^{p}} - \sqrt{\gamma_{sv}^{AB}} \right)^2 + \left(\sqrt{\gamma_{lv}^{d}} - \sqrt{\gamma_{sv}^{LW}} \right)^2 \qquad (8.9)$$

where:
γ_{sl} is the solid–liquid interfacial tension

In the same context, according to Equation 8.10, the work of spreading of liquid over a polymer surface, W_s, takes positive or negative values, as the adhesion work, W_a, is higher (for hydrophilic materials) or lower (for hydrophobic materials) than the cohesive work, W_c, of the liquid, respectively:

$$W_s = W_a - W_c = 2\left[\left(\gamma_{sv}^{LW} \gamma_{lv}^{d} \right)^{0.5} + \left(\gamma_{sv}^{+} \gamma_{lv}^{-} \right)^{0.5} + \left(\gamma_{sv}^{-} \gamma_{lv}^{+} \right)^{0.5} \right] - 2\gamma_{lv} \qquad (8.10)$$

Figures 8.1 through 8.4 show that surface analysis of some functionalized polysulfones was performed for a better understanding of the interfacial chemistry of adhesion not only with water but also with blood components and plasma proteins [32,63,64,66].

The blood–polymer surface interactions depend on the physicochemical properties of the polymer surface (crystallinity, hydrophilicity, and chemical functional groups) and protein properties (such as toxicological properties, electrical charge, hydrophobicity, available chemical functional groups, stability of the protein structure, interactions between proteins in the adsorbed layer, relative concentration in bulk phase, and molecular size) [27,63,73,74]. Blood components are implicated in several of the above-mentioned complex physiological processes [such as transport of gases, nutrients, waste products, processed molecules, regulatory molecules, regulation of pH

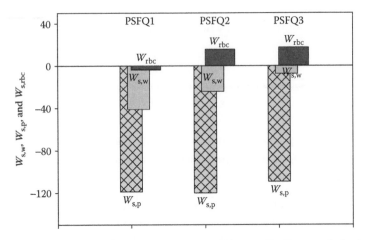

FIGURE 8.1 Work of spreading of water, $W_{s,w}$, red blood cells, $W_{s,rbc}$, and platelets, $W_{s,p}$, (mN m^{-1}) over the surface of quaternized polysulfones (PSFQ1, PSFQ2, and PSFQ3—with different ionic chlorine content) obtained by the quaternization reaction with N,N-dimethylethanolamine. (Data from Ioan, S., and Filimon, A., *A Search for Antibacterial Agents*, InTech, Rijeka, Croatia, 2012.)

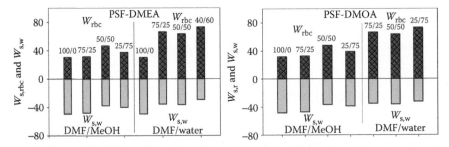

FIGURE 8.2 Work of spreading of water, $W_{s,w}$, red blood cells, $W_{s,rbc}$, and platelets, $W_{s,p}$, (mN m^{-1}) over the surface of quaternized polysulfones [obtained by the quaternization reaction with N,N-dimethylethylamine (PSF-DMEA), or N,N-dimethyloctylamine (PSF-DMOA)] films prepared at different compositions of N,N-dimethylformamide/methanol and N,N-dimethylformamide/water. (Data from Ioan, S. et al., *J. Appl. Polym. Sci.*, 121, 127–137, 2011; Albu, R. M. et al., *J. Biomater. Nanobiotechnol.*, 2, 114–123, 2011.)

and osmosis, maintenance of body temperature, protection against foreign substances (complement system), and clot formation, for preventing bleeding after injury (coagulation cascade)] [30]. Also, assuring the biocompatibility of blood-contacting devices, it is important to avoid the phenomenon of thrombotic response induced by the materials. In this respect, worth mentioning are the scientific investigations on blood compatibility based on polysulfone complex structures; analyzing the different blood components, such as red blood cells, platelets, and plasma proteins, such as albumin, immunoglobulin G (IgG), and fibrinogen. The interfacial tension of solid blood components or plasma proteins, γ_{sl}, and the interfacial free energy between two material particles in the blood phase, ΔG_{sls}, (Equations 8.7 and 8.8) show that either attraction

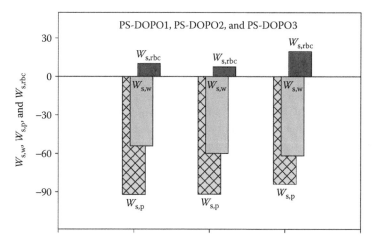

FIGURE 8.3 Work of spreading of water, $W_{s,w}$, red blood cells, $W_{s,rbc}$, and platelets, $W_{s,p}$, (mN m^{-1}) over the surface of the phosphorus-modified polysulfones (PSF-DOPO) (subscripts 1, 2, and 3 correspond to different substitution degrees: 0.59, 0.72, and 1.85, respectively), obtained by the chemical modification of the chloromethylated polysulfone by reacting the chloromethyl group with the P—H bond of 9,10-dihydro-oxa-10-phosphophenanthrene-10-oxide. (Data from Ioan, S., and Filimon, A., *A Search for Antibacterial Agents*, InTech, Rijeka, Croatia, 2012.)

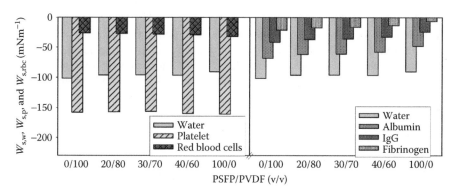

FIGURE 8.4 Work of spreading of water, $W_{s,w}$, and plasma proteins ($W_{s,albumin}$, $W_{s,IgG}$, and $W_{s,fibrinogen}$), over the surface of 0/100, 20/80, 30/70, 40/60, and 100/0 v/v quaternized polysulfone/poly(vinylidene fluoride) blend films (PSFP/PVDF). (Data from Buruiana, L. I. et al., *Polym. Plast. Technol. Eng.*, Doi:10.1080/03602559.2014.979496.)

or rejection occurs between the two material surfaces, s, immersed in the various components of blood. In addition, the work of spreading of blood components ($W_{s,rbc}$, $W_{s,p}$) and plasma proteins ($W_{s,albumin}$, $W_{s,IgG}$, and $W_{s,fibrinogen}$) over the material surfaces can be evaluated with Equation 8.9, using the surface energy parameters (γ_{lv}, γ_{lv}^d, γ_{lv}^+, and γ_{lv}^-) for biological materials [68,72]. According to the negative or positive values of the interfacial free energy of a complex material, the work of spreading of the different blood components (Figures 8.1 through 8.4) takes either negative or positive values, suggesting a lower or higher work of adhesion, comparatively with that of cohesion.

Exposure of plasma proteins to polymer films can generate high albumin cohesion, followed by lower values of IgG and fibrinogen cohesion.

An important problem in the evaluation of biocompatibility refers to the analysis of the competitive or selective adsorption of blood proteins onto the biomaterial surface. Predictions about these interactions can only be formulated if the exact structure of the biomaterial is known. Initially, the surface of an implanted material is mainly coated with albumin and immunoglobulins, especially IgG and fibrinogen from the plasma. Sanguine plasma proteins are selected for the study of the affinity of polymer blends toward physiological fluid media, due to their presence in the biological events from blood.

On the other hand, considering that blood is exposed to a biomaterial surface, cell adhesion decides the life of the implanted biomaterials. Cellular adhesion onto the biomaterial surfaces can activate coagulation and immunological cascade, having a direct impact on the thrombogenicity and immunogenicity of a biomaterial, thus influencing its blood compatibility [32,63,64,66]. Consequently, blood compatibility requires prevention of platelet adhesion and deactivation of the intrinsic coagulation system, generated by the competitive blood protein adsorption on the polymer surface.

Blood platelets are essential in maintaining hemostasis, as they are highly sensitive to the changes in the blood microenvironment. Platelet aggregation is used as a marker for materials' thrombogenic properties, the polymer–platelet interaction being an important step toward the understanding of their hematocompatibility [75,76].

Adhesion of platelets is promoted by the adsorbed fibrinogen and γ-globulin, whereas the adsorbed albumin inhibits platelet adhesion. It is also demonstrated that albumin adheres to a hydrophilic surface rather than to a hydrophobic one, whereas fibrinogen adheres to a hydrophobic surface [77,78]. Moreover, the literature shows that the adhesion of the red blood cells onto a surface requires knowledge of the interactions with the vascular components [79]. Polymer interaction with red blood cells is mediated mostly by the hydrophobic interaction with the lipid bilayer (the red blood cell hydrophobic layer containing transmembrane proteins), the electrostatic interaction with the surface charges, and/or the direct interaction with membrane proteins, depending on polymer characteristics. Thus, endothelial glycocalyx, together with the mucopolysaccharides adsorbed onto the endothelial surface of the vascular endothelium, reject the clotting factors and platelets, known as playing a significant role in thrombus formation. In this context, such results can be applied for the encapsulation of some implantable biosensors to form a biocompatible interface between the probe and the brain tissue [80], being equally useful for evaluating bacterial adhesion on the polymer surface, in the study of some possible infections induced by implanted devices.

8.5   GENERAL REMARKS

The field of biomaterials is an interdisciplinary one, including aspects of materials science, chemistry, biology, and medicine. Experience in testing the biocompatibility of the complex structure of polysulfone showed the need for a careful characterization of these materials in accordance with the individual biological properties required by specific applications. The evaluation depends on the category of medical device employed, selected in accordance with the nature of the body contact, and its duration. In this context, the ISO 10993 guideline is generally accepted worldwide. For some endpoints and studies, differences in the different designs are required by international authorities, for example, Ministry of Health, Labour and Welfare, Japan, and the U.S. Food and Drug Administration. Biomaterials in contact with biological systems are enabling tools for many advances in the biomedical research.

Biocompatible polysulfones are a critical functional element in a variety of bioartificial areas, such as implants, diagnosis, bioprocessing, and therapeutics. Reactions of biocellular response caused by the presence of polysulfone foreign materials are major subjects, related to fundamental biomedical polymer research for superior results in biomedical applications.

To conclude, polysulfonic systems are shown with blood-contacting applications with a highly superior *in situ* fabrication concept, in which the biocompatibility by reorientation of the diblock copolymer entrapped on an ultrathin surface was successfully achieved using self-transformable fabrication processes. Both blood and compatible cell determination demonstrated that modified polysulfones can be biocompatible, being desirable candidates for biomaterials.

REFERENCES

1. Park, J. and Lakes, R. S., *Biomaterials: An Introduction*, 3rd ed., Springer Press, New York, 2007.
2. Ratner, B. D. and Bryant, S. J., Biomaterials: Where we have been and where we are going. *Annu. Rev. Biomed. Eng.*, 6, 41–75, 2004.
3. Nair, L. S. and Laurencin, C. T., Biodegradable polymers as biomaterials. *Progr. Polym. Sci.*, 32(12), 762–798, 2007.
4. Ratner, B. D., The catastrophe revisited: Blood compatibility in the 21st century. *Biomaterials*, 28(34), 5144–5147, 2007.
5. Seo, J. H., Matsuno, R., Konno, T., Takai, M., and Ishihara, K., Surface tethering of phosphorylcholine groups onto poly(dimethylsiloxane) through swelling—deswelling methods with phospholipids moiety containing ABA-type block copolymers. *Biomaterials*, 29(10), 1367–1376, 2007.
6. Liu, P.-S., Chena, Q., Wu, S.-S., Shena, J., and Lin, S.-C., Surface modification of cellulose membranes with zwitterionic polymers for resistance to protein adsorption and platelet adhesion. *J. Membrane Sci.*, 350(1/2), 387–394, 2010.
7. Kim, Y.-W., Kim, J.-J., and Kim, Y. H., Surface characterization of biocompatible polysulfone membranes modified with poly(ethylene glycol) derivatives. *Korean J. Chem. Eng.*, 20(6), 1158–1165, 2003.
8. Väisänen, P. and Nyström, M., Comparison of polysulfone membranes and polysulfone films. *Acta Polytechnica Scandinavica*, 247, 25–34, 1997.
9. Higuchi, A., Shirano, K., Harashima, M., Yoon, B. O., Hara, M., Hattori, M., and Imamura, K., Chemical modification hollow fibers with vinylpyrrolidone having improved blood compatibility. *Biomaterials*, 23(13), 2659–2666, 2002.
10. Tomaszewska, M., Jarosiewicz, A., and Karakulski, K., Physical and chemical characteristics of polymer coatings in CRF formulation. *Desalination*, 146(1–3), 319–323, 2002.
11. Guan, R., Zou, H., Lu, D., Gong, C., and Liu, Y., Polyethersulfone sulfonated by chlorosulfonic acid and its membrane characteristics. *Eur. Polym. J.*, 41(7), 1554–1560, 2005.

12. Yu, H., Huang, Y., Ying, H., and Xiao, C., Preparation and characterization of a quaternary ammonium derivative of konjac glucomannan. *Carbohydrate Polym.*, 69(1), 29–40, 2007.

13. Ioan, S., Filimon, A., and Avram, E., Influence of the degree of substitution on the solution properties of chloromethylated polysulfone. *J. Appl. Polym. Sci.*, 101(1), 524–531, 2006.

14. Filimon, A., Avram, E., and Ioan, S., Influence of mixed solvents and temperature on the solution properties of quaternized polysulfones. *J. Macromol. Sci. Phys. Part B*, 46(3), 503–520, 2007.

15. Idris, A. and Zain, N. M., Effect of heat treatment on the performance and structural details of polyethersulfone ultrafiltration membranes. *J. Teknol.*, 44(F), 27–43, 2006.

16. Kochkodan, V., Tsarenko, S., Potapchenko, N., Kosinova, V., and Goncharuk, V., Adhesion of microorganisms to polymer membranes: A photobactericidal effect of surface treatment with TiO_2. *Desalination*, 220(1–3), 380–385, 2008.

17. Guiver, M. D., Black, P., Tam, C. M., and Deslandes, Y., Functionalized polysulfone membranes by heterogeneous lithiation. *J. Appl. Polym. Sci.*, 48(9), 1597–1606, 1993.

18. James, B. and Post, M. D., Thrombocytopenia associated with use of a biocompatible hemodialysis membrane: A case report. *Am. J. Kidney Dis.*, 55(6), e25–e28, 2010.

19. Chenoweth, D. E. and Henderson, L. W., Complement activation during hemodialysis: Laboratory evaluation of hemodialyzers. *Artif. Organs*, 11(2), 155–162, 1987.

20. Brendolan, A., Nalesso, F., Fortunato, A, Crepaldi, C., De Cal, M., Cazzavillan, S., Cruz, D., Techawathanawanna, N., and Ronco, C., Dialytic performance evaluation of Rexeed: A new polysulfone-based dialyzer with improved flow distributions. *Int. J. Artif. Organs*, 28(10), 966–975, 2005.

21. Hakim, R. M., Clinical implications of hemodialysis membrane biocompatibility. *Kidney Int.*, 44(3) 484–494, 1993.

22. Su, B., Fu, P., Li, Q., Tao, Y., Li, Z., Zao, H., and Zhao, C., Evaluation of polyethersulfone highflux hemodialysis membrane *in vitro* and *in vivo*. *J. Mater. Sci. Mater. Med.*, 19(2), 745–751, 2008.

23. Park, J. Y., Acar, M. H., Akthakul, A., Kuhlman, W., and Mayes, A. M., Polysulfone-graft-poly(ethylene glycol) graft copolymers for surface modification of polysulfone membranes. *Biomaterials*, 27(6), 856–865, 2006.

24. Tathe A., Ghodke M., and Nikalje A. P., A brief review: Biomaterials and their application. *Int. J. Pharmacy Pharm. Sci.*, 2(4), 19–23, 2010.

25. Caldorera-Moore, M. and Peppas, N. A., Micro- and nanotechnologies for inteligent and responsive biomaterial-based medical systems. *Adv. Drug Delivery Rev.*, 61(15), 1391–1401, 2009.

26. Xiang, T., Zhang, L. S., Wang, R., Xia J., Su, B. H., and Zhao, C. S., Blood compatibility comparison for polysulfone membranes modified by grafting block and random zwitterionic copolymers via surface-initiated ATRP. *J. Colloid. Interface Sci.*, 432, 47–56, 2014.

27. Farag, A. A., *Biomedical Image Analysis Statistical and Variational Methods*. Manchester Metropolitan University, Manchester, UK, 2014.

28. Slevin, M., Current advances in the medical application of nanotechnology, Manchester Metropolitan University, Manchester, UK, 2012.

29. Ratner, B. D. A., Surface properties and surface characterization of materials. In *Biomaterials Science. An Introduction to Materials in Medicine*, eds., Ratner, B. D., Hoffman, A. S., Schoen, F. J., Lemons, J. E., Elsevier/Academic Press, San Diego, CA, pp. 40–59, 2004.

30. Salvagnini, C., Bodybuilding: The bionic human. *Nature*, 295, 995–1033, 2002.

31. Wenz, L. M., Merritt, K., Brown, S. A., Moet, A., and Steffee, A. D., *In vitro* biocompatibility of polyetheretherketone and polysulfone composites. *J. Biomed. Mat. Res. Part A*, 24(1), 207–215, 1990.

32. Ioan, S., Albu, R. M., Avram, E., Stoica, I., and Ioanid, E. G., Surface characterization of quaternized polysulfone films and biocompatibility studies. *J. Appl. Polym. Sci.*, 121(1), 127–137, 2011.

33. Baumann, H. and Kokott, A., Surface modification of the polymers present in a polysulfone hollow fiber hemodialyser by covalent binding of heparin or endothelial cell surface heparan sulfate: Flow characteristics and platelet adhesion. *J. Biomater. Sci. Polym. Ed.*, 11(3), 245–272, 2000.

34. Dahe, G. J., Kadam, S. S., Sabale, S. S., Kadam, D. P., Sarkate, L. B., and Bellare, J. R., *In vivo* evaluation of the biocompatibility of surface modified hemodialysis polysulfone hollow fibers in rat. *PLoS One*, 6(10), e25236, 2011.

35. Mangindaan, D., Yared, I., Kurniawan, H., Sheu, J. R., and Wang, M. J., Modulation of biocompatibility on poly(vinylidene fluoride) and polysulfone by oxygen plasma treatment and dopamine coating. *J. Biomed. Mater. Res. Part A*, 100(11), 3177–3188, 2012.

36. Liu, Z., Deng, X., Wang, M., Chen, J., Zhang, A., Gub, Z., and Zhao, C., BSA-modified polyethersulfone membrane: Preparation, characterization and biocompatibility. *J. Biomater. Sci. Polym. Ed.*, 20(3), 377–397, 2009.

37. Pavanatti, S. L., Zavaglia, C. A. C., Belangero, W. D., and Kawano, Y., Study of biocompatibility of particles and rods of polysulfone. *Acta Ortop. Bras.*, 9(3), 11–18, 2001.

38. Hörl, W. H., Hemodialysis membranes: Interleukins, biocompatibility, and middle molecules, *J. Am. Soc. Nephrol.*, 13(Suppl 1), S62–S71, 2002.

39. Gautham, A., Muhammed Javad, M., Murugan, M., and Mansoor, S. N., Hemodialisis membranes: Past, present and future trends. *Int. Res. J. Pharm.*, 4(5), 16–19, 2013.

40. Gastaldello, K., Melot, C., Kahn, R. J., Vanherweghem, J. L., Vincent, J. L., and Tielemans, C., Comparison of cellulose diacetate and polysulfone membranes in the outcome of acute renal failure. A prospective randomized study. *Nephrol. Dial. Transplant.*, 15(2), 224–230, 2001.

41. Rahimy, M. H., Peyman, G. A., Chin, S. Y., Golshani, R., Aras, C., Borhani, H., and Thompson, H., Polysulfone capillary fiber for intraocular drug delivery: *In vitro* and *in vivo* evaluations. *J. Drug Target*, 2(4), 289–2298, 1994.

42. Sivaraman, K. M., Kellenberger, C., Pané, S., Ergeneman, O., Lühmann, T., Luechinger, N. A., Hall, H., Stark, W. J., and Nelson, B. J., Porous polysulfone coatings for enhanced drug delivery. *Biomed. Microdevices*, 14(3), 603–612, 2012.

43. Chanard, J., Lavaud, S., Randoux, C., and Rieu, P., New insights in dialysis membrane biocompatibility: Relevance of adsorption properties and heparin binding. *Nephrol. Dial. Transplant.*, 18(2), 252–257, 2003.

44. Huang, X.-J., Guduru, D., Xu, Z.-K., Vienken, J., and Groth, T., Blood compatibility and permeability of heparin-modified polysulfone as potential membrane for simultaneous hemodialysis and LDL removal. *Macromol. Biosci.*, 11(1), 131–140, 2011.

45. Huang, X.-J., Guduru, D., Xu, Z.-K., Vienken, J., and Groth, T., Immobilization of heparin on polysulfone surface for selective adsorption of low-density lipoprotein (LDL). *Acta Biomater.*, 6(3), 1099–1106, 2010.

46. Huang, X.-J., Xu, Z.-K., Wan, L. S., Wang, Z. G., Wang, J. L., Surface modification of polyacrylonitrile-based membranes by chemical reactions to generate phospholipid moieties. *Langmuir*, 21(7), 2941–2947, 2005.

47. Dufresne, M., Bacchin, P., Cerino, G., Remigy, J. C., Adrianus, G. N, Aima, P., and Legallais, C., Human hepatic cell behavior on polysulfone membrane with double porosity level. *J. Membrane Sci.*, 428, 454–461, 2013.

48. Granicka, L., Kawiak, J., Werynski, A., The biocompatibility of membranes for immunoisolation. *Biocyb. Biomed. Eng.*, 28(2), 59–68, 2008.

49. Clark, W. R. and Gao, D., Properties of membranes used for hemodialysis therapy. *Semin. Dial.*, 15(3), 191–195, 2002.

50. Saito, A., Definition of high-performance membranes—From a clinical point of view. In *High Performance Membrane Dialyzers. Contributions to Nephrology*, eds., Saito, A, Kawanishi, H., Yamashita, A. C., and Mineshima, M., Karger, Basel, Switzerland, Vol. 173, 2011, pp. 1–10.

51. Liu, Z. H., Janzen, J., and Brooks, D. E., Adsorption of amphiphilic hyperbranched polyglycerol derivatives onto human red blood cells. *Biomaterials*, 31(12), 3364–3373, 2010.

52. Jain, K., Kesharwani, P., Gupta, U., and Jain, N. K., Dendrimer toxicity: Let's meet the challenge. *Int. J. Pharm.*, 394(1/2), 122–142, 2010.

53. Ware, J. A., Kang, J., DeCenzo, M. T., Smith, M., Watkins, S. C., Slayter, H. S., and Saitoh, M., Platelet activation by a synthetic hydrophobic polymer, polymethylmethacrylate. *Blood*, 78(7), 1713–1721, 1991.

54. Vesel, A., Eleršič, K., Modic, M., Junkar, I., and Mozetič, M., Formation of nanocones on highly oriented pyrolytic graphite by oxygen plasma. *Materials*, 7(3), 2014–2029, 2014.

55. Yang, C. Y., Huang, L. Y., Shen, T. L., and Yeh, J. A., Cell adhesion, morphology and biochemistry on nano-topographic oxidized silicon surfaces. *Eur. Cells Mater.*, 20, 415–430, 2010.

56. Koh, L. B., Rodriguez, I., and Venkatraman, S. S., The effect of topography of polymer surfaces on platelet adhesion. *Biomaterials*, 31(7), 1533–1545, 2010.

57. Dolatshahi-Pirouz, A., Foss, M., and Besenbacher, F., Interfacial fibrin polymerization and fibrillation kinetics is influenced by nanoscale roughness and fibrinogen-fibrin cleavage in solution. *J. Phys. Chem. C*, 115(28), 13617–13623, 2011.

58. Curtis, A. and Wilkinson, C., New depths in cell behaviour: Reactions of cells to nano-topography. *Biochem. Soc. Symp.*, 66, 15–26, 1999.

59. Ferraz, N., Carlsson, J., Hong, J., and Ott, M. K., Influence of nanoporesize on platelet adhesion and activation. *J. Mater. Sci. Mater. Med.*, 19(9), 3115–3121, 2008

60. Dalby, M. J., Riehle, M. O., Johnstone, H., Affrossman, S., and Curtis, A. S. G., *In vitro* reaction of endothelial cells to polymer demixed nanotopography. *Biomaterials*, 23(10), 2945–2954, 2002.

61. Goodman, S. L., Grasel, T. G., Cooper, S. L., and Albrecht, R. M., Platelet shape change and cytoskeletal reorganization on polyurethaneureas. *J. Biomed. Mater. Res.*, 23(1), 105–123, 1989.

62. Khang, G., Lee, H. B., and Park, J. B., Biocompatibility of polysulfone. I. Surface modifications and characterizations. *Biomed. Mater. Eng.*, 5(4), 245–258, 1995.

63. Ioan, S. and Filimon, A., Biocompatibility and antimicrobial activity of some quaternized polysulfones. In *A Search for Antibacterial Agents.*, Book 2, eds., Bobbarala, V., InTech, Rijeka, Croatia, Chapter 13, pp. 249–274, 2012.

64. Albu, R. M., Avram, E., Stoica, I., Ioanid, E. G., Popovici, D., and Ioan S., Surface properties and compatibility with blood of new quaternized polysulfones. *J. Biomater. Nanobiotechnol.*, 2(2), 114–123, 2011.

65. Ioan, S., Filimon, A., Hulubei, C., Stoica, I., and Dunca, S., Origin of rheological behavior and surface/interfacial properties of some semi-alicyclic polyimides for biomedical applications. *Polym. Bull.*, 70(10), 2873–2893, 2013.

66. Buruiana, L. I., Avram, E., Popa, P., and Ioan, S., Impact of some properties of quaternized polysulfone/poly(vinylidene fluoride) blend on the potential biomedical applications. *Polym. Plast. Technol. Eng.*, 2015. doi:10.1080/03602559.2014.979496.

67. Rankl, M., Laib, S., and Seeger, S., Surface tension properties of surface-coatings for application in biodiagnostics determined by contact angle measurements. *Colloid Surf. B Biointer.*, 30(3), 177–186, 2003.

68. Vijayanand, K., Deepak, K., Pattanayak, D. K., Rama Mohan, T. R., and Banerjee, R., Interpreting blood-biomaterial interactions from surface free energy and work of adhesion. *Trends Biomater. Artif. Organs*, 18(2), 73–83, 2005.
69. Kwok, S. C. H., Wang, J., and Chu, P. K., Surface energy, wettability, and blood compatibility phosphorus doped diamond-like carbon films. *Diamond Relat. Mater.*, 14(1), 78–85, 2005.
70. Agathopoulos, S. and Nikolopoulos, P., Wettability and interfacial interactions in bioceramic-body-liquid systems. *J. Biomed. Mater. Res. Part A*, 29(4), 421–429, 1995.
71. van Oss, C. J., Surface properties of fibrinogen and fibrin. *J. Protein Chem.*, 9(4), 487–491, 1990.
72. van Oss, C. J., Long-range and short-range mechanisms of hydrophobic attraction and hydrophilic repulsion in specific and aspecific interactions. *J. Mol. Recognit.*, 16(4), 177–190, 2003.
73. Labarre, D., Improving blood-compatibility of polymeric surfaces. *Trends Biomater. Artif. Organs*, 15(1), 1–3, 2001.
74. Anderson, J. M., Biological responses to materials. *Annu. Rev. Mater. Res.*, 31, 81–110, 2001.
75. Dobrovolskaia, M. A., Patri, A. K., Simak, J., Hall, J. B., Semberova, J., De Paoli Lacerda, S. H., and McNeil, S. E., Nanoparticle size and surface charge determine effects of PAMAM dendrimers on human platelets in vitro. *Mol. Pharm.*, 9(3), 382–393, 2012.
76. Michanetzis, G. P. A. K., Missirlis, Y. F., and Antimisiaris, S. G., Haemocompatibility of nanosized drug delivery systems: Has it been adequately considered? *J. Biomed. Nanotechnol.* 4(3), 218–233, 2008.
77. Kawakami, H., Takahashi, H., Nagaoka, S., and Nakayama, Y., Albumin adsorption to surface of annealed fluorinated polyimide. *Polym. Adv. Technol.*, 12(3/4), 244–252, 2001.
78. Nagaoka, S., Ashiba, K., and Kawakami, H., Interaction between biocomponents and surface modified fluorinated polyimide. *Mater. Sci. Eng. Part C*, 20(1/2), 181–185, 2002.
79. Reitsma, S., Slaaf, D. W., Vink, H., van Zandvoort, M. A. M. J., and oude Egbrink, M. G. A., The endothelial glycocalyx: Composition, functions, and visualization. *Pflugers Arch.*, 454(3), 345–359, 2007.
80. Hajj Hassan, M., Chodavarapu, V., and Musallam, S., NeuroMEMS: Neural probe microtechnologies. *Sensors*, 8(8), 6704–6726, 2008.

9 Antimicrobial Activity of Polysulfone Structures

Anca Filimon and Silvia Ioan

CONTENTS

9.1 INTRODUCTION

In recent decades, modern medicine has been challenged with complex problems that have led to technological advancements in the area of healthcare [1]. However, in the domain of tissue engineering, a multidisciplinary field combining the principles of biology, medicine, and engineering, which aims at replacing damaged, injured, or missing organs and tissues with a functional artificial substitute, numerous complex problems still remain. Besides the cell-material interaction, the antibacterial properties also play an important role in medical implants.

Both antibacterial and antimicrobial are similar concepts and are sometimes used interchangeably; however, there are some differences between them. Thus, antibacterial represents anything that destroys bacteria or suppresses their growth or their ability to reproduce. Heat and chemicals, such as chlorine and antibiotic drugs, have antibacterial properties. The term *antibacterial* is often used synonymously with that of antibiotic(s); today, however, with the increased knowledge on the causative agents of various infectious diseases, antibiotic(s) has come to denote a broader range of antimicrobial compounds, including antifungal and other compounds.

On the other hand, antimicrobial is a substance that kills or inhibits the growth of microorganisms such as bacteria, fungi, and protozoans. Antimicrobial drugs either kill microbes (microbiocidal) or prevent their growth (microbiostatic). Disinfectants are antimicrobial substances used on nonliving objects or outside the body.

In the above-mentioned context, when an acellular scaffold is implanted, both cells and bacteria compete to adhere and grow onto the surface. This process is called the *race for the surface* [2]. If the tissue cells win the race, the surface of the implant is covered by tissue, whereas when the situation is in favor of bacteria, the attached and growing bacterial colonies soon produce an extracellular polymeric matrix (EPM) [1]. This protects the bacteria against antibiotics and the body's defense system, and allows them to form a biofilm. Depending on the bacterial species involved, the biofilm may be composed of 10%–25% bacterial cells and 75%–90% EPM, also called *slime* [3]. This EPM helps bacterial cells to adhere and trap nutrients from the contacting medium. It also provides a safety cover that protects bacteria from host immunization, predators, as well as antibacterial agents. Antibiotics are thus much less efficient in destroying the bacterial biofilms than circulating bacteria. In most cases, this biofilm leads to further infections and inflammations, which can result in the (partial) removal of the infected implant [2,4,5].

Infections caused by pathogenic microorganisms are of a great concern in many fields, particularly for medical devices, drugs, hospital surfaces/furniture, dental restoration and surgical equipment, healthcare products and hygienic applications, water purification systems, textiles, food packaging and storage, major or domestic appliances, aeronautics, and so on [6,7]. Infectious diseases causes more deaths than any other single cause worldwide. These diseases are of a particular significance in hospitals, where great efforts and important overheads are consumed for struggling against infections triggered by germs (bacteria, viruses, fungi, and protozoa), which are found everywhere, in air, soil, and water.

Generally, these infections are combated with antimicrobial agents, which are susceptible to their action. Particularly problematic is the resistant microorganisms that rapidly and easily mutate their genes, making their elimination difficult.

In brief, the use of potent and/or specific antimicrobial systems will help to mitigate, combat, and/or eradicate these infections, which means an improvement in the state of well-being. In this respect, polymers, due to their intrinsic properties, are extensively and efficiently employed in all these fields. Therefore, the use of polymeric materials with antimicrobial properties gains an increasing interest from both academic and industrial perspectives (Scheme 9.1).

Polymers can act as a matrix for the materials holding antimicrobial agents. In this case, the characteristics of the polymer, such as its hydrophilicity or molecular weight, have a great influence on the final antimicrobial activity, starting from the rate of biocide release up to even conferring synergistic activities. In addition, the development of polymers with antimicrobial activity themselves is also an important area of research, focused on solving the problem of contamination by microorganisms. This alternative avoids the inconvenience of the diffusion of the low-molecular-weight biocides through the polymeric matrix, which often causes toxicity to the human body. Besides, antimicrobial polymers usually present longer-term activity [8–18].

Consequently, this chapter reviews the recent notable problems concerning the field of polymeric materials with antimicrobial activity, such as polysulfones (PSFs): from general aspects to perspective applications.

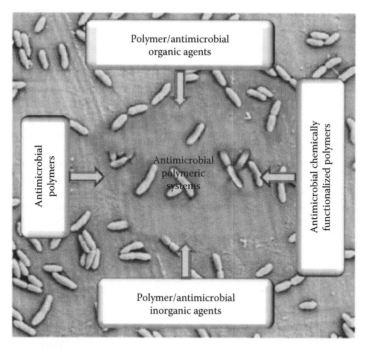

SCHEME 9.1 Illustration of polymeric materials with antimicrobial properties applicable in various fields.

9.2 OVERVIEW OF THE MICROORGANISMS WORLD

Bacteria are nonchlorophyllated unicellular organisms that reproduce themselves by fission and do not present nuclear envelope. Gram's stain is a staining technique used to classify bacteria based on the different characteristics of their cell walls. It is known that the component of Gram-positive bacteria cell walls is peptidoglycan, which confers to them a hydrophobic character, whereas the major constituent of Gram-negative bacteria cell walls is peptidoglycan, together with other membranes, such as lipopolysaccharides and proteins, assuring their hydrophilic character of bacteria [19]. In this context, the specific compositions of the cell wall of both Gram-negative and Gram-positive bacteria induce different antimicrobial activity. Therefore, Gram-positive and Gram-negative bacteria are determined by the amount and the location of peptidoglycan in the cell wall, exhibiting different chemical compositions and structures, cell-wall permeabilities, physiologies, metabolisms, and pathogenicities [20].

In recent years, several Gram-negative and Gram-positive bacteria species have posed overwhelming threats to the healthcare-associated infections [21,22] (Table 9.1).

Such a situation is primarily due to the fact that the bacterial resistance to multidrug has been increasing up to global dimensions and at an alarming magnitude. In this respect, the predominant resistance issues are those related to Gram-negative bacteria species, including Enterobacteriaceae [23], *Klebsiella pneumoniae, Pseudomonas*

TABLE 9.1
Classification of Some Microorganisms as a Function of Strain Type

Strain Type	Bacteria Name
Gram-negative	*Bacteroides forsythus, Enterobacter aerogenes, Escherichia coli, Haemophilus influenzae, Klebsiella pneumoniae, Proteus mirabilis, Proteus vulgaris, Pseudomonas aeruginosa, Salmonella enteritidis, S. typhi, S. typhimurium, Spiroplasma citri,* and *Yersinia pseudotuberculosis*
Gram-positive	*Acholeplasma laidlawii, Actinomyces viscosus, Bacillus coagulans, B. cereus, B. macroides, B. megaterium Bifidobacterium bifidum, B. breve, Enterococcus faecalis, E. faecium, Lactobacillus salivarius, Listeria monocytogenes, Staphylococcus aureus, Staphylococcus epidermidis, Staphylococcus haemolyticus, Staphylococcus hominis, S. saprophyticus, Streptococcus mutans,* and *Streptococcus pneumoniae*
Fungi	*Alternaria alternata, Aspergillus niger, A. terreus, Cladosporium cladosporioides, Eurotium tonophilum, Fusarium moniliforme, Microsporum gypseum, Mucor circinelloides, Penicillium digitatum, Sporotrichum pulverulentum, Stachybotrys chartarum, Trichoderma lignorum,* and *Trichoderma viride*
Yeasts	*Aureobasidium pullulans, Candida albicans, C. parapsilosis, Hanseniaspora guilliermondii, Kluyveromyces fragilis, Pichia jadinii, Rhodotorula rubra,* and *Saccharomyces cerevisiae*
Algae	*Amphora coffeaeformis, Dunaliella tertiolecta,* and *Navicula incerta*
Viruses	Herpes simplex, Human Immunodeficiency, Influenza A, and Varicella zoster

aeruginosa, and *Acinetobacter baumannii.* These circulating isolates have created serious problems in the treatment of nosocomial infection, because they carry highly transmissible elements encoding multiple resistance genes, for example, extended spectrum beta-lactamases—which inactivate different classes of first-line antibiotics [24]—metallo-beta-lactamases—which hydrolyze penicillins, cephalosporins, and carbapenems—efflux pumps—which decrease the bacterial-transporting ability to almost all antibiotics and natural antimicrobial products [25]—and promoters—which ensure the transcription of these genes.

Moreover, microbial diseases present a significant clinical interest, because some bacteria species are more virulent than others and show alteration in sensibility to conventional antimicrobial drugs, mainly the species of the *Staphylococcus, Pseudomonas, Enterococcus,* and *Pneumococcus* genera.

The extensive use of penicillin since World War II promoted the appearance of the first strains of penicillin-resistant Gram-positive bacteria [26]. Vancomycin and methicillin showed a large spectrum of bactericidal actions against many Gram-positive bacteria. However, some strains also presented resistance to these compounds, vancomycin-resistant to *Enterococcus* and methicillin-resistant to *Staphylococcus aureus,* respectively. As a consequence, the resistance of pathogenic microorganisms to antibiotics has stimulated the search of new antimicrobial drugs [27,28].

Worth mentioning is also the fact that transmissions of infectious diseases in healthcare facilities, particularly the drug-resistant species, have been an important and urgent challenge to the infection-control community. For instance, the bacterium *P. aeruginosa*, one of the most common causes of healthcare-associated infections, is increasingly resistant to many antibiotics. *Staphylococcus aureus* is also a bacterium that commonly colonizes human skin and mucosa, without causing severe problems. However, serious diseases, ranging from mild to life-threatening ones, such as skin infections, infected eczema, abscesses, heart valves infections or endocarditis, pneumonia, and blood stream infection or bacteremia, as illustrated in Figure 9.1, can be developed if the bacteria enter the body. Nasal carriage of *S. aureus* represents the most important way of transmitting infections of the microorganism. Some *S. aureus* bacterial strains are resistant to the antibiotic methicillin and often require different types of antibiotics to treat them.

A supergerm called *carbapenem-resistant* Enterobacteriaceae, resistant to the last line of antibiotics, was first detected in 2001 in 41 states in the United States. Enterobacteriaceae is mostly transmitted among the elderly ones, with a weak immune system, by surface contacts, but so far it has only occurred in hospitals or nursing homes, rather than in the community.

On the other hand, fungal infections in humans can range from common, mild superficial ones, such as athlete's foot and candidiasis or thrush (both vaginal and oral) to serious life-threatening diseases, such as invasive aspergillosis, derived from the diversity of *Aspergillus* fungi. In this respect, humans are daily exposed to molds belonging to the kingdom fungi and yeasts, eukaryotic unicellular microorganisms, and pluricellular molds, simply by touching or inhaling them. Because molds naturally exist both outdoors and indoors, their excessive growth is also a health concern. Thus, *Candida* represents the third leading cause of infections in intensive care units (ICUs) worldwide [29]. The increasing prevalence of invasive fungal infections in critically ill patients [30–33] is due to a variety of factors, including the widespread use of broad-spectrum antibiotics [34]. Crude and attributable mortality associated with invasive candidiasis have been reported to be as high as 58% and 43%, respectively [34–36]. Various independent risk factors of mortality in invasive

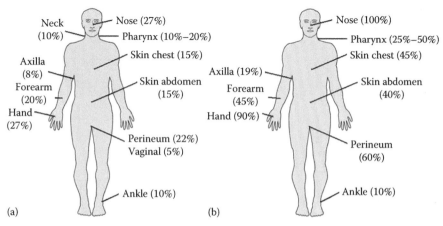

FIGURE 9.1 Carriage rates of *Staphylococcus aureus* on human body site: (a) noninfested and (b) infested.

candidiasis have been identified, including the lack of prescription of an appropriate antifungal agent, and the failure to initiate early antifungal prophylaxis [34,37]. Inadequate doses may also contribute not only to treatment failure [38,39] but also to the emergence of resistance. With the increasing prevalence of nonalbicans *Candida* species [36] and their reduced susceptibility to some antifungal agents, appropriate choice and dosing of antifungals are essential for optimizing clinical outcomes and minimizing resistance. Rational dosing can only be achieved by considering the relevant pharmacokinetics and pharmacodynamics of the selected antifungal agents in critically ill patients.

In fact, microorganisms can be transmitted from sources onto different material surfaces by contacts and aerosol deposition, and can survive on them for weeks and even months in hospital environments. During their survival on such surfaces, the germs can undergo several growth stages, leading to the formation of biofilms (Figure 9.2), if sufficient time is given.

The biofilms formed on the surfaces of materials cannot be easily eradicated by spraying regular biocides, except for the use of chlorine bleach or of a solution of glutaraldehyde. The microorganisms on the surfaces of the materials can directly transmit diseases by contacts, or they can serve in the aerosol source at any stage of growth.

The discovery and introduction of antibiotics revolutionized the human therapy, the veterinary, and plant medicine. Despite the obtained spectacular results, several problems have subsequently appeared. Emergence of antibiotic resistance is an enormous clinical and public health concern. Thus, methicillin-resistant to *S. aureus*, streptomycin-resistant to *Erwinia amylovora* and Rosaceae, the emergence of extended spectrum beta-lactamase, producing the carbapenem-resistant to

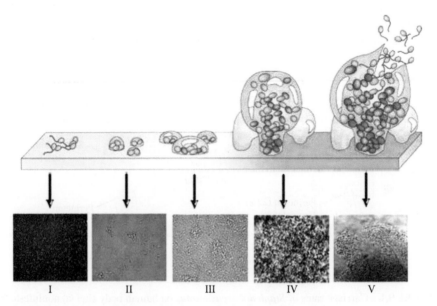

FIGURE 9.2 Stages of biofilms forming on the surfaces of materials.

Enterobacteriaceae and *Klebsiella pneumoniae*, and polyresistant to *Pseudomonas* and *Acinetobacter* cause serious difficulties in the treatment of severe infections [40]; therefore, a comprehensive strategy, a multidisciplinary effort, is required to combat them infections. The new strategy includes compliance with infection control principles: antimicrobial stewardship and the development of new antimicrobial agents effective against multiresistant Gram-negative and Gram-positive pathogens. Therefore, the antimicrobial functions on the novel materials have been considered as a potential tool in reducing the transmission of diseases, assuming that they could reduce the population of microorganisms. Considering such a speculation and the urgent need in the control of infectious diseases, numerous antimicrobial polymers, coating, fibers, and fabrics have been developed in recent decades.

9.3 ANTIMICROBIAL AGENTS: FROM CONCEPT TO THERAPEUTIC PERSPECTIVES

The treatment of infectious diseases still remains an important and challenging problem because of a combination of factors, including emerging infectious diseases and the increasing number of multidrug-resistant microbial pathogens [41]. In spite of the large number of antibiotics and chemotherapeutics available for medical use, the concomitant emergence of antibiotic resistance requires a substantial medical need for new classes of antimicrobial agents. There is a really perceived need for the discovery of new compounds possessing antimicrobial activity, possibly acting through various mechanisms, distinct from those of well-known classes of antimicrobial agents to which many clinically relevant pathogens are now resistant.

Due to the outbreak of infectious diseases caused by different pathogenic bacteria and the development of antibiotic resistance, researchers are searching for new antibacterial agents. Most antimicrobial agents used for the treatment of bacterial infections may be categorized according to their main mechanism of action. Thus, there are five major modes of action: (1) interference with cell wall synthesis (betalactams and glycopeptides); (2) inhibition of protein synthesis (bacterial ribosomes); (3) interference with the nucleic acid synthesis (deoxyribonucleic acid, DNA, and ribonucleic acid, RNA); (4) inhibition of a metabolic pathway; and (5) disruption of bacterial membrane structure [42].

Therefore, many recent events have attracted an increased interest for the development of new microbicidal polymers, which are both bactericidal and biocompatible, as well as nanotechnological materials [43].

9.3.1 PSFs with Quaternary Ammonium Compounds

Polymeric materials with intrinsic antimicrobial properties have become highly important as coatings and adhesives used in many domains, such as environmental and hospital disinfection, and equipment surfaces [44–48]. In this regard, polymers with quaternary ammonium groups are the most explored kind of polymeric biocides. Therefore, quaternary ammonium compounds belong to this group of compounds, which exhibit high antimicrobial activity and appear as safer than the chemically active disinfectants, such as chlorine and glutaraldehyde. However, the irritating and cytotoxic effects of these compounds on human cells/tissues such as keratinocytes, fibroblasts, cornea, and respiratory mucosa [49,50] have been also shown, so that the improvement of quaternary ammonium compounds is necessary not only for their antimicrobial activity but also for the safety of human cells. To overcome these problems, anchoring the quaternary ammonium compounds to a polymer backbone might be promising in developing materials that would have antimicrobial activity.

Starting from the literature data, a variety of PSFs have been molecularly designed [51–56] to enhance their performance, becoming biologically inert and nontoxic compounds, exhibiting stable mechanical, morphological, and adhesion characteristics during their exploitation. The combination of these factors assures the biocompatibility of PSFs and, implicitly, the possibility of their action inside a living organism or in contact with living systems, without negative consequences.

Conjugated polymers are organic macromolecules with a backbone of alternating single and double bonds functionalized with side groups, to facilitate their solubility in organic solvents. Water-soluble conjugated polymers or polyelectrolytes are obtained when functionalized with ionic side groups. The family of cationic conjugated polyelectrolytes includes quaternized polysulfones (PSFQs), which are antimicrobial polymers with complex properties. Therefore, the chemical modification of PSFs, especially quaternization with ammonium groups [57], is an efficient method to obtain some properties recommended in multiple applications, for example, as biomaterials and semipermeable membranes [56]. It was shown that these groups can modify hydrophilicity and increase water permeability (of special interest for biomedical applications) [58,59], antimicrobial action [7,56], and solubility characteristics [60–63], while also improving separation [64,65].

Accordingly, quaternary ammonium salts are known as effective antimicrobial compounds against a plethora of Gram-negative and Gram-positive bacteria, fungi, and certain types of viruses [66], so that they can be included in the composition of polymers, to impart antibacterial properties. Their antimicrobial effectiveness is strongly correlated with the length of the adjacent alkyl chain and the size and number of cationic ammonium groups in the molecule.

As generally known, the biological activity of quaternary ammonium compounds depends on the nature of the organic groups attached to nitrogen, the number of nitrogen atoms present, and counterion [67]. They usually contain four organic groups linked to nitrogen, with similar or different chemistry and structure. The organic substituents are alkyl, aryl, or heterocyclic compounds. It has been shown that an increase in the alkyl chain length of an amphiphilic compound is followed by an increase in the hydrophobic interaction with the lipid bilayer of the cell wall, which in turn increases the antimicrobial activity of the compound. Quaternary ammonium compounds containing one long alkyl substituent of at least eight carbon atoms were shown to be very active biocides in water [68]. Moreover, the nature of the counterions can affect the antimicrobial activity. Recently, a series of new bioactive polymers with pendant chlorine analogous groups were prepared to demonstrate this effect [56,69,70].

Two main hypotheses for the mode of action of antimicrobial substances based on quaternary ammonium salts are discussed in the literature [44]. In this respect, it is well known that most bacterial cell walls are negatively charged, containing phosphatidylethanolamine (70%) as the major component; hence, most antimicrobial polymers are positively charged. It is generally accepted that the mechanism of bactericidal action of the polycationic biocides involves destructive interactions with the cell wall and/or cytoplasmic membranes [71]. Macromolecules may interact more effectively with the cells of Gram-positive bacteria, as their polyglycane outer layer is sufficiently loosely packed to facilitate the deep penetration of the polymer chain inside the cell, to interact with the cytoplasmic membrane.

On the other hand, a Gram-negative bacterial cell has an additional membrane with a bilayer phospholipid structure, which protects the inner cytoplasmic membrane to a higher extent against the adverse action of the polymeric biocide.

The antimicrobial function arises from the attractive interactions between the cationic ammonium group of the quaternary amine (positive charge) and the negatively charged cell membrane of the bacteria; these interactions consequently result in the formation of a cationic surface–microbe complex, which, in turn, causes an interruption of all essential functions of the cell membrane and thus the interruption of protein activity [72]. Several authors explain that the prime stage of bacterial adhesion process is called the *docking phase*, when bacteria come close to the material surface by Brownian motion, sedimentation, and convective mass transport as driving forces. Once the bacteria are close to the surface, the interactions, such as van der Waals, electrostatic, hydrophobic, and steric, occur in another stage, called the *locking phase*. In this stage, bacteria still show Brownian motion. However, the second, crucial locking stage includes mediated binding, for example, a specific ligand–receptor interaction which, in turn, incites the process of bacterial adhesion to the material surfaces [73]. After the *docking* of the salt on a bacterium, a sufficiently long hydrophobic alkyl chain can penetrate the bacterial phospholipid membrane and disturb it [1,73,74]. Dunne elucidates that the adhesion process is dictated by a number of variables, including bacterial species, surface composition, and environmental factors [75].

The adhesion mechanism is a reversible one, which means that bacteria can firmly attach onto the surface, due to the existence of adhesion and the absence of physical and chemical interventions. This will subsequently lead to biofilm formation and might cause biofouling onto membrane surfaces. In addition, the quaternary ammonium groups can reduce the multiplication ability [76]. If the long hydrocarbon chain is bonded to cationic ammonium in the structure of the quaternary ammonium salts, two types of interactions can occur between the agent and the microorganism: a polar interaction, with the cationic nitrogen of the ammonium group, and a nonpolar interaction, with the hydrophobic chain. Penetration of the hydrophobic group of the microorganism consequently occurs, enabling the alkylammonium group to physically interrupt all key cell functions [77].

Finally, the incorporation of the hydrophilic and biocompatible quaternary groups has been suggested to improve both antimicrobial efficiency and biocompatibility. Therefore, due to the bactericidal efficacy of PSFQs, they show maximal biocompatibility, which extends their use in biomaterial applications.

9.3.2 PSFs Containing Phosphorium Derivatives

Despite their numerous positive properties, the antimicrobial activity of polymers with quaternary ammonium salts is not just as efficient against a wide range of bacteria compared to other polymeric compounds. PSFQs exhibit less intense antimicrobial effects generated by the quaternary nitrogen, which is pendant, away from the backbone chain. Therefore, for an enhanced biocidal effect, it is necessary to introduce hydrophobic groups with high charge density. To solve this, another successful antimicrobial system is formed by polymers containing nonsoluble quaternary phosphonium salts grafted on the backbone chain [78,79].

This assertion was supported by the hydrophobic nature of the polymer, the enlargement of the polymeric coil, and increase of the charge density - generated by the active cationic centers present on a single polyelectrolyte molecule. Consequently, these polymers exhibit quite a high biocidal activity as long as the polymeric chain retains positive charge density, whereas some active phosphorous centers unscreened by counterions are also present. On the other hand, usually, cell membranes carry excessive negative charges and the counterions do not interact with membranes under physiological conditions. In a slightly acidic medium, the phospholipids of the cell wall are protonated and the counterions can interact with the membrane. In addition to the electrostatic ones, these interactions also involve hydrogen bonds and hydrophobic bindings [80].

For many years, phosphorous derivatives with antimicrobial activity have been investigated as medicals and antiseptics [73,79]. Recently, the use of antiseptics and disinfectants has been questioned, because of the possibility of hospital-acquired infections [79]. Besides that, bacteria can be altered with respect to their susceptibility toward other antiseptics and antibiotics. Moreover, phosphorous compounds have been designed to prevent virus-cell fusion/attachment, principally in sexually transmitted diseases [7].

The action mechanism of antimicrobial PSF-bearing quaternary phosphonium compounds on killing bacteria by damaging the cell wall membrane is similar to that for PSF-containing quaternary ammonium.

In conclusion, traditional antimicrobial drugs target only a few cellular processes and are derived from a few distinct chemical classes. Meanwhile, antimicrobial strategies offer timely therapeutic countermeasures, which are urgently required for possible outbreaks of new superbug infections. One promising strategy—the development of new biomaterials as antibacterial agents (e.g., PSFQs with ammonium and phosphorous compounds)—provides an opportunity for enhancing broad spectrum therapeutics against upgrading infections caused by multidrug resistant pathogenic species, where many successful compounds have failed. This advantage is unique, having the potential to selectively kill target pathogens with specific species and even strains. Of particular interest are the possibilities to tailor the antimicrobial spectrum to the use of conventional antibiotics by potentiating their activity and reverse resistance.

9.3.3 Antimicrobial Inorganic Compounds

The field of bioinorganic chemistry, which reflects the impact of metal complexes in biological systems, has opened a new horizon for the scientific research, due to its richness in metal- or metalloid-based drugs, including Paul Erlich's organoarsenic compounds for the treatment of antiarthritic syphilis [81]. A large number of compounds are biologically important. Some metals, essential for their biological functions, are found in enzymes and cofactors required for various processes. For example, hemoglobin from red blood cells contains an iron–porphyrin complex, which is used for oxygen transport and storage in the body, whereas chlorophyll from green plants, responsible for photosynthetic process, contains a magnesium–porphyrin complex. Cobalt is found in coenzyme B_{12}, which is essential in the biological systems for the transfer of alkyl groups from one molecule to another. Metals such as copper, zinc, iron, and manganese are incorporated into catalytic proteins (the metalloenzymes), which facilitate a multitude of chemical reactions needed for life [41].

Today, medicinal inorganic chemistry remains a field of great promise with many challenges. The potential for a major expansion of chemical diversity into new structural and reactivity materials with high therapeutic impact is unquestionable. Therefore, metal ions may be introduced into a biological system for therapeutic or diagnostic purposes. Several metal complexes are known to accelerate the drug action and the efficacy of the organic therapeutic agent. The efficiency of the various organic therapeutic agents can often be enhanced by coordinating with a suitable metal ion. The pharmacological activity of metal complexes is highly dependent on the nature of metal ions and the donor sequence of ligands, because different ligands exhibit different biological properties. There is a really perceived need for the discovery of new compounds endowed with antimicrobial activities. The newly prepared compounds should be more effective, and should act through a mechanism distinct from those of well-known classes of antimicrobial agents to which many clinically relevant pathogens are now resistant. Materials obtained on the basis of inorganic active agents with good potential for antimicrobial activity can be categorized in two main groups: inorganic materials and their nanocomposites (including titanium dioxide, silver, zinc oxide, copper, gallium, gold nanoparticles, carbon nanotubes, and nanolayered clay) and inorganic materials loaded in organic carriers (including polymers loaded with inorganic materials, nano- and microcapsules having inorganic nanoparticles, metallic dendrimer nano-composites, and inorganic nanoparticles loaded in liposomes) (Scheme 9.2) [81].

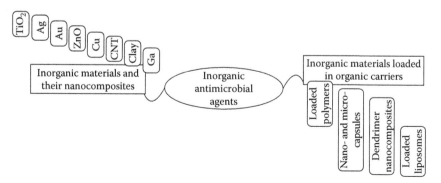

SCHEME 9.2 Classification of antimicrobial materials on the basis of inorganic active agents.

In order to establish the efficiency of their antimicrobial activity, many organic materials require the interaction with metals. These materials interact with metals at their target site or during their metabolism, or disturb the balance of metal–ion uptake and distribution in cells and tissue. Consequently, the unique properties of metal complexes tend to offer advantages in the discovery and development of new drugs. Metal complexes are amenable to combinatorial synthetic methods, and an immense diversity of structural scaffolds can be thus achieved. Metal centers are capable of organizing the surrounding atoms to achieve pharmacophore geometries that are not readily achieved by other means. Additionally, the effects of metals can be highly specific and can be modulated by recruiting cellular processes that recognize specific types of metal–macromolecules interactions. Understanding these interactions can lead the way toward a rational design of metallopharmaceuticals and the implementation of new cotherapies.

Finally, organic materials–metal combinations have proven to be essential in antimicrobial treatment, due to a number of important considerations: (1) they increase activity through the use of compounds with synergistic or additive activity; (2) they thwart drug resistance; (3) they decrease the required doses, reducing both cost and the chances of toxic side effects; and (4) they increase the spectrum of antimicrobial activity.

Currently, TiO_2 nanoparticles have created a new approach for remarkable applications, as an attractive multifunctional material. TiO_2 nanoparticles possess unique properties, such as a high, long-lasting stability, and act as a safe broad-spectrum antibiotic. This makes TiO_2 nanoparticles applicable in many fields, such as self-cleaning, antibacterial, and ultraviolet-protecting agents.

Since ancient times, among various antimicrobial agents, silver has been most extensively studied and has been used to control infections and prevent spoilage. At present, many researchers have focused on antibacterial and multifunctional properties of silver nanoparticles [82]. In particular, there is an increasing interest toward the exploitation of silver nanoparticles technology in the development of bioactive biomaterials, aiming at combining the relevant antibacterial properties of the metal with the peculiar performance of the biomaterial [83,84]. Silver is a safer antimicrobial agent in comparison with some organic antimicrobial agents that have been avoided because of their possible harmful effects on the human body. Silver has been described as being *oligodynamic* because of its ability to exert a bactericidal effect on products containing silver, principally due to its antimicrobial activities and low toxicity to human cells. Its therapeutic property has been proven against a broad range of microorganisms, over 650 disease-causing organisms in the body, even at low concentrations. The antimicrobial mechanism is illustrated in Scheme 9.3 [81]. Generally, metal ions destroy or pass through the cell membrane and bind to the −SH group of the cellular wall. The subsequent decrease of enzymatic activity modifies the metabolism of microorganisms and inhibits their growth, up to cell death. Metal ions also catalyze by generating oxygen radicals that oxidize the molecular structure of bacteria. Formation of active oxygen occurs according to the following chemical reaction:

$$H_2O + 1/2\ O_2 \rightarrow H_2O_2 \rightarrow H_2O + (O)$$

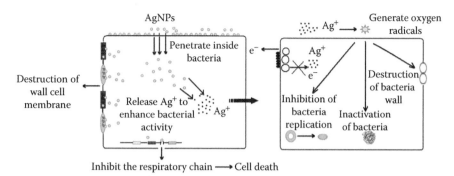

SCHEME 9.3   General representation of the antimicrobial mechanism of silver nanoparticles.

Such a mechanism does not need any direct contact between the antimicrobial agent and bacteria, because the produced active oxygen diffuses from the fiber to the surrounding environment. Silver ions can lead to protein denaturation and cell death, because of their reaction with the nucleophilic amino acid residues in proteins, and can be attached to the sulfhydryl, amino, imidazole, phosphate and carboxyl groups of the membrane or enzyme proteins. Respiration blocking and cell death may also be caused by R—S—S—R bonds formation.

In the case of polyelectrolytes (e.g., functionalized PSFs), the stabilization of metal nanoparticles is explained by the electronic interaction of the polymer functional groups with the metal particles [82]. In fact, their nucleophilic character is sufficient to bind the metal particles by donating electrons. Protective polymers can coordinate metal ions before reduction, forming a polymer–metal ion complex; such a complex can be then reduced under mild conditions, resulting in a smaller and a narrower size distribution than those obtained without protective polymers. Once reduction occurs, the stabilizing effect of these macromolecules is attributable to the fact that either the particles are attached to the much larger protecting polymers or the protecting molecules cover or encapsulate the metal particles. To find applications in the biomaterials field, both the stabilizing and the reducing agents should not represent a biological hazard [82].

Gold nanoparticles are known as a novel biomedical application. Their potent antibacterial effectiveness against acne and the lack of tolerance to the antibiotic have caused their commercial usage in soap and cosmetic industries. They can remove waste materials from the skin and control sebum.

Among the many types of antimicrobial metal and metal oxide nanoparticles, including silver, gold, aluminum, TiO_2, MgO, and CuO nanoparticles, ZnO nanoparticles also represent the well-known and very prominent antimicrobial metal oxide structures, because of their spectacular properties [85]. Although the antibacterial mechanism of ZnO is still under investigation, ZnO nanomaterials present a good antimicrobial activity in various applications and products [85,86]. Sawai et al. [87] found out that the most important mechanism for killing microorganisms by ZnO was the production of hydrogen peroxide from photocatalytic generation. Some studies have also evidenced that the production of reactive oxygen species by ZnO nanoparticles could interact with the bacterial cells and cause the death of cells [88,89]. Brayner et al. [90] and Huang et al. [91] reported that ZnO diffusion through the cell wall and the disorganization of the bacterial membrane upon contact with ZnO nanoparticles could reduce bacterial growth. Another mechanism for killing microorganisms is the larger accumulation of nanoparticles within the cell membrane and cytoplasm [92].

In conclusion, the use of metal and/or metal oxide nanoparticles to impart antimicrobial activities to various kinds of materials is an increasing research area for many fields, including polymeric materials, textiles, in the medical field, and in the production of some medicines [81,85,86].

9.4 RELATIONSHIPS BETWEEN CHEMICAL STRUCTURE AND ACTIVITY OF PSFs AGAINST GRAM-POSITIVE AND GRAM-NEGATIVE BACTERIA

Intensive research into antibacterial agents continues to be a necessity, due to microbial resistance and infectious diseases. Microorganisms continue to contaminate the surfaces of medical devices, hospital and dental equipment, water purification systems, food packaging, and textiles [93]. Hence, there exists a strong demand for the development of a broad spectrum of antibacterial materials that can deliver such agents. Because bacterial colonization and subsequent biofilm formation occurs on virtually any surface, the antibacterial materials should be robust and readily applicable to a variety of surface topographies.

In this context, the development of new polymers, which are both bactericidal and biocompatible, represents a substantial research interest for many applications. Literature highlights that PSFs are widely used as biomaterials due to several outstanding properties, such as high mechanical strength, resistance to acids and alkalis, thermal and chemical stability, and, most importantly, film-forming properties and excellent biocompatibility [94].

Currently, PSFs application is focused on blood-contact devices (e.g., hemodialysis, hemodiafiltration, and hemofiltration in the form of membranes) [95,96], cell- and tissue-contact devices (e.g., bioreactors made of hollow-fiber membranes) [97,98], and nerve generation (through semipermeable, hollow PSF membranes) [99,100]. On the other hand, biomedical PSFs have been widely used in extracorporeal and biomedical devices. Therefore, a thorough understanding of the relationships between polymer surface and blood components is very important for the development of novel biomedical polymers.

Although these materials have excellent overall properties, their intrinsic hydrophobic nature often restricts their utility in membrane applications, such as saline solution perfusions, artificial kidney membranes, and cell culture bioreactors, all requiring hydrophilic characteristics. To meet these demands, the structural modification of conventional materials is often essential. Therefore, the functionalization of PSFs represents an efficient method to attain some properties recommended in various fields, for example, in biomedicine, as antimicrobial agents with an important role in medical implants.

Literature [1,10,101] discusses different possible approaches that prevent the adhesion of bacteria onto the surface. One way is to deposit a coating that offers resistance against bacterial colonization on the implant surface. However, it should be kept in mind that the antibacterial properties of the surface should not compromise the attachment of cells from the surrounding tissue. Some antibacterial polymers, which kill bacteria or prevent their attachment, may be used for such a coating [56]. In this regard, polymers with quaternary ammonium groups—positively charged— are the most explored kind of polymeric biocides. It is generally accepted that the mechanism of bactericidal action of polycationic biocides involves destructive inter- actions with the cell wall and/or cytoplasmic membranes [71]. In this context, the performance of a bactericidal polymer is measured by its ability to strike the balance between the microbicidal and biocompatible properties, maximizing the selectiv- ity of the material [43]. Therefore, the literature [56] has reported the bioactivity dependence on the pendant chain size of quaternary ammonium salts, allowing the establishment of a structure–bioactivity relationship for PSFQs with different ionic chlorine contents (PSFQ). The results showed that the new PSFQs have higher anti- bacterial properties, which makes them promising candidates as semipermeable membranes for clinical and industrial applications.

The antimicrobial efficiency of PSFQs was examined against two representative microorganisms of clinical interest: *Escherichia coli* (Gram-negative) and *S. aureus* (Gram-positive). It is well known that *E. coli* can cause gastroenteritis, urinary tract infections, and neonatal meningitis, whereas *S. aureus* is part of human flora, being mainly present in the nose and skin. These bacteria are a leading cause of food poisoning, resulting from the consumption of food contaminated with enterotoxins [102,103].

As shown in Figure 9.3, PSFQs inhibit the growth of microorganisms, inhibition becoming stronger with increasing the polycationic nature of the modified PSFs. Also, for all solutions, the inhibition is intense compared to dimethyl sulfoxide (DMSO), which was used as a control sample [56]. These conclusions are evaluated in terms of the diameter of the inhibition zone presented in Figure 9.3.

Worth mentioning here is that cationic PSFs modified with quaternary ammo- nium groups interfere with the bacterial metabolism by electrostatic stacking at the cell surface of bacteria [104]. In this context, the specific compositions of the cell wall of Gram-negative (*E. coli*) and Gram-positive (*S. aureus*) bacteria induce differ- ent antimicrobial activity. It is known that the component of Gram-positive bacteria cell walls is peptidoglycan, which confers the hydrophobic character of *S. aureus*, whereas the major constituent of Gram-negative bacteria cell walls is peptidoglycan, together with other membranes, such as lipopolysaccharides and proteins, assuring the hydrophilic character of *E. coli* [19]. Thus, it was found out that the inhibition of the hydrophilic *E. coli* to the hydrophilic PSFQs is higher than the inhibition of hydrophobic *S. aureus* cells; in other words, *E. coli* was found to be much more sen- sitive to the investigated polymers than *S. aureus*.

Finally, the general analysis of the relationship between the chemical structure and the activity of PSFQs against Gram-positive and Gram-negative bacteria indi- cates that the antimicrobial activity of PSFQs depended not only on the nature of the functionalized groups of PSFQs but also on the hydrophilic or hydrophobic character of microorganisms, generating different interactions of the quaternary ammonium salt groups with the bacterial cell membrane.

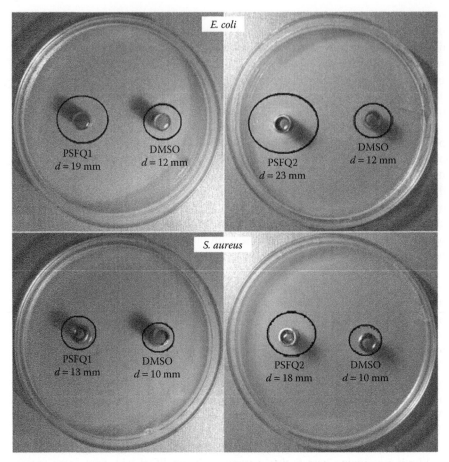

FIGURE 9.3 Antimicrobial screening tests for PSFQ1 and PSFQ2 in DMSO against *E. coli* and *S. aureus* bacteria, expressed by the inhibition zone diameter, *d*. In each figure, the inhibition area on the right side was recorded for DMSO (control sample).

On the other hand, recent studies [70,74,105,106] were focused on the bactericidal effect of silver (Ag) nanoparticles against a wide range of microorganisms. By utilizing polymers (i.e., PSFs), it is possible to create composite materials that maximize the bactericidal properties of active agents, such as silver nanoparticles. In this respect, PSF has appeared to be a more promising material, as it is an easy handling polymeric structure, soluble in organic solvents and resistant to chemical attack [107,108]. Thus, the combination of polymer and Ag particles may enhance the antibacterial property, due to the protection offered by polymer-hosting [109]. The high antibacterial activity with very low loading and the improved distribution of silver particles in the polymer matrix are the essential properties that should be taken into account during the fabrication of this composite [106].

Basri et al. have reported that polyethersulfone (PES)-silver composite membranes, prepared using silver nitrate ($AgNO_3$) as antibacterial agent and polyvinylpyrrolidone

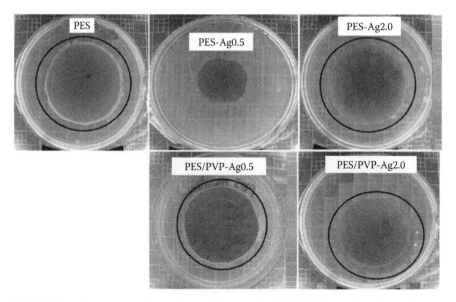

FIGURE 9.4   Results of antimicrobial activity tests for PES/PVP-Ag composite membranes with different dosage of diffusible inhibitory compounds from silver particles.

(PVP) as a dispersant in dope formulation, possess inhibition zones against Gram-negative bacteria, *E. coli* (Figure 9.4) [106].

Release of a higher dosage of diffusible inhibitory compounds from silver particles into the surrounding medium (PES-Ag2.0 and PES/PVP-Ag2.0), and the uniform distribution of Ag particles have significantly contributed to 100% inhibition against *E. coli* within 24 h incubation. Based on these findings, it can be concluded that PES-silver composite membranes with PVP offers a huge potential as membranes for bacteria removal and disinfection.

Later, Basri et al. [73] studied a new type of antibacterial and antiadhesion membrane, obtained by blending PES with 2,4,6-triaminopyrimidine (TAP) as a compatibilizer, and $AgNO_3$ as an antibacterial agent, which results in better hydrophilicity, high tensile strength, and a smoother surface with antiadhesion properties. In addition, the PES/TAP/Ag membrane prepared via the simple phase-inversion technique evidenced antiadhesion properties when tested on *E. coli* bacteria (Figure 9.5). These properties are prominent factors in preventing or minimizing bioactivity problems in membrane applications.

The analysis of results states, beyond any doubt, that PES/TAP/Ag membranes showed much fewer *E. coli* microorganisms adhering on the surfaces. In contrast, PES/Ag and PES/PVP/Ag membranes exhibited a significant amount of *E. coli* on the surface. Furthermore, PES/Ag and PES/PVP/Ag membrane surfaces appeared as good templates for the proliferation of *E. coli* and the formation of a biofilm, which might easily occur on such surfaces upon contact with *E. coli*. Moreover, silver particle attachment and distribution in the polymer host induce the effective removal of bacteria.

Moreover, the incorporation of silver nanoparticles (AgNPs) into polymeric nanofibers fabricated by the electrospinning process has attracted a great deal of attention due to the strong antimicrobial activity generated by the resulting fibers [105].

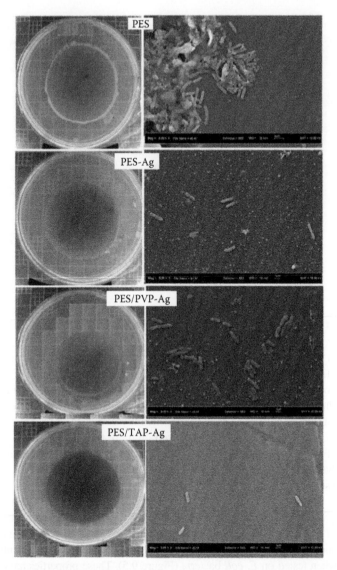

FIGURE 9.5 Results of the antibacterial activity on *E. coli* for PES, PES-Ag, PES/PVP-Ag, and PES/TAP-Ag composite membranes. In the right side of each figure, adhesion tests of microorganism (field-emission scanning electron microscope—FESEM scanning) are illustrated.

This technique can yield flexible composite mats, which can then be applied as a thin coating for any surface. Due to their high surface area-to-volume ratio, electrospun mats exhibit higher antimicrobial activity than conventional microfibers [110].

Literature [105] presents researches on the antibacterial activity of PSF fibers whose surfaces were functionalized with cationic polyethylenimine (PEI)-coated silver nanoparticles (AgNPs) via electrostatic interactions, following an oxygen plasma treatment (Figure 9.6a–c).

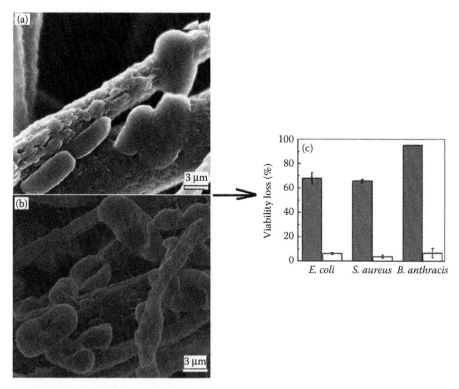

FIGURE 9.6 FESEM micrographs of PSF-AgNP mats displaying *E. coli* cells incubated for (a) 5 min and (b) 180 min. Toxicity assay results for various bacteria in contact PSF-AgNP mats incubated for 15 min in an isotonic solution (0.9% NaCl, pH 5.7) at 37°C. (c) Error bars indicate standard deviation.

Plasma-treated PSF-AgNP mats display high bioactivity against *E. coli*, *S. aureus*, and *Bacillus anthracis* microorganisms (Figure 9.6b). Thus, plasma treatment for 60 s represented the shortest time required for maximum loss of bacteria (*E. coli*) viability. Time-dependent bacterial cytotoxicity studies indicate that PSF-AgNP mats exhibit a high level of inactivation against both Gram-negative bacteria, *E. coli*, and Gram-positive bacteria, *B. anthracis* and *S. aureus*. Therefore, it is demonstrated that electrospun PSF mats whose surface had been modified with PEI-coated AgNPs offer potential applicability as broad-spectrum biocidal coatings.

Research into composite systems, which maximize the efficiency of active bactericidal agents, continues to be a necessity because infectious diseases and bacterial outbreaks remain.

9.5 CONCLUSIONS AND FUTURE PERSPECTIVES

Synthetic antimicrobial polymers offer a wide range of possibilities in application areas of medicine, pharmacy, food, aeronautics, and so on. This is due to their nontoxic and nonirritant properties and prolonged antimicrobial activities, compared with the ordinary low-molecular-weight antibacterial agents, which present some disadvantages, such as toxicity and short-term antimicrobial ability. In addition, the increased use of antibiotics in human and veterinary medicine is provoking microbial resistance, with serious impact on public health. Conventional antibiotics penetrate microorganisms without damaging the bacteria cell wall. In contrast, antimicrobial polymers can destroy the bacterial membrane that may help to prevent antibiotic resistance. The exponential increase in the development/performance of these antimicrobial materials demonstrates their great potential and the significance of bolstering the research regarding the improvement of their synthesis, as well as on their activity and mechanisms of action. It is crucial to achieve innocuous materials, non-cytotoxic to the human organisms, with potent and a broad range of antimicrobial activity, long-lasting response, and even reusable to maintain the activity, while never neglecting the environmental and recycling aspects.

As shown throughout this chapter, there are many strategies to design synthetic antimicrobial polymers with diverse manners of action over microorganisms. Their activity may be inherent in their original structure, but the chemical modification or the introduction of organic or inorganic antimicrobial agents confers the biocidal behavior.

Most research has been focused on polycationic systems, more straightforward and synthetically flexible. Therefore, progress will be concentrated on the increment of their selectivity and durability. However, systems based on the combination of organic and inorganic antimicrobial agents present a special commercial interest. In this respect, their improvement will be assured through antimicrobial agent incorporation, so that toxicity will be reduced, while the activity is maintained or enhanced. In addition, special efforts will be done in the area of nanotechnology, in which a small amount of active components, less than 5 wt%, renders the whole system effective.

Cytotoxicity reduction will be another goal, which is not a problem in the areas of decontamination or antifouling, where they are expected to have a great potential. Efforts will be also focused to reduce costs, by investigating inexpensive systems. In short, the future of these materials will go through a combination of different approaches, along with a continuous investigation on the killing action of these promising systems.

ACKNOWLEDGMENT

This work was supported by a grant of the Romanian National Authority for Scientific Research, CNCS–UEFISCDI (project number PN-II-RU-TE-2012-3-143).

REFERENCES

1. Vasilev, K., Cook, J., and Griesser, H. J. Antibacterial surfaces for biomedical devices. *Expert Rev. Med. Devices*, 6(5), 553–567, 2009.
2. Jacobs, T., Morent, R., De Geyter, N., Dubruel, P., and Leys, C. Plasma surface modification of biomedical polymers: Influence on cell-material interaction. *Plasma Chem. Plasma Process*, 32(5), 1039–1073, 2012.

3. Kumar, V., Rauscher, H., Bretagnol, F., Arefi-Khonsari, F., Pulpytel, J., Colpo, P., and Rossi, F. Preventing biofilm formation on biomedical surfaces. In *Plasma Technology for Hyper Functional Surfaces: Food, Biomedical and Textile Applications*, Rauscher, H., Perucca, M., and Buyle, G. ed., Wiley, Weinheim, Germany, Chapter 7, p. 184, 2010.
4. Subbiahdoss, G., Kuijer, R., Grijpma, D. W., van der Mei, H. C., and Busscher, H. J. Microbial biofilm growth vs. tissue integration: "The race for the surface" experimentally studied. *Acta Biomater.*, 5(5), 1399–1404, 2009.
5. Bazaka, K., Jacob, M. V., Crawford, R. J., and Ivanova, E. P. Plasma-assisted surface modification of organic biopolymers to prevent bacterial attachment. *Acta Biomater.*, 7(5), 2015–2028, 2011.
6. Muñoz-Bonilla, A., Cerrada, M., and Fernández-García, M. *Polymeric Materials with Antimicrobial Activity: From Synthesis to Applications*. Royal Society of Chemistry, Cambridge, UK, 2013.
7. Muñoz-Bonilla, A. and Fernández-García, M. Polymeric materials with antimicrobial activity. *Prog. Polym. Sci.*, 37(2), 281–339, 2012.
8. Tashiro, T. Antibacterial and bacterium adsorbing macromolecules. *Macromol. Mater. Eng.*, 286(2), 63–87, 2001.
9. Pascual, A. Pathogenesis of catheter-related infections: Lessons for new designs. *Clin. Microbiol. Infect.*, 8(5), 256–264, 2002.
10. Hetrick, E. M. and Schoenfisch, M. H. Reducing implant-related infections: Active release strategies. *Chem. Soc. Rev.*, 35(9), 780–789, 2006.
11. Kenawy, E. R., Worley, S. D., and Broughton, R. The chemistry and applications of antimicrobial polymers: A state-of-the-art review. *Biomacromolecules*, 8(5), 1359–1384, 2007.
12. Chen, S. and Jiang, S. A new avenue to nonfouling materials. *Adv. Mater.*, 20(2), 335–338, 2008.
13. Ferreira, L. and Zumbuehl, A. Non-leaching surfaces capable of killing microorganisms on contact. *J. Mater. Chem.*, 19(42), 7796–7806, 2009.
14. Lichter, J. A. and Rubner, M. F. Polyelectrolyte multilayers with intrinsic antimicrobial functionality: The importance of mobile polycations. *Langmuir*, 25(13), 7686–7694, 2009.
15. Lichter, J. A., Van Vliet, K. J., and Rubner, M. F. Design of antibacterial surfaces and interfaces: Polyelectrolyte multilayers as a multifunctional platform. *Macromolecules*, 42(22), 8573–8586, 2009.
16. Jaeger, W., Bohrisch, J., and Laschewsky, A. Synthetic polymers with quaternary nitrogen atoms-synthesis and structure of the most used type of cationic polyelectrolytes. *Prog. Polym. Sci.*, 35(5), 511–577, 2010.
17. Timofeeva, L. and Kleshcheva, N. Antimicrobial polymers: Mechanism of action, factors of activity, and applications. *Appl. Microbiol. Biotechnol.*, 89(3), 475–492, 2011.
18. Charnley, M., Textor, M., and Acikgoz, C. Designed polymer structures with antifouling-antimicrobial properties. *React. Funct. Polym.*, 71(3), 329–334, 2011.
19. Ong, Y.-L., Razatos, A., Georgiou, G., and Sharma, M. M. Adhesion forces between *E. coli* bacteria and biomaterial surfaces. *Langmuir*, 15(8), 2719–2725, 1999.
20. Pacheco, A. G., Alcântara, A. F. C., Abreu, V. G. C., and Corrêa, G. M. Relationships between chemical structure and activity of triterpenes against gram-positive and gram-negative bacteria. In *A Search for Antibacterial Agents*, Bobbarala, V. ed., InTech, Rijeka, Croatia, Chapter 1, p. 1, 2012.
21. Engel, L. S. The dilemma of multidrug-resistant gram-negative bacteria. *Am. J. Med. Sci.*, 340(3), 232–237, 2010.
22. Peleg, A. Y. and Hooper, D. C. Hospital-acquired infections due to gram-negative bacteria. *New Eng. J. Med.*, 362(19), 1804–1813, 2010.

23. Deshpande, P., Rodrigues, C., Shetty, A., Kapadia, F., Hedge, A., and Soman, R. New Delhi Metallo-beta lactamase (NDM-1) in Enterobacteriaceae: Treatment options with carbapenems compromised. *J. Assoc. Physicians India*, 58, 147–149, 2010.
24. Bush, K. Alarming beta-lactamase-mediated resistance in multidrug-resistant Enterobacteriaceae. *Curr. Opin. Microbiol.*, 13(5), 558–564, 2010.
25. Pages, J. M., Alibert-Franco, S., Mahamoud, A., Bolla, J. M., Davin-Regli, A., Chevalier, J., and Garnotel, E. Efflux pumps of gram-negative bacteria, a new target for new molecules. *Curr. Top. Med. Chem.*, 10(18), 1848–1857, 2010.
26. Silveira, G. P., Nome, F., Gesser, J. C., Sá, M. M., and Terenzi, H. Recent achievements to combat bacterial resistance. *Quim. Nova*, 29(4), 844–855, 2006.
27. Al-Fatimi, M., Wurster, M., Schroder, G., and Lindequist, U. Antioxidant, antimicrobial and cytotoxic activities of selected medicinal plants from Yemen. *J. Ethnopharmacol.*, 111(3), 657–666, 2007.
28. Rahman, A. U., Zareen, S., Choudhary, M. I., Ngounou, F. N., Yasin, A., and Parvez, M. *Terminalin A*, a novel triterpenoid from *Terminalia glaucescens*. *Tetrahedron Lett.*, 43(35), 6233–6236, 2002.
29. Vincent, J. L., Rello, J., Marshall, J., Silva, E., Anzueto, A., Martin, C. D, Moreno, R. et al. International study of the prevalence and outcomes of infection in intensive care units. *JAMA*, 302(21), 2323–2329, 2009.
30. Luzzati, R., Allegranzi, B., Antozzi, L., Masala, L., Pegoraro, E, Azzini, A, and Concia, E. Secular trends in nosocomial candidaemia in non-neutropenic patients in an Italian tertiary hospital. *Clin. Microbiol. Infect.*, 11(11), 908–913, 2005.
31. Playford, E. G., Lipman, J., and Sorrell, T. C. Management of invasive candidiasis in the intensive care unit. *Drugs*, 70(7), 823–839, 2010.
32. Pfaller, M. A. and Diekema, D. J. Epidemiology of invasive candidiasis: A persistent public health problem. *Clin. Microbiol. Rev.*, 20(1), 133–163, 2007.
33. Alberti, C., Brun-Buisson, C., Burchardi, H., Martin, C., Goodman, S., Artigas, A., Sicignano, A. et al. Epidemiology of sepsis and infection in ICU patients from an international multicentre cohort study. *Intensive Care Med.*, 28(1), 108–121, 2002.
34. Eggimann, P., Garbino, J., and Pittet, D. Epidemiology of Candida species infections in critically ill non-immunosuppressed patients. *Lancet Infect. Dis.*, 3(1), 685–702, 2003.
35. Lepak, A. and Andes, D. Fungal sepsis: Optimizing antifungal therapy in the critical care setting. *Crit. Care Clin.*, 27(1), 123–147, 2011.
36. Smith, J. A. and Kauffman, C. A. Recognition and prevention of nosocomial invasive fungal infections in the intensive care unit. *Crit. Care Med.*, 38(8 Suppl), S380–S387, 2010.
37. Marriott, D. J. E., Playford, E. G., Chen, S., Slavin, M., Nquyen, Q., Ellis, D., Sorrell, T. C.; Australian Candidaemia Study. Determinants of mortality in non-neutropenic ICU patients with candidaemia. *Crit. Care*, 13(4), R115 (1–8), 2009.
38. Zilberberg, M. D., Kollef, M. H., Arnold, H., Labelle, A., Micek, S. T., Kothari, S., and Andrew, F. S. Inappropriate empiric antifungal therapy for candidemia in the ICU and hospital resource utilization: A retrospective cohort study. *BMC Infect. Dis.*, 10(1), 150–157, 2010.
39. Labelle, A. J., Micek, S. T., Roubinian, N., and Kollef, M. H. Treatment-related risk factors for hospital mortality in Candida bloodstream infections. *Crit. Care Med.*, 36(11), 2967–2972, 2008.
40. Fodor, A., Hevesi, M., Fodor, A. M., Racsko, J., and Hogan, J. A. Novel anti-microbial peptides of xenorhabdus origin against multidrug resistant plant pathogens. In *A Search for Antibacterial Agents*, Bobbarala, V. ed., InTech, Rijeka, Croatia, Chapter 9, p. 147, 2012.
41. Rizzotto, M. Metal complexes as antimicrobial agents. In *A Search for Antibacterial Agents*, Bobbarala, V. ed., InTech, Rijeka, Croatia, Chapter 5, p. 73, 2012.
42. Neu, H. C. (1992). The crisis in antibiotic resistance. *Science*, 257(5073), 1064–1073, 1992.

43. Stratton, T. R., Applegate, B. M., and Youngblood, J. P. Effect of steric hindrance on the properties of antibacterial and biocompatible copolymers. *Biomacromolecules*, 12(1), 50–56, 2011.
44. Mondrzyk, A., Fischer J., and Ritter, H. Antibacterial materials: Structure–bioactivity relationship of epoxy–amine resins containing quaternary ammonium compounds covalently attached. *Polym. Int.*, 63(7), 1192–1196, 2014.
45. Gao, Y. and Cranston, R. Recent advances in antimicrobial treatments of textile. *Text. Res. J.*, 78(1), 60–72, 2008.
46. Schindler, W. D. and Hauser, P. J. *Chemical Finishing of Textiles*, Woodhead Publishing Ltd, Cambridge, UK, 2004.
47. Dring, I. Anti-microbial, rotproofing and hygiene finishes. In *Textile Finishing*, Heywood, D. ed., Society of Dyers and Colourists, Bradford, UK, pp. 351–371, 2003.
48. Purwar, R. and Joshi, M. Recent developments in antimicrobial finishing of textiles. *AATCC Rev.*, 4(1), 22–26, 2004.
49. Augustin, C. and Damour, O. Phannacotoxicological applications of an equivalent dermis: Three measurements of cytotoxicity. *Cell Biol. Toxicol.*, 11(1), 167–171, 1995.
50. Steinsvag, S. K., Bjerknes, R., and Berg, O. H. Effects of topical nasal steroids on human respiratory mucosa and human granulocytes *in vitro*. *Acta Otolaryngol.*, 116(2), 868–875, 1996.
51. Takashi, H., Yasuhiko, I., and Kazuhiko, I. Preparation and performance of protein adsorption-resistant asymmetric porous membrane composed of polysulfone/phospholipid polymer blend. *Biomaterials*, 22(3), 243–251, 2001.
52. Yuan, J., Zhang, J., Zang, X. P., Shen, J., and Lin, S. Improvement of blood compatibility on cellulose membrane surface by grafting betaines. *Colloids Surf. B Biointerfaces*, 30(1/2), 147–155, 2003.
53. Ye, S. H., Watanabe, J. I., Iwasaki, Y., and Ishihara, K. Novel cellulose acetate membrane blended with phospholipid polymer for hemocompatible filtration system. *J. Membr. Sci.*, 210(2), 411–421, 2002.
54. Park, J. Y., Acar, M. H., Akthakul, A., Kuhlman, W., and Mayes, A. M. Polysulfone-graft-poly(ethylene glycol) graft copolymers for surface modification of polysulfone membranes. *Biomaterials*, 27(6), 856–865, 2006.
55. Ioan, S. and Filimon, A. Biocompatibility and antimicrobial activity of some quaternized polysulfones. In *A Search for Antibacterial Agents*, Bobbarala, V. ed., InTech, Rijeka, Croatia, Chapter 13, p. 249, 2012.
56. Filimon, A., Avram, E., Dunca, S., Stoica, I., and Ioan, S. Surface properties and antibacterial activity of quaternized polysulfones. *J. Appl. Polym. Sci.*, 112(3), 1808–1816, 2009.
57. Luca, C., Avram, E., and Petrariu, I. Quaternary ammonium polyelectrolytes. V. Amination studies of chloromethylated polystyrene with *N,N*-dimethylalkylamines. *J. Macromol. Sci., Part A Chem.*, 25(4), 345–361, 1988.
58. Guan, R., Zou, H., Lu, D., Gong, C., and Liu, Y. Polyethersulfone sulfonated by chlorosulfonic acid and its membrane characteristics. *Eur. Polym. J.*, 41(7), 1554–1560, 2005.
59. Yu, H., Huang, Y., Ying, H., and Xiao, C. Preparation and characterization of a quaternary ammonium derivative of konjac glucomannan. *Carbohydr. Polym.*, 69(1), 29–40, 2007.
60. Ioan, S., Filimon, A., and Avram, E. Influence of the degree of substitution on the solution properties of chloromethylated polysulfone. *J. Appl. Polym. Sci.*, 101(1), 524–531, 2006.
61. Ioan, S., Filimon, A., and Avram, E. Conformational and visometric behavior of quaternized polysulfone in dilute solution. *Polym. Eng. Sci.*, 46(7), 827–836, 2006.
62. Filimon, A., Avram, E., and Ioan, S. Influence of mixed solvents and temperature on the solution properties of quaternized polysulfones. *J. Macromol. Sci. Part B Phys.*, 46(3), 503–520, 2007.

63. Filimon, A., Albu, R. M., Avram, E., and Ioan, S. Effect of alkyl side chain on the conformational properties of polysulfones with quaternary groups. *J. Macromol. Sci. Part B Phys.*, 49(1), 207–217, 2010.

64. Idris, A. and Zain, N. M. Effect of heat treatment on the performance and structural details of polyethersulfone ultrafiltration membranes. *J. Teknol.*, 44(1), 27–40, 2006.

65. Kochkodan, V., Tsarenko, S., Potapchenko, N., Kosinova, V., and Goncharuk, V. Adhesion of microorganisms to polymer membranes: A photobactericidal effect of surface treatment with TiO₂. *Desalination*, 220(1–3), 380–385, 2008.

66. Ahlström, B., Chelminska-Bertilsson, M., Thompson, R. A., and Edebo, L. Long-chain alkanoylcholines, a new category of soft antimicrobial agents that are enzymatically degradable. *Antimicrob. Agents Chemother.*, 39(1), 50–55, 1995.

67. Li, G., Shen, J., and Zhu, Y. A study of pyridinium-type functional polymers. III. Preparation and characterization of insoluble pyridinium-type polymers. *J. Appl. Polym. Sci.*, 78(3), 668–675, 2000.

68. Abel, T., Cohen, J. I., Engel, R., Filshtinskaya, M., Melkonian, A., and Melkonian, K. Preparation and investigation of antibacterial carbohydrate-based surfaces. *Carbohydr. Res.*, 337(24), 2495–2499, 2002.

69. Derya, Y. K.-I., Borte, K., Mahmut, A., and Ismail, K. The production of polysulfone (PS) membrane with silver nanoparticles (AgNP): Physical properties, filtration performances, and biofouling resistances of membranes. *J. Membr. Sci.*, 428, 620–628, 2013.

70. Panisello, C., Peña, B., Oriol, G. G., Constantí, M., Gumí, T., and Garcia-Valls, R. Polysulfone/vanillin microcapsules for antibacterial and aromatic finishing of fabrics. *Ind. Eng. Chem. Res.*, 52(29), 9995–10003, 2013.

71. Kenawy, E. R., Abdel-Hay, F. I., El-Shanshoury, A. E. R. R., and El-Newehy, M. H. Biologically active polymers. V. Synthesis and antimicrobial activity of modified poly(glycidyl methacrylate-co-2-hydroxyethyl methacrylate) derivatives with quaternary ammonium and phosphonium salts. *J. Polym. Sci. Part A Polym. Chem.*, 40(14), 2384–2393, 2002.

72. Gilbert, P. and Moore, L. E. Cationic antiseptics: Diversity of action under a common epithet. *J. Appl. Microbiol.*, 99(4), 703–715, 2005.

73. Basri, H., Ismail, A. F., and Aziz, M. Microstructure and anti-adhesion properties of PES/TAP/Ag hybrid ultrafiltration membrane. *Desalination*, 287(1), 71–77, 2012.

74. Harris, L. G. and Richards, R. G. Staphylococci and implant surfaces: A review. *Injury*, 37(2 Suppl), S3–S14, 2006.

75. Dunne Jr., W. M. Bacterial adhesion: Seen any good biofilms lately? *Clin. Microbiol. Rev.* 15(2), 155–166, 2002.

76. Marini, M., Bondi, M., Iseppi, R., Toselli, M., and Pilati, F. Preparation and antibacterial activity of hybrid materials containing quaternary ammonium salts via sol-gel process. *Eur. Polym. J.*, 43(8), 3621–3628, 2007.

77. Kügler, R., Bouloussa, O., and Rondelez, F. Evidence of a charge-density threshold for optimum efficiency of biocidal cationic surfaces. *Microbiology*, 151(5), 1341–1348, 2005,

78. Popa, A., Davidescu, C. M., Trif, R., Ilia, G., Iliescu, S., and Dehelean, G. Study of quaternary "onium" salts grafted on polymers: Antibacterial activity of quaternary phosphonium salts grafted on "gel-type" styrene-divinylbenzene copolymers. *React. Funct. Polym.*, 55(2), 151–158, 2003.

79. Gorbunova, M. Novel guanidinium and phosphonium polysulfones: Synthesis and antimicrobial activity, *J. Chem. Pharmaceutical Res.*, 5(1), 185–192, 2013.

80. Berkovich, A., Orlov, V., and Melik-Nubarov, N. Interaction of polyanions with electroneutral liposomes in a slightly acidic medium. *Polym. Sci. Seria A*, 51(2), 648–657, 2009.

81. Moustafa, M. and Fouda, G. Antibacterial modification of textiles using nanotechnology. In *A Search for Antibacterial Agents*, Bobbarala, V. ed., InTech, Rijeka, Croatia, Chapter 4, p. 47, 2012.

82. Travan, A., Pelillo, C., Donati, I., Marsich, E., Benincasa, M., Scarpa, T., Semeraro, S., Turco, G., Gennaro, R., and Paoletti, S. Non-cytotoxic silver nanoparticle-polysaccharide nancomposites with antimicrobial activity. *Biomacromolecules*, 10(6), 1429–1435, 2009.

83. Fu, J., Ji, J., Fan, D., and Shen, J. Construction of antibacterial multilayer films containing nanosilver via layer-by-layer assembly of heparin and chitosan-silver ions complex. *J. Biomed. Mater. Res. Part A*, 79(3), 665–674, 2006.

84. Sanpui, P., Murugadoss, A., Prasad, P. V. D., Ghosh, S. S., and Chattopadhyay, A. The antibacterial properties of a novel chitosan–Ag-nanoparticle composite. *Int. J. Food Microbiol.*, 124(2), 142–146, 2008.

85. Rathnayake, W. G. I. U., Ismail, H., Baharin, A., Bandara, I. M. C. C. D., and Rajapakse, S. Enhancement of the antibacterial activity of natural rubber latex foam by the incorporation of zinc oxide nanoparticles. *J. Appl. Polym. Sci.*, 131(1), 39601–39609, 2014.

86. Rajendra, R., Balakumar, C., Ahammed, H. A. M., Jayakumar, S., Vaideki, K., and Rajesh, E. Use of zinc oxide nano particles for production of antimicrobial textiles. *Int. J. Eng. Sci. Technol.*, 2(1), 202–208, 2010.

87. Sawai, J., Shoji, S., Igarashi, H., Hashimoto, A., Kokugan, T., Shimizu, M., and Kojima, H. Hydrogen peroxide as an antibacterial factor in zinc oxide powder slurry. *J. Ferment. Bioeng.*, 86(5), 521–522, 1998.

88. Applerot, G., Lipovsky, A., Dror, R., Perkas, N., Nitzan, Y., Lubart, R., and Gedanken, A. Enhanced antibacterial activity of nanocrystalline ZnO due to increased ROS-mediated cell injury. *Adv. Funct. Mater.*, 19(6), 842–852, 2009.

89. Zhang, L., Jiang, Y., Ding, Y., Daskalakis, N., Jeuken, L., Povey, M., O'Neill, A. J., York, D. W. Mechanistic investigation into antibacterial behaviour of suspensions of ZnO nanoparticles against *E. coli*. *J. Nanopart. Res.*, 12(5), 1625–1636, 2010.

90. Brayner, R., Ferrari-Iliou, R., Brivois, N., Djediat, S., Benedetti, M. F., and Fievet, F. Toxicological impact studies based on *Escherichia coli* bacteria in ultrafine ZnO nanoparticles colloidal medium. *Nano Lett.*, 6(4), 866–870, 2006.

91. Huang, Z., Zheng, X., Yan, D., Yin, G., Liao, X., Kang, Y., Yao, Y., Di Huang, A., and Hao, B. Toxicological effect of ZnO nanoparticles based on bacteria. *Langmuir*, 24(8), 4140–4144, 2008.

92. Jones, N., Ray, B., Ranjit, K. T., and Manna, A. C. Antibacterial activity of ZnO nanoparticle suspensions on a broad spectrum of microorganisms. *FEMS Microbiol. Lett.*, 279(1), 71–76, 2008.

93. Spellberg, B., Guidos, R., Gilbert, D., Bradley, J., Boucher, H. W., Scheld, W. M., Bartlett, J. G., and Edwards, J. The epidemic of antibiotic-resistant infections: A call to action for the medical community from the infectious diseases society of America. *Clin. Infect. Dis.*, 46(2), 155–164, 2008.

94. Nie, S., Xue, J., Lu, Y., Liu, Y., Wang, D., Sun, S., Ran, F., and Zhao, C. Improved blood compatibility of polyethersulfone membrane with a hydrophilic and anionic surface. *Colloid Surf. B Biointerfaces*, 100(1), 116–125, 2012.

95. Vanholder, R. Biocompatibility issues in hemodialysis. *Clin. Mater.*, 10(1), 87–133, 1992.

96. Cases, A., Reverter, C., Escolar, G., Sanz, C., Lopez-Pedret, J., Revert, L., and Ordinas, A. Platelet activation on hemodialysis: Influence of dialysis membranes. *Kidney Int.*, 41(6 Suppl), S217–S220, 1993.

97. Tharakan, J. P. and Chau, P. C. A radial flow hollow fiber bioreactor for the large-scale culture of mammalian cells. *Biotech. Bioeng.*, 28(3), 329–342, 1986.

98. Alsuler, G. L., Dziewulski, D. M., Sowek, J. A., and Belfort, G., Continuous hybridoma growth and monoclonal antibody production in hollow fiber reactors–separators. *Biotech. Bioeng.*, 28(5), 646–658, 1986.

99. Aebischer, P., Guenard, V., Winn, S. R., Valentini, R. F., and Galletti, P. M. Blind-ended semipermeable guidance channels support peripheral nerve regeneration in the absence of a distal nerve stump. *Brain Res.*, 454(1/2), 179–187, 1988.

100. Aebischer, P., Guenard, V., and Brace, S. Peripheral nerve regeneration through blindended semipermeable guidance channels: Effect of the molecular weight cutoff. *J. Neurosci.*, 9(10), 3590–3595, 1989.

101. Martin, T. P., Kooi, S. E., Chang, S. H., Sedrans, K. L., and Gleason, K. K. Initiated chemical vapor deposition of antimicrobial polymer coatings. *Biomaterials*, 28(6), 909–915, 2007.

102. Giammanco, A., Maggio, M., Giammanco, G., Morelli, R., Minelli, F., Scheutz, F., and Caprioli, A. Characteristics of *Escherichia coli* strains belonging to enteropathogenic *E. coli* serogroups isolated in Italy from children with diarrhea. *J. Clin. Microbiol.*, 34(3), 689–694, 1996.

103. Jaggi, P., Paule, S. M., Peterson, L. R., and Tan, T. Q. Characteristics of *Staphylococcus aureus* infections, Chicago pediatric hospital. *Emerg. Infect. Dis.*, 13(2), 311–314, 2007.

104. Xu, X., Li, S., Jia, F., and Liu, P. Synthesis and antimicrobial activity of nano-fumed silica derivative with *N,N*-dimethyl-*n*-hexadecylamine. *Life Sci. J.*, 3(1), 59–62, 2006.

105. Schiffman, J. D., Wang, Y., Giannelis, E. P., and Elimelech, M. Biocidal activity of plasma modified electrospun polysulfone mats functionalized with polyethyleneiminecapped silver nanoparticles. *Langmuir*, 27(21), 13159–13164, 2011.

106. Basri, H., Ismail, A. F., and Aziz, M. Polyethersulfone (PES)–silver composite UF membrane: Effect of silver loading and PVP molecular weight on membrane morphology and antibacterial activity. *Desalination*, 273(1), 72–80, 2011.

107. Wang, Y., Yang, Q., Shan, G., Wang, C., Du, J., Wang, S., Li, Y., Chen, X., Jing, X., and Wei, Y. Preparation of silver nanoparticles dispersed in polyacrylonitrile nanofiber film spun by electrospinning. *Mater. Lett.*, 59(24/25), 3046–3049, 2005.

108. Susanto, H. and Ulbricht, M. Characteristics, performance and stability of polyethersulfone ultrafiltration membranes prepared by phase separation method using different macromolecular additives. *J. Membr. Sci.*, 327(1), 125–135, 2009.

109. Babu, V. R., Kim, C., Kim, S., Ahn, C., and Lee, Y.-I. Development of semi-interpenetrating carbohydrate polymeric hydrogels embedded silver nanoparticles and its facile studies on *E. coli. Carbohydr. Polym.*, 81(1), 196–202, 2010.

110. Lee, H. K., Jeong, E. H., Baek, C. K., and Youk, J. H. One-step preparation of ultrafine poly(acrylonitrile) fibers containing silver nanoparticles. *Mater. Lett.*, 59(23), 2977–2980, 2005.

10 Potential Biomedical Applications of Functionalized Polysulfones

Luminita-Ioana Buruiana

CONTENTS

10.1 INTRODUCTION

The technological progress of medicine, as well as of other scientific fields, brings to light new challenging discoveries, which explains the constant motivation for an objective evaluation of new techniques. In recent years, the main scientific interest has been focused not only on the synthesis of new types of polymeric materials but also on the modification of the existing polymers and their properties, to meet requirements for new applications, especially biomedical ones [1].

Biodegradable polymers have been widely used and promoted for the development of biomedical fields due to their biocompatibility and biodegradability. The progress of medical technology has set higher requirements for biomedical materials. Synthetic biodegradable polymers have been found to be more versatile and suitable for diverse biomedical applications, owing to their tailorable designs or modifications. The general criteria of materials used in medical applications include special mechanical properties and a degradation time appropriate to the medical purpose.

At the same time, the materials should not present toxic or immune responses and they should be immediately metabolized in the body. According to these demands, various biodegradable and biocompatible polymers have been designed and used, due to their interesting characteristics for potential biomedical applications.

Polysulfone (PSF) polymers, as biocompatible and bioinert materials, have been proposed for a variety of bio-applications, such as tissue engineering [2–4], hemodialysis [5], ultrafiltration [6,7], bioreactor technology [8], as well as drug delivery [9] and cell culture applications [10].

Tissue engineering represents an interdisciplinary field based on the development and application of the principles from chemistry, physics, engineering, life, and clinical sciences, to the solutions for clinical medical issues, such as tissue injury and organ failure [11]. The fundamentals of this application are represented by a proper understanding of the structure–function relationships in normal and pathological tissue, along with the development of biological substitutes expected to restore, maintain, and improve tissue function.

For *in vitro* engineering of living tissues, cells are cultured on a scaffold—a bioactive degradable substrate—that provides the physical and chemical directions to guide their differentiation and assembly into three-dimensional (3D) structures [12].

One of the important issues in tissue engineering is obtaining porous scaffolds with specific physical, mechanical, and biological properties; scaffolds act like a substrate for cellular growth and support new tissue formation. Materials used for tissue engineering applications must be designed to stimulate specific cell response at the molecular level, inducing specific attachment, proliferation, and differentiation of cells. Selection of biomaterials constitutes the most important factor for the success of tissue engineering practice. The essential claims of the biomaterials used in tissue regeneration are biocompatible surfaces and advantageous mechanical properties. Because a single-component polymer material cannot satisfy all requirements, the design and preparation of multicomponent polymer systems constitute a viable strategy, assuring the progress in the multifunctional biomaterials domain. On the other hand, nanotechnology deals with systems that mimic the complex structure of the original tissue. Consequently, a confluence of nanotechnology and biology can solve many biomedical problems, representing an important tool in health and medicine field [13].

Polymer nanocomposites are formed by the combination of polymers and inorganic/organic fillers in the nanometer domain [14,15]. The interaction between nanostructures and the polymer matrix represents the basis for favorable functional properties, as compared to common microcomposites. Nanocomposite materials exhibit a proper balance between strength and toughness and improved characteristics, compared to their individual components [16]. As an example, one can mention composite materials based on functionalized PSFs with special architecture—an excellent choice as bone tissue engineering scaffolds [17–19].

In *drug delivery* and *control release applications*, polymers with reactive pendant groups can conjugate drugs to form a macromolecular prodrug that reduces the side effects of free drugs. Thus, the main function of polymeric carriers is to transport drugs to the specific site of action. Ideally, the polymeric structure should be biodegradable, for an easy renal elimination of the complex; if the polymeric structure is not biodegradable, then the nano-sized polymers must be used. An important feature of the polymers used in drug delivery is represented by the mechanism through which they are removed from the body: they may be excreted directly by kidneys (renal clearance) or biodegraded into smaller molecules (metabolic clearance). Molecular weight is especially relevant for substances that are not biodegradable, so that macromolecules with a molecular weight lower than the glomerular limit (under 50 KDa) can be safely removed from the body, thus preventing their accumulation and potential toxicity.

In the design of biodegradable polymers, one can control the chemical structure (hydrophobicity degree, covalent bonds between monomers, etc.), because the speed, degradation conditions, and the rate and site of the drug release can be modulated as a function of the chemical structure of the polymer used.

For nonbiodegradable polymers, the drug can be covalently attached to the polymeric structure by a linker that can be degraded under different conditions (i.e., in acidic medium or by different enzymes).

The objective of controlled release systems is to improve the drug therapy effectiveness, by modifying several parameters of the drug: release profile, capacity to pass over biological carriers, biodistribution, clearance, and stability. Thus, the pharmacokinetics and pharmacodynamics of the drug are modified by these formulations. This process offers many advantages over the conventional dosage forms, such as increased therapeutic activity and reduced side effects, so that a lower drug dosage may be applied during the treatment. The method also offers an appropriate tool for site-specific and controlled drug delivery. Different kinds of drugs—antibiotics [20–23]—chemotherapeutic drugs [24,25], anti-inflammatory agents [26], and vaccines [27,28], can benefit from distribution or time-controlled delivery.

Hemodialysis is a life-sustaining procedure that can be, sometimes associated with complications, responsible for diminishing the quality of life. However, in recent years, it has become clear that hemodialysis can no longer be considered a simple process, whereby blood and the dialysate are separated by an inert semipermeable membrane. The side effects may be due to the interactions of blood with different components of the hemodialysis equipment. Biocompatibility—as it relates to hemodialysis—can be defined as the sum of specific interactions between blood and the artificial materials of the hemodialysis circuit. When this interaction, described as an inflammatory response, is well tolerated by the material, it is considered to be biocompatible; at the same time, the intensity of the interaction may determine adverse effects to the patients or lead to other deleterious outcomes. Also, some important aspects on the hemodialysis biocompatibility are crucial to the success of the dialysate biocompatibility (sodium concentration, acetate/bicarbonate, etc.), the dialytic procedure (which can be intermittent, sequential, or continuous), and the other dialysis components (blood access or blood line). Also, other aspects on hemodialysis biocompatibility procedure should be taken into account: the sterilant used in the process (ethylene oxide, steam, or gamma rays), the reuse procedure (which can be manual or automated), as well as the residual materials from the manufacturing process (soluble phthalate) [29,30].

Cellulose-based materials, used since the beginning of hemodialysis membranes manufacturing, still remain the most commonly used materials in the field. But, besides that, several synthetic materials have been introduced into clinical practice, due to advantages such as decreasing the intensity and specificity of blood–membrane interactions. The synthetic polymers used in this type of applications can be hydrophilic or hydrophobic.

In general, the hydrophobic membranes are apolar, have a low energy of interaction with water, adsorb proteins, are more porous, and have high ultrafiltration coefficients. This category of membranes includes PSF membranes, along with polymethylmethacrylate, and polyacrylonitrile membranes. The ability of these membranes to adsorb proteins may be a determinant for their biocompatibility. Still, the main disadvantage that remains is their hydrophobic character; therefore, many studies being focused on membrane fouling—caused by the adsorption of nonpolar solutes, hydrophobic particles, or bacteria—poses a serious problem in membrane filtration that requires a higher quantity of energy, shorter membrane lifetime, and unpredictable separation performance. Considering all these concerns, PSF membranes used in hemodialysis are usually modified by hydrophilic polymers. There are several approaches for the modification of PSF membranes, the most common one being surface modification (i.e., blending with some hydrophilic additive or membrane forming agent, surface-coating, or grafting methods) [31,32].

The modification procedures allow a compromise between hydrophobicity and hydrophilicity, and localize the hydrophilic materials in the membrane pores, where they have an important effect on flux and fouling reduction, and improving blood compatibility. All modifications rely on the premise that the materials used for modification increase hydrophilicity and absorb less protein than the base substrate.

Protein adsorption on material surface represents an important event during thrombogenic formation; the amount of protein adsorbed on the membrane is being considered as one of the most important factors in evaluating blood compatibility. Platelet adhesion to blood-contacting medical devices is a key phenomenon in thrombus formation on the material surface. The clearance of small molecules—urea, creatinine, and phosphate—must be also evaluated for testing the safety and efficiency of hemodialysis membranes. To conclude, the hemodialysis membranes showed a good blood compatibility and solute clearance for becoming a viable commercial product [33].

At the same time, an important domain in which polymers are found to be applicable is represented by *sensor applications*. In recent years, research developments have focused on the fabrication of different types of sensors, including biosensors, immunosensors, and electrochemical sensors. A *biosensor* is considered as a combination of a bioreceptor, biological component, and a transducer. The main effect of a biosensor is to transform a biological event into an electrical signal. Biosensors found extensive applications in medical diagnosis, environmental pollution control, and for measuring toxic gases in the atmosphere and toxic soluble compounds in river water. Estimation of organic compounds concentration is important for the control of food manufacturing and for the evaluation of food quality. *Electrochemical sensors* are ideally suited for the measurement of *in situ* analyses, such as measuring analytes of interest in clinical chemistry, due to their high sensitivity and selectivity, portable field-based size, rapid response time, and low cost. Demanded by modern medical diagnosis, recent trends in microfabrication technology have led to the development of fast, sensitive, and selective electrochemical sensors for clinical analysis. Electrochemical sensors have improved the performance of the conventional analytical tools, eliminated slow preparation and the use of expensive reagents, and provided low-cost analytical tools. Also, they have been successfully applied in clinical diagnosis, environmental monitoring, and food analysis. On the other hand, electrochemical sensors evidence several disadvantages, such as a weak long-term stability and electrochemical interferences in the samples [34].

Nanotechnology provides new opportunities for biosensors construction and for the development of novel electrochemical bioassays. Nanoscale materials have been used to accomplish direct gripping of enzyme to the electrode surface, to promote electrochemical reactions, and to amplify the signal of biorecognition events. Electrochemical nanobiosensors were applied especially in the areas of cancer diagnostic and the detection of infectious organism [35]. Literature mentioned various studies made on carbon nanotube/PSF biocomposite-based sensors that immobilize specific enzymes [36].

During the last decade, many research groups have directed part of their efforts to the development and optimization of electrochemical *immunosensors*—which combine specific immunoreactions with electrochemical transduction—preferred because of their quick and sensitive response [37]. Also, this type of sensor has optimized the premises of immunoassays to obtain better performances, such as the possibility to use very small volumes and miniaturized arrays of electrochemical sensors. At the same time, the design of this type of immunosensor displayed the immobilization of immunoreagents onto the electrode surface that determines its quality and reproducibility. Some of the immunoreagents immobilization strategies include physical adsorption, enzyme entrapment, and encapsulation or covalent attachment [38–41]. The reason for which the enzymes are analytically preferred for immobilization is their repetitive use and easier product recovery, enzymes being also known for their biocatalyst applications.

The low level of electrochemical interferences in complex clinical applications represent a relevant advantage over the optical approaches, which makes this technique suitable for the detection of some important analytes (biological and chemical pathogens or contaminants). All these reasons make the electrochemical sensor for antibody detection a perfect tool for diagnosis, prevention, and treatment of specific illness, including infections and autoimmune diseases. In this context, PSFs—as attractive immunomaterial carriers—act not only as a membrane but also as a reservoir for immunological materials (enzymes and antibodies) [42,43].

10.2 FUNCTIONALIZED PSFs AND THEIR POTENTIAL MEDICAL APPLICATIONS

The suitable combination of properties of PSFs—high-performance thermoplastic materials with chemical and biological inertness, excellent thermal and hydrolytic stabilities, mechanical strength, and film-forming properties, with unique long life under sterilization procedures and resistance to most common hospital chemicals—makes them especially attractive for the manufacture of commercial membranes and in biomedical applications (gas separation, hemodialysis, nano/ultrafiltration, drug delivery, tissue engineering, bio-artificial devices, etc.). However, there are some drawbacks that inhibit the use of PSFs as biomaterial membranes in filtration and blood-contact applications. In this context, their hydrophobic properties are often responsible for the protein fouling of membranes, which reduces the permeation flux and the selectivity of the membrane [44]; moreover, in blood-contact applications, the adsorption of serum protein onto PSF membranes induces some life-threatening complications. Thus, modification procedures allow a compromise between hydrophobicity and hydrophilicity; moreover, to improve the blood compatibility of biomedical materials, many studies have focused on the hydrophilic modification of the hydrophobic membranes of conventional PSFs.

On the other hand, since their introduction in practice, PSFs have replaced glass, stainless steel, and other plastics. Over the years, functionalized PSFs have proven their utility in typical medical applications, including surgical and lab equipments, life-support parts, autoclavable tray systems, orthopedic implants, tissue culture bottles, sheet/lenses, and artificial heart. Due to their unique performances, PSFs also found usefulness in a host of components for ultrasonic nebulizers, humidifiers, as well as bacteria or expiratory filter housings. One of the important advantages over other polymers is their ability to participate to repeated sterilization cycles, and their resistance to cleaning compounds—especially ammonia-based products.

In hospital laboratories, the classical medical equipment can suffer by repeated cleaning or by hard usage. From that reason, PSF medical bottles—transparent and unbreakable—were proved to be highly resistant to clouding, as observed for other plastics also exposed to steam. They contribute to the good image of the hospital by withstanding detergents and high cleaning temperatures, without losing their clean appearance. In other cases, PSFs have successfully replaced glass in funnels as lab devices. The flexibility of the thermoplastic polymer assures a superior seal, resulting in a lower chance of breaking vacuum and losing sterility—besides easier processability and low cost.

Another possibility to use PSFs is in special medical devices from the operating room; the most common example is represented by the microsurgical knives that can be used either as received or can be sterilized for reutilization by standard methods. The knives are designed as integral units or as tips in different configurations, such as screw into PSFs handles.

Latest biomedical researchers have some new alternatives to tissue culture bottles. PSFs offer a better utility as favorable substrates for tissue culture cell attachment and growth, with no obvious breakage problems.

In the following part of the chapter, the potential applications of functionalized PSFs in medicine will be particularized, pointing out the latest discoveries in every specific domain.

10.2.1 SCAFFOLDING MATERIALS FOR TISSUE ENGINEERING

Tissue engineering is being known as a mean to replace diseased or damaged organs using tissue-specific cells grown on a scaffold material to give a 3D structure with the goal of creating a functional organ. Different compounds were being examined for use as scaffolds in tissue engineering, including both synthetic and natural materials. Scaffolds with high porosity are preferred, as their cells can penetrate the pores, then fill the support, and grow into 3D tissues. Once implanted, the cells recreate the organ or tissue functions, whereas blood vessels attach to and penetrate the new tissue. The use of synthetic polymers as scaffolds becomes interesting as they can be easily produced and then modified for specific applications [3].

Also, 3D structures with excellent cell growth capacity could be used in the bioreactor technology. In this context, new open-cell hollow fibers made of polyethersulfones (PESs) with small pore diameters and homogenous pore size distribution were described [45]. The advantage of PSF membrane preparation is that the applied technique requires no organic solvents and, consequently, no residual solvent—which could be harmful to cell growth and function—which is not present in the final product. Until now, synthetic porous PES membranes have been used in hemodialysis, filtration, and ultrafiltration applications [46–48], but few studies have been focused on determining the ability of cell growth on a PES support. In the literature, rat fibroblast and osteoblast cells have demonstrated to grow on PES, as well as a human astrocytoma cell line onto the ion-beam irradiated PES films [49,50].

In addition, analyses regarding the blood compatibility of PES pointed out values within acceptable ranges; PES hollow fibers subcutaneously implanted in rats evidenced intense neovascularization within the fibrotic overgrowth that surrounded these implants [51,52].

10.2.2 Substrates for Growth of Different Human Cells

Due to the many advantages exhibited by this type of biomaterial scaffold, they aroused much interest for tissue engineering applications. To determine the ability of PES fibers to serve as a scaffold material, a variety of human cell types of different tissue origins, including endothelial, epithelial, fibroblast, glial, keratinocyte, and osteoblast cells, was examined. Analyses showed that porous PES fibers possess properties that fulfill many of the requirements of a biomaterial scaffold [53]. The specificity of these fibers consists in a homogenous open-porous morphology with interconnecting pores and a rough surface; at the same time, depending on some manufacture parameters—for example, melt temperature, concentration of carbon dioxide in the polymer, and temperature of the die during the process—structures with closed or open cells, with a dense or a porous rough surface may be formed [45]. These special characteristics are very important not only for the permeability of liquids but also for the attachment and growth of cells and as the direction for the transport of nutrients and the removal of metabolites. In this context, it is worth mentioning that the problems associated with residual solvents do not exist in the final product, as no organic solvents are involved in PES preparation. All these features make the studied PSFs a potential substrate for different biomedical applications—scaffolds for implant biomaterials (especially bones), biological fluid-filtering systems, controlled drug delivery systems, and cell bioreactors. As a biomaterial for bone regeneration, PESs display many characteristics necessary for a favorable growth of osteoblasts and bone formation [54]. Until now, rat fibroblast and osteoblast cell growth have been proved to occur on PES, as well as on an astrocyte cell line [50]. In this study it was proved that PES fibers support the attachment, spread, and the growth of different types of human cells with various tissue origins—from epithelial to glial cells. In this way, PES fibers can support the major cell type forming the vascular system on all surfaces, including cut surfaces. Also, PES can be modified to include macromolecules—by the fluorination method to improve the blood compatibility and chemical stability, or after preparation by a special type of irradiation, to alter the surface [50,55]—to optimally design surfaces for specific tissue engineering applications.

Summarizing, PES hollow-fiber materials constitute an excellent substrate for the growth of human cells, while also evidencing a large part of the desired properties of a biomaterial scaffold. However, further studies must be made to establish whether the specific cell types that grow on this material present normal phenotypes and functions. All the above aspects guarantee the continuation of PES studies to fully determine their applicability as a biological material.

10.2.3 Bio-Artificial Organs

Implantable bio-artificial liver has been studied for patients that suffer from liver insufficiency after acute liver failure. The experimental method consists of an implantable device with hepatic cells [56]. Several different cell types have been investigated for the treatment of liver insufficiency, including primary human hepatocytes or cells derived from stem cells [57]. Hepatocytes attached to microcarriers or cultures on scaffolds appear as an alternative to direct cell transplantation. In this context, hepatic cells—including cell derived from human liver tumors—differentiate into 3D culture conditions [58].

Hepatic cell growth on a 3D scaffold has the advantage of being more similar to physiologic conditions than a simple monolayer culture. Implantable membranes/scaffolds made of PES have been studied for allowing cell growth on an extracellular matrix protein; at the same time, they permit implantation in patients with liver failure. The investigations evaluated the *in vivo* spongy PES membrane as a synthetic support for hepatic cells grown to 3D structures and then transplanted into mice [2]. As a result, PES was proved to be well tolerated by mice cells, no toxic effects being noticed, as well.

10.2.4 Neuronal Cell Culture Scaffolds

In vitro studies of neurobiological systems include, as recent advances, the development of substrates that can control specific arrangements of neuronal axon growth and synaptic connectivity in neuronal networks. Information deduced from studying these cell cultures allows the manipulation of some important events, such as axonal regeneration [10].

Several years ago, a research group managed to realize a pattern substrate that could control axonal growth for *in vitro* neuronal cell cultures. Since then, many groups have tested different methods for designing structured biomaterial surfaces for controlling axonal guidance. Some important aspects described in these studies were the nerve guide conduit, material properties, dimensions, and the configuration of the biomaterial [59–62].

In order to improve the initially obtained results, surface modification or matrix incorporation of collagen or fibrin gel was realized, to enhance cell adhesion, growth factor immobilization to conduit walls, and microcarrier incorporation, along with the use of novel biomaterial surfaces, such as electrically conducting polymers [63–66].

In order to devise methods for improving *in vivo* nerve regeneration, researches were focused on the topography of biomaterial surfaces used for controlling neurite outgrowth. In this context, the literature mentions multiple methods for generating these structures:

- Microfabrication technology of photolithography—applied to create different topographical structures on a surface to construct grooved pathways for specific axonal growth [67–69]
- Technique of microcontact printing—used to direct hippocampal neuronal growth on lysine- and laminin-patterned surfaces [70]
- Creation of a microcontact printing surface with more complex patterns using adhesive proteins and molecules [71–73]
- Photolithography combined with microcontact printing to create a microfluidic device for continued *in vitro* growth of specific neuronal cell arrangements [74]
- Achieving *in vitro* 3D neuronal scaffolds of the polymer/extracellular matrix protein by inkjet printing [75]

The above-mentioned studies helped to establish the proper scaffolds used for generating *in vitro* systems to control neuronal cell networks. Recent researches point out the development of a scaffold for controlling specific neuronal cell body and *in vitro* axonal process outgrowth through modification by excimer laser ablation in microporous PES hollow fibers. The method was used to generate specific channels in the walls of PES fibers in order to sort the growth of neuronal cell bodies from their axonal processes, and subsequently facilitate directed growth into the 3D space of the fiber lumens; this process may determine a synaptic network between cell bodies within a 3D space. The idea is to incorporate these scaffolds into a hollow fiber-based bioreactor, an implement meant at establishing high-density 3D *in vitro* neuronal cell cultures with axonal pathways in the direction of the scaffolds lumens. The growth of neuronal axons into the fiber scaffolds enables a direct method of analyzing neurite outgrowth within a 3D space at high densities, which mimics more accurately the *in vivo* environment [10]. Therefore, laser-modified PES fibers serve as scaffolds with channels, supporting the direct neuronal cell process growth. These hollow-fiber scaffolds can be used in combination with the perfusion and oxygenation of fiber membrane for the preparation of a hollow fiber-based 3D bioreactor appropriate for the study of *in vitro* neuronal networking between compartmentalized cultures.

10.2.5 Bone Tissue Engineering Scaffolds

The strategy in biomaterial research began to shift from developing biomaterials with a bio-inert tissue response to producing bioactive components that could elicit a controlled action and reaction in the physiological environment. From the beginning

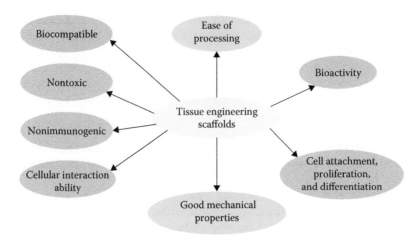

FIGURE 10.1   Key factors involved in the design of optimal scaffolds for bone tissue engineering.

of the new millennium, a great potential has been attributed to the application of bioactive glasses in tissue engineering and regenerative medicine [76,77].

Bone tissue engineering is one of the most exciting future clinical applications of bioactive glasses. The most important function of a bone tissue engineering scaffold is that of a template that allows cells to attach, proliferate, differentiate, and organize into a normal, healthy bone as the scaffold degrades. Figure 10.1 illustrates the most important factors involved in the design of scaffolds and their interdependencies.

On the other hand, it is well known that bioceramics are the most widely used bioactive materials; besides many benefits, there is also a major disadvantage of bioactive ceramics generated by their low fracture toughness and brittleness. For that reason, for bone tissue scaffold applications, bioceramics are used in combination with biodegradable polymers to accomplish proper mechanical and biological performance [78,79].

Thus, the development of composite materials in this field of application is very attractive, due to their interesting properties suitable to physiologic demands of the host tissue by controlling the volume fraction, morphology, and the arrangement of the reinforcing phase. At the same time, the structure and morphology of the scaffold, characterized by a highly interconnected 3D pore network and tailored surface characteristics, determine the suitability of a scaffold for specific applications. For bone tissue engineering, high pore interconnectivity, for a better attachment and proliferation of cells; ingrowths; and vascularization of the newly formed tissue are desired [53].

Composites used in tissue engineering must show special properties, such as high initial strength and tailored elastic modulus close to that of bones. Polymers, by themselves, exhibit a relatively low mechanical strength and stiffness, and can be easily fabricated into complex shapes and porous structures; on the other hand, they do not have a bioactive function—such as strong bonding to bone—as they are too flexible for mechanical demands in bone regeneration processes [80].

Starting from all these considerations, bioactive glass fibers were investigated for application as a fixation vehicle among a low modulus, polymeric composite, and bone tissue [81]. In an initial study, bioactive glass fiber/PSF composites and PSF control rods were implanted into rabbit tibia; subsequently, the study was extended to implantation into rabbit femur. The result recorded after several weeks of implantation showed that the bone tissue displayed a direct contact to the glass fibers and adjacent polymer matrix and a mechanical bond between the composite and bone tissue. The composite material realizes the fixation to bone tissue by a triple mechanism:

- A chemical bond between the bioactive glass fiber and the calcified tissue
- A close apposition and a possible chemical bond between some portions of the polymer and calcified bone tissue
- A mechanical interlocking between the calcified tissue and the composite, by partial resorption of the bioactive glass fibers and their replacement by the calcified tissue [82]

This elaborated study proved that bioactive glass fiber/PSF composites were able to be resorbed to different degrees and replaced by calcified tissue through a complex, three-stage fixation mechanism, resulting in interfacial bond strength significantly higher after several weeks of implantation.

10.2.6 BIO-ARTIFICIAL PANCREAS DEVICE FOR *IN VITRO* STUDIES

Insulin-dependent diabetes mellitus is a chronic disease characterized by high blood–glucose levels and long-term complications, such as micro- and macroangiopathic lesions that may lead to retinopathy, neuropathy, and nephropathy. It is an autoimmune disease, usually manifested in children and young people, resulting from the destruction of the patients' own immune system of cell clusters, called *islets of Langerhans*, known as responsible for insulin production and secretion. In recent years, researchers have been trying to develop bio-artificial pancreas devices, containing β-cells or islets of Langerhans restricted by a synthetic biocompatible semipermeable membrane, that separates the foreign tissue from the host immune system, which otherwise would rapidly be destroyed.

An essential characteristic of a successful bio-artificial pancreas device is a fast response to a high glucose concentration in blood, which means that diffusion must occur fast and efficiently throughout the device. Although extravascular devices are easier to implant and fabricate, they are usually difficult to recover, and the diffusion of nutrients and metabolites occurs slowly. Intravascular devices have also an important disadvantage: the tendency to form blood clots near the anastomosed ends of the device. However, if this problem can be overcome, they present faster diffusion rates than any extravascular device [83]. Preliminary experiments made for this type of application should test and optimize the operational conditions of the device, cytotoxicity, and blood-clotting induction.

By now, some experiments performed with PSFs have established the *in vitro* performance of hydroxylated PSF membranes in perfusion assays [84], whereas other investigations determined their immunoisolation ability against viruses [85].

Recent studies in this application domain presented an *in vitro* setup for preliminary testing of a microporous membrane with immobilized biologic material, determining its tolerability as a bioprotective membrane for a future bio-artificial pancreas construction. Performance of the device with pancreatic islets and encapsulated insulinoma cells was tested for evaluating insulin release and device longevity, as well as cell viability and adherence to the membrane. Beta TC-3 cells were used due to higher control and reproducibility of cell number and behavior, whereas the addition of hemoglobin was beneficial for sustained cell viability, especially during cell insertion in the device; at the same time, the cells did not adhere to the PSF membranes [86].

10.2.7   DRUG DELIVERY SYSTEMS

Human health is threatened by autoimmune, neurodegenerative, metabolic, and cancer diseases, very difficult to treat with systemically delivered drugs. Conventional pharmacotherapy involves the use of drugs whose absorption and bioavailability depend on several factors, such as solubility, acid dissociation constant (pKa), molecular weight, number of bonds per hydrogen atom of the molecule, and chemical stability. Thus, the latest research is being conducted into new formulations that provide a better pharmacological response that would lead to lower drug doses and minimization of side effects—consequently improving drugs bioavailability. In this context, intense researches have been lately made on the modification of drug absorption and release, the new developments offering additional advantages to the above-mentioned ones and facilitating the release of poorly soluble drugs. Also, these systems will facilitate more patient-friendly drug administration, thus resulting in an increased patient satisfaction [87].

Drug delivery systems are designed to enhance the efficacy of therapeutic agents by enabling their targeting and controlled release; ideally, these systems release medication exclusively to the diseased part of the body and deliver it in a controlled manner (Figure 10.2).

Recent trends in this field pointed out the miniaturization to the micro/nanoscale with the purpose of improving the pharmacokinetics, biodistribution, and solubility of drugs [88]. These features have brought to light some challenges: the devices must be able to host a clinically relevant amount of drug, to meet the biocompatibility and nontoxicity standards, and so on. Drug delivery has become a multidisciplinary

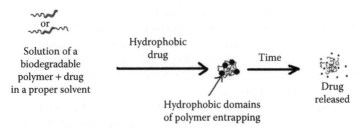

FIGURE 10.2   Biodegradable drug delivery system—a polymer–drug complex.

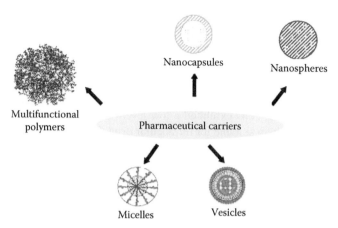

Multifunctional polymers · Nanocapsules · Nanospheres · Pharmaceutical carriers · Micelles · Vesicles

FIGURE 10.3 Pharmaceutical carriers used as drug release systems.

science, in which biology, medicine, nanotechnology, chemistry, and microfabrication are closely related to one another.

Apart from the therapeutic agents, other molecules can be also attached to these particles; their role is to help in targeting specific tissues and to stay in circulation for a longer time inside the body. Nanoparticle-based drug delivery systems, made of liposomes and biodegradable polymers, are drawing much attention because of their efficiency in penetrating the tumors endothelium, due to their enhanced permeability and retention effect [89]. Different pharmaceutical carriers have been studied lately for their role as drug release systems, nanocapsules, nanospheres, micelles, and vesicles; equally, multifunctional polymers received most attention in this context (Figure 10.3).

The particles, once they get access to tumors, release their contents and raise local drug concentrations inside them. There are still concerns about the toxicity of nanoparticle-based systems. Due to the very small size—ranging between 1 and 100 nm—their long-term effects on the body are not very well understood, thereby restricting their commercial use [90].

Advances in microelectromechanical systems technology has resulted in the commercialization of lab-on-a-chip devices for medical diagnosis and extended development of scaffolds for tissue engineering, stents, or implantable drug delivery devices [91]. Most of these systems demonstrate the use of polymers and their attractive properties at micro/nanoscale levels.

The use of a wireless guided microrobot was proposed for performing robotic surgery and targeted drug delivery [92]; initially, it was intended to use for intraocular applications, later on being envisaged for use in other parts of the human body, as well. A porous coating made of PSF was proposed in targeted drug delivery applications using a microrobot. PSFs have found so far usefulness in medical equipment, such as blood dialysis membranes [93], or in intraocular drug delivery as capillary fibers [94].

In a recent research, a porous, biocompatible, and nontoxic polymer coating of PSFs was evolved for drug delivery by solving $CaCO_3$ nanoparticles embedded in bulk PSF coatings; the coating was obtained by dip or spin coating. The difference observed in the morphology of bulk and porous PSF certified that porosity is a result of a selective dissolving process. The suitability of the porous coating for enhanced drug loading and delivery was tested using Rhodamine B as a model drug. Tests regarding the cell viability using fibroblast cell types have pointed out that this parameter is comparable with that of other biocompatible coatings, for example, gold. At the same time, cells exhibited a low level of adhesion on the porous PSF coatings that makes them suitable for intraocular drug delivery [95].

The eye represents a complex organ where drug delivery is difficult, in right amounts at the desired sites, because of the presence of some anatomical, physiological, and physiochemical barriers. To overcome these shortcomings and to achieve the desired ophthalmologic levels, scientists and ocular pharmacologists have developed two strategies for drug delivery, considering an efficient drug administration mode. The first approach involves using alternate delivery routes to the conventional ones, allowing for a more direct access to the target sites; the second approach implies the development of novel drug delivery systems, providing better permeability, treatability, and controlled release at target site. A combination of these approaches is being employed and optimized in order to accomplish optimal therapy with minimal adverse effects. Along with advances in delivering dosage form by different routes, important progress has been recorded in the design of dosage forms permitting better targeting and controlled release [96].

In this context, implants appear as devices that control drug release kinetics using various degradable or nonbiodegradable polymeric membranes. In this context, PSF capillary fibers are among the most commonly used nonbiodegradable implant polymers for intraocular drug delivery, applicable to lipophilic as well as to hydrophilic compounds. The advantage in the use of PSF is due to the presence of deep macrovoids in the membrane that determine the increase of surface area for drug diffusion and release. Drug bioactivity is maintained if the fabrication process does not require the presence of chemical reactions, heat, or solvent. Implants based on PSF capillary fibers can be sterilized, but they have to be subsequently removed. Kinetic studies of carboxyfluorescein release from the PSF capillary fiber—carried out in the rabbit eye—exhibited a constant intravitreal level for up to several days, and no signs of ocular toxicity [94,97].

Collagen gel-based 3D cultures of hepatocytes have been suggested for the evaluation of drug hepatotoxicity, due to their reliability, higher than that of a traditional monolayer culture. Collagen gel entrapment of hepatocytes in hollow fibers has been shown to evidence *in vivo* drug hepatotoxicity, being still limited by hydrophobic drugs adsorption onto hollow fibers [98,99].

Researchers have investigated the impact of hollow fibers on hepatocyte performance and drug hepatotoxicity. To this end, a polysulfone-*g*-poly(ethylene glycol) (PSF-*g*-PEG) hollow fiber was prepared and applied to suppress drug adsorption. The obtained results highlight that these fibers are very important for maintaining cell functions and the toxicological response of gel-entrapped hepatocytes, rather than being only a supporting scaffold. Tetracycline, acetaminophen, rifampicin, chloroquine, and amiodarone are some of the drugs used as model medication; the PSF-*g*-PEG hollow fiber largely suppressed drug adsorption, which improved the application of a gel-entrapment culture for predicting drug hepatotoxicity. Thereby, gel-entrapped hepatocytes within the PSF-*g*-PEG hollow fiber would provide a promising tool for *in vitro* drug investigations [100].

Heparin, known as a common anticoagulant used to impede thrombi formations, is a highly sulfated glycosaminoglycan with the highest negatively charged density in biomacromolecules [101]. Still, it is difficult to use heparin directly as a blood-compatible material because of its water solubility, which calls for an alternative anticoagulant material, based on diverse approaches for modifying hemodialysis membranes. Several investigations on heparin-like polymers have been carried out to develop new materials that contain ionic polymers, including sulfate, sulfamide, and carboxylate groups; this is a consequence of the idea that the anticoagulant activity of heparin was produced by the presence of the ionic functional groups [102,103].

Heparin-like PES was synthesized by a combination of polycondensation and postcarboxylation methods, and then mixed with PES at any ratio to prepare a membrane. Microscopy results suggest that the presence of heparin alters the morphology of membranes and has a considerable effect on increasing hydrophilicity. Comparatively, with the PES membrane, the one containing heparin presented low values of bovine serum albumin (BSA) and bovine serum fibrinogen (BSF) adsorption, good blood compatibility, low platelet adhesion, and low activation of platelets and leukocytes, as well. The obtained membranes delayed blood clotting due to the existence of their functional groups ($-SO_3Na$, $-COONa$) as heparin, whereas cytocompatibility was enhanced [104]. All these results indicate that the modified membranes had the potential to be used for blood purification, hemodialysis, or as bio-artificial liver supports, and might be applied in the industry due to the ease of their preparation.

Other studies showed that heparin could be immobilized on PSF membranes to act as a ligand for the adsorption of low-density lipoprotein (LDL) in human blood. The hydrophilicity of PSF membranes was estimated by the decrease of the water contact angle after the binding of heparin to PSF membranes. At the same time, zeta-potential measurements revealed that, under physiological conditions, heparin-modified PSF possessed a negative potential. The results exhibited an increase of LDL adsorption due to heparin immobilization. The longer thrombin time, partial thromboplastin time, and platelet adhesion on the heparin-modified PSF surface showed that the blood compatibility of the membrane was considerably improved after heparin immobilization. Also, results for BSA solution permeation suggest that the manufactured membranes possess protein antifouling properties [105,106]. Thus, it can be concluded that heparin-modified membranes have a huge potential for simultaneous applications in LDL removal, in the treatment of patients with kidney failure, and hypercholesterolemia, as well as in hemodialysis.

10.2.8 Hemodialysis Membranes Applications

Hemodialysis membranes stand for a major part of artificial kidney systems, advancing in time both quantitatively and qualitatively. Lately, besides simply serving as a life-saving treatment, this procedure is viewed as a means of improving the quality of life. The complications appearing after a prolonged hemodialysis become a

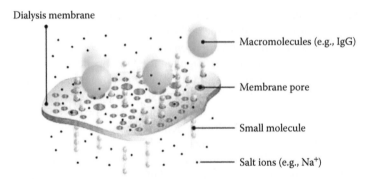

FIGURE 10.4 Schematic representation of a dialysis membrane.

problem that needs to be solved by introducing some high-performance dialyzers; they have to suppress complement activation and, due to their antithrombotic activity, they become more compatible than ever. PSF membranes have the capacity to remove a large range of uremic toxins, to retain endotoxins, and to provide intrinsic biocompatibility and low cytotoxicity. A schematic representation of a dialysis membrane is given in Figure 10.4.

Usually, to impart to each type of membranes its specific characteristics, PSF had to be blended with other polymers. Differences observed among PSF membranes were caused by the variation in the relative amounts of copolymer used in the blend and by the fiber spinning process employed. New generation of PSF dialysis membranes has been described using a process of fiber spinning that produces larger, uniformly sized, and densely distributed pores; these attributes improve membrane permselectivity by creating a steeper sieving curve for low-molecular-weight proteins and a sharp cut-off. Due to these important characteristics, the PSF membrane is capable of achieving an outstanding middle molecule removal with minimal albumin loss; at the same time, its biocompatibility and capacity of endotoxin retention attain maximum levels [107]. The older type of membranes required a much higher albumin loss for an efficient treatment using dialysis membranes with low permselectivity [108].

Other studies have attempted at binding vitamin E to a PSF membrane [109]. Vitamin E is known for its different pharmacological actions, the most important being the antioxidative ones; at the same time, it is known that PSF membranes presented excellent properties as hemodialysis membranes. Thus, vitamin E-modified PSF membrane dialyzer was proposed to serve as a novel dialyzer that can utilize the advantage of vitamin E and exert antioxidative activity. This type of membrane was expected to protect hemodialysis patients through the physiological actions of vitamin E and cytokine. The effects of this type of membrane on complement activation and on cytokines were comparable to those of PSF membranes, whereas granulocyte elastase following dialysis with vitamin E-modified PSF membranes tended to be lower than that noticed for PSF membranes. The effects of PSF–vitamin E-induced methemoglobin, lipid peroxide, and oxygen radicals were lower than those of the PSF membrane, indicating the antioxidative activity of this new type of membranes. Also, vitamin E-modified PSF membrane dialyzers were proved to have favorable effects on the immune system and to manifest antithrombotic and antioxidative actions.

Polyether sulfone hollow-fiber membranes for hemodialysis were prepared by a dry–wet spinning technique based on a liquid–liquid phase separation method. Even when using this preparation technique, the blood compatibility of membranes is not adequate, a coagulant being needed during hemodialysis. Several methods are in use for modifying PES membranes, with the aim of improving their biocompatibility and protein antifouling properties. The simplest and most frequently used technique to modify PES membranes for flat-sheet and hollow-fiber membranes is blending with hydrophilic polymers, such as polyvinylpyrrolidone [110,111] and polyethylene glycol [112], also used as pore-forming agents. This method enhances membranes hydrophilicity, antifouling properties, and blood compatibility [110,112]. Recently, amphiphilic copolymers have been synthesized for blending with PES to prepare membranes with improved properties [113,114].

In some research, high-molecular-weight polyvinylpyrrolidone was blended with PES for the preparation of hollow-fiber hemodialysis membranes, following their *in vitro* and *in vivo* performances [110]. Thus, the biocompatibility profiles of the membranes showed slight neutropenia and platelet adhesion in the initial stage of hemodialysis, although the clearance and reduction ratios after hemodialysis of small molecules (urea, creatinine, and phosphate) were higher *in vitro* than that *in vivo*.

Other studies in this field evaluated dialysis membrane hemocompatibility [115]. In this respect, a series of hepatocompatible parameters (i.e., the generation of complement factor 5a, thrombin–antithrombin III-complex, release of platelet factor 4, and platelet count) was estimated for comparing different polymers used in the manufacturing of dialysis membranes. Results proved that membrane hemocompatibility improved when blending polyarylate with PES; at the same time, they also provided issues that facilitate the selection of membrane polymers with an appropriate hemocompatibility pattern for dialysis therapy.

Membrane fouling represents an essential problem for hollow-fiber membranes. To overcome this shortcoming, researches in the domain have tried to improve the antifouling properties of the membrane by increasing its hydrophilicity. Thereby, a modified PES hollow-fiber membrane was manufactured by blending with Tetronic 1307 as a hydrophilic surfactant [116]. The fouling properties of the obtained membranes were lower than those of the original PES membrane for BSA filtration. In another study, a functional terpolymer of poly(methyl methacrylate–acrylic acid–vinyl pyrrolidone) was synthesized by a free radical solution polymerization using dimethylacetamide as a solvent [117]. The obtained results evidenced that the hydrophilicity of the blended membranes increased and, consequently, membranes showed good protein antifouling properties.

Many other methods can be used for the modification of PES hollow-fiber hemodialysis membranes, the best known being:

- Surface coating [118]
- Photo-induced surface grafting [10,119,120]
- Plasma treatment and plasma-induced grafting polymerization [121]
- Thermal-induced grafting and immobilization [32]

10.3 FINAL REMARKS AND FUTURE PERSPECTIVES

Important progresses have been made lately in medical technology, especially as to an improved participation of a biomaterial to potential clinical applications. This chapter focuses on functionalized PSFs used for complex medical uses, special emphasis being laid on drug delivery applications and tissue engineering. However, technological and scientific challenges have still to be overcome for a better fulfillment of the demands necessary to more accurately mimic the *in vivo* environment. By optimizing the above-discussed complex parameters, drug delivery systems and tissue engineering based on polymeric biomaterials will act as future therapeutic alternatives to the classical medical methods.

Future directions of study should exploit the latest discoveries recorded in biomedical fields. Also, the next generation of polymer-based delivery systems containing growth factors, hormones, antibodies, genes, and peptides should enhance their efficiency and, at the same time, minimize the unwanted effects.

REFERENCES

1. Yilmaz G., Toiserkani H., Odaci Demirkol D., Sakarya S., Timur S., Yagci Y., and Torun L., Modification of polysulfones by click chemistry: Amphiphilic graft copolymers and their protein adsorption and cell adhesion properties. *J. Polym. Sci. Polym. Chem.*, 49(1), 110–117, 2011.
2. Kinasiewicz A., Dudzinski K., Chwojnowski A., Werynski A., and Kawiak J., Three-dimensional culture of hepatocytes on spongy polyethersulfone membrane developed for cell transplantation. *Transplant. Proc.*, 39(9), 2914–2916, 2007.
3. Unger R. E., Huang Q., Peters K., Protzer D., Paul D., and Kirkpatrick C. J., Growth of human cells on polyethersulfone (PES) hollow fiber membranes. *Biomaterials*, 26(1), 1877–1884, 2005.
4. Ulbricht M., Advanced functional polymer membranes. *Polymer*, 47(7), 2217–2262, 2006.
5. Yoon K., Hsiao B. S., and Chu B., Formation of functional polyethersulfone electrospun membrane for water purification by mixed solvent and oxidation processes. *Polymer*, 50(13), 2893–2899, 2009.
6. Yadav K. and Morison K., Effects of hypochlorite exposure on flux through polyethersulphone ultrafiltration membranes. *Food Bioprod. Process.*, 88(4), 419–424, 2009.
7. Boussu K., Vandecasteele C., and Van der Bruggen B., Study of the characteristics and the performance of self-made nanoporous polyethersulfone membranes. *Polymer*, 47(10), 3464–3476, 2006.
8. Hancock L. F., Fagan S. M., and Ziolo M. S., Hydrophilic, semipermeable membranes fabricated with poly(ethylene oxide)-polysulfone block copolymer. *Biomaterials*, 21(7), 725–733, 2000.
9. Unger R. E., Peters K., Huang Q., Funk A., Paul D., and Kirkpatrick C. J., Vascularization and gene regulation of human endothelial cells growing on porous polyethersulfone (PES) hollow fiber membranes. *Biomaterials*, 26(17), 3461–3469, 2005.
10. Brayfield C. A., Marra K. G., Leonard J. P., Cui X. T., and Gerlach J. C., Excimer laser channel creation in polyethersulfone hollow fibers for compartmentalized in vitro neuronal cell culture scaffolds. *Acta Biomater.*, 4(2), 244–255, 2008.
11. Armentano I., Dottori M., Fortunati E., Mattioli S., and Kenny J. M., Biodegradable polymer matrix nanocomposites for tissue engineering: A review. *Polym. Degrad. Stab.*, 95(2), 2126–2146, 2010.

12. Place E. S., George J. H., Williams C. K., and Stevens M. M., Synthetic polymer scaffolds for tissue engineering. *Chem. Soc. Rev.*, 38(4), 1139–1151, 2009.
13. Gleiter H., Nanostructured materials, basic concepts and microstructure. *Acta Mater.*, 48(1), 1–29, 2000.
14. Gorrasi G., Vittoria V., Murariu M., Ferreira A. S., Alexandre M., and Dubois P., Effect of filler content and size on transport properties of water vapor in PLA/calcium sulfate composites. *Biomacromolecules*, 9(3), 984–990, 2008.
15. Peponi L., Tercjak A., Torre L., Mondragon I., and Kenny J. M., Nanostructured physical gel of SBS block copolymer and Ag/DT/SBS nanocomposites. *J. Mater. Sci.*, 44(5), 1287–1293, 2009.
16. Tjong S. C., Structural and mechanical properties of polymer nanocomposites. *Mater. Sci. Eng.*, 53(3/4), 73–197, 2006.
17. Szaraniec B., Rosol P., and Chlopek J., Carbon composite material and polysulfone modified by nano- hydroxyapatite. *E-Polymers*, 30(1), 1–7, 2005.
18. Murugan R. and Ramakrishna S., Development of nanocomposites for bone grafting. *Compos. Sci. Technol.*, 65(15/16), 2385–2406, 2005.
19. Hule R. A. and Pochan D. J., Polymer nanocomposites for biomedical applications. *MRS Bull.*, 32(4), 354–358, 2007.
20. Italia J. L., Yahya M. M., Singh D., and Ravi Kumar M. N., Biodegradable nanoparticles improve oral bioavailability of amphotericin B and show reduced nephrotoxicity compared to intravenous Fungizone. *Pharm. Res.*, 26(6), 1324–1331, 2009.
21. Nahar M. and Jain N. K., Preparation, characterization and evaluation of targeting potential of amphotericin B-loaded engineered PLGA nanoparticles. *Pharm. Res.*, 26(12), 2588–2598, 2009.
22. Pandey R. and Khuller G. K., Nanoparticle-based oral drug delivery system for an injectable antibiotic-streptomycin. *Chemotherapy*, 53(6), 437–441, 2007.
23. Jeong Y. I., Na H. S., Seo D. H., Kim D. G., Lee H. C., Jang M. K., Na S. K., Roh S. H., Kim S. I., and Nah J. W., Ciprofloxacin-encapsulated poly(DL-lactide-co-glycolide) nanoparticles and its antibacterial activity. *Int. J. Pharm.*, 352(1/2), 317–323, 2008.
24. Huo D., Deng S., Li L., and Ji J., Studies on the poly(lactic-co-glycolic) acid microspheres of cisplatin for lung-targeting. *Int. J. Pharm.*, 289(1/2), 63–67, 2005.
25. Nagarwal R. C., Singh P. N., Kant S., Maiti P., and Pandit J. K., Chitosan coated PLA nanoparticles for ophthalmic delivery: Characterization, in-vitro and in-vivo study in rabbit eye. *J. Biomed. Nanotechnol.*, 6(6), 648–657, 2010.
26. Varshosaz J. and Koopaie N., Cross-linked poly (vinyl alcohol) hydrogel: Study of swelling and drug release behaviour. *Iran. Polym. J.*, 11(2), 123–131, 2002.
27. DeMuth P. C., Min Y., Huang B., Kramer J. A., Miller A. D., Barouch D. H., Hammond P. T., and Irvine D. J., Polymer multilayer tattooing for enhanced DNA vaccination. *Nat. Mater.*, 12(4), 367–376, 2013.
28. Adams J. R. and Mallapragada S. K., Enhancing the immune response through next generation polymeric vaccine adjuvants. *Technology*, 2(1), 1–12, 2014.
29. Khulbe K. C., Feng C., and Matsuura T., The art of surface modification of synthetic polymeric membranes. *J. Appl. Polym. Sci.*, 115(2), 855–895, 2010.
30. Van der Bruggen B., Chemical modification of polyethersulfone nanofiltration membranes: A review. *J. Appl. Polym. Sci.*, 114(1), 630–642, 2009.
31. Krieter D. H., Morgenroth A., Barasinski A., Lemke H. D., Schuster O., von Harten B., and Wanner C., Effects of a polyelectrolyte additive on the selective dialysis membrane permeability for low-molecular-weight proteins. *Nephrol. Dial. Transplant.*, 22(2), 491–499, 2007.
32. Kroll S., Meyer L., Graf A. M., Beutel S., Glökler J., Döring S., Klaus U., and Scheper T., Heterogeneous surface modification of hollow fiber membranes for use in micro-reactor systems. *J. Membr. Sci.*, 299(1/2), 181–189, 2007.

33. Yang Q., Chung T. S., and Weber M., Microscopic behavior of polyvinylpyrrolidone hydrophilizing agents on phase inversion polyethersulfone hollow fiber membranes for hemofiltration. *J. Membr. Sci.*, 326(2), 322–331, 2009.

34. Wang Y., Xu H., Zhang J., and Li G., Electrochemical sensors for clinic analysis. *Sensors*, 8(4), 2043–2081, 2008.

35. Sánchez S., Pumera M., and Fàbregas E., Carbon nanotube/polysulfone screen-printed electrochemical immunosensor. *Biosens. Bioelectron.*, 23(3), 332–340, 2007.

36. Sánchez S., Pumera M., Cabruja E., and Fàbregas E., Carbon nanotube/polysulfone composite screen-printed electrochemical enzyme biosensors. *Analyst*, 132(2), 142–147, 2007.

37. Ricci F., Volpe G., Micheli L., and Palleschi G., A review on novel developments and applications of immunosensors in food analysis. *Anal. Chim. Acta*, 605(2), 111–129, 2007.

38. Deng H. T., Xu Z. K., Liu Z. M., Wu J., and Ye P., Adsorption immobilization of Candida rugosa lipases on polypropylene hollow fiber microfiltration membranes modified by hydrophobic polypeptides. *Enzyme Microb. Technol.*, 35(5), 437–443, 2004.

39. Knežević Z., Milosavić N., Bezbradica D., Jakovljević Z., and Prodanović R., Immobilization of lipase from *Candida rugosa* on Eupergit®C supports by covalent attachment. *Biochem. Eng. J.*, 30(2), 269–278, 2006.

40. Palomo J. M., Segura R. L., Fernández-Lorente G., Pernas M., Rua M. L., Guisán J. M., and Fernández-Lafuente R., Purification, immobilization, and stabilization of a lipase from *Bacillus thermocatenulatus* by interfacial adsorption on hydrophobic supports. *Biotechnol. Progr.*, 20(2), 630–635, 2004.

41. Gupta S., Yogesh, Javiya S., Bhambi M., Pundir C. S., Singh K., and Bhattacharya A., Comparative study of performances of lipase immobilized asymmetric polysulfone and polyether sulfone membranes in olive oil hydrolysis. *Int. J. Biol. Macromol.*, 42(2), 145–151, 2008.

42. Edward V. A., Pillay V. L., Swart P., and Singh S., Localisation of *Thermomyces lanuginosus* SSBP xylanase on polysulphone membranes using immunogold labelling and environmental scanning electron microscopy (ESEM). *Process Biochem.*, 38(6), 939–943, 2003.

43. Sanchez S. and Fàbregas E., New antibodies immobilization system into a graphite-polysulfone membrane for amperometric immunosensors. *Biosens. Bioelectron.*, 22(6), 965–972, 2007.

44. Wang J. Y., Xu Y. Y., Zhu L. P., Li J. H., and Zhu B. K., Amphiphilic ABA copolymers used for surface modification of polysulfone membranes, Part 1: Molecular design, synthesis, and characterization. *Polymer*, 49(15), 3256–3264, 2008.

45. Huang Q., Paul D., and Seibig G., Advances in solvent-free manufacturing of polymer membranes. *Membrane Technol.*, 140, 6–9, 2001.

46. David S., Gerra D., De Nitti C., Bussolati B., Teatini U., Longhena G. R., Guastoni C., Bellotti N., Combarnous F., and Tetta C., Hemodiafiltration and high-flux hemodialysis with polyethersulfone membranes. *Contrib. Nephrol.*, 138, 43–54, 2003.

47. Locatelli F., Di Filippo S., and Manzoni C., Efficiency in hemodialysis with polyethersulfone membrane (DIAPES). *Contrib. Nephrol.*, 138, 55–58, 2003.

48. Mocé-Llivina L., Jofre J., and Muniesa M., Comparison of polyvinylidene fluoride and polyether sulfone membranes in filtering viral suspensions. *J. Virol. Methods*, 109(1), 99–101, 2003.

49. Hunter A., Archer C. W., Walker P. S., and Blunn G. W., Attachment and proliferation of osteoblasts and fibroblasts on biomaterials for orthopaedic use. *Biomaterials*, 16(4), 287–295, 1995.

50. Pignataro B., Conte E., Scandurra A., and Marletta G., Improved cell adhesion to ion beam-irradiated polymer surfaces. *Biomaterials*, 18(22), 1461–1470, 1997.

51. Stefoni S., Coli L., Cianciolo G., Donati G., Dalmastri V., Orlandi V., D'Addio F., and Ramazzotti E., In vivo evaluation of cellular and inflammatory response to a new polyethersulfone membrane. *Contrib. Nephrol.*, 138, 68–79, 2003.

52. Zhao C. S., Liu T., Lu Z. P., Cheng L. P., and Huang J., An evaluation of a polyethersulfone hollow fiber plasma separator by animal experiment. *Artif. Organs*, 25(1), 60–63, 2001.

53. Hutmacher D. W., Scaffolds in tissue engineering bone and cartilage. *Biomaterials*, 21(24), 2529–2543, 2000.

54. Rose F. R. and Oreffo R. O., Bone tissue engineering: Hope vs. hype. *Biochem. Biophys. Res. Commun.*, 292(1), 1–7, 2002.

55. Ho J. Y., Matsuura T., and Santerre J. P., The effect of fluorinated surface modifying macromolecules on the surface morphology of polyethersulfone membranes. *J. Biomater. Sci. Polym. Ed.*, 11(10), 1085–1104, 2000.

56. Gupta S. and Chowdhury J. R., Therapeutic potential of hepatocyte transplantation. *Semin. Cell. Dev. Biol.*, 13(6), 439–446, 2002.

57. Chamuleau R. A., Deurholt T., and Hoekstra R., Which are the right cells to be used in a bioartificial liver? *Metab. Brain Dis.*, 20(4), 327–335, 2005.

58. Kinasiewicz A., Kawiak J., and Werynski A., 3D Matrigel culture improves differentiated functions of HepG2 cells *in vitro*. *Biocyber. Biomed. Eng.*, 26(4), 47–54, 2006.

59. Flynn L., Dalton P. D., and Shoichet M. S., Fiber templating of poly(2-hydroxyethyl methacrylate) for neural tissue engineering. *Biomaterials*, 24(23), 4265–4272, 2003.

60. Blacher S., Maquet V., Schils F., Martin D., Schoenen J., Moonen G., Jerome R., and Pirard J. P., Image analysis of the axonal ingrowth into poly(D,L-lactide) porous scaffolds in relation to the 3-D porous structure. *Biomaterials*, 24(6), 1033–1040, 2003.

61. Dodla M. and Bellamkonda R., Anisotropic scaffolds facilitate enhanced neurite extension in vitro. *J. Biomed. Mater. Res. A*, 78A(2), 213–221, 2006.

62. Cai J., Peng X., Nelson K. D., Eberhart R., and Smith G. M., Permeable guidance channels containing microfilament scaffolds enhance axon growth and maturation. *J. Biomed. Mater. Res. A*, 75(2), 374–386, 2005.

63. Rafiuddin A. M. and Jayakumar R., Peripheral nerve regeneration in cell adhesive peptide incorporated collagen tubes in rat sciatic nerve—early and better functional regain. *J. Peripher. Nerv. Syst.*, 10(4), 390–391, 2005.

64. Rafiuddin A. M. and Jayakumar R., Peripheral nerve regeneration in RGD peptide incorporated collagen tubes. *Brain Res.*, 993(1–2), 208–216, 2003.

65. Cao X. and Shoichet M. S., Defining the concentration gradient of nerve growth factor for guided neurite outgrowth. *Neuroscience*, 103(3), 831–840, 2001.

66. Kotwal A. and Schmidt C. E., Electrical stimulation alters protein adsorption and nerve cell interactions with electrically conducting biomaterials. *Biomaterials*, 22(10), 1055–1064, 2001.

67. Dowell-Mesfin N. M., Abdul-Karim M. A., Turner A. M. P., Schanz S., Craighead H. G., Roysam B., Turner J. N., and Shain W., Topographically modified surfaces affect orientation and growth of hippocampal neurons. *J. Neural Eng.*, 1(2), 78–90, 2004.

68. Claverol-Tinture E., Ghirardi M., Fiumara F., Rosell X., and Cabestany J., Multielectrode arrays with elastomeric microstructured overlays for extracellular recordings from patterned neurons. *J. Neural Eng.*, 2(2), L1–L7, 2005.

69. Mahoney M. J., Chen R. R., Tan J., and Saltzman W. M., The influence of microchannels on neurite growth and architecture. *Biomaterials*, 26(7), 771–778, 2005.

70. Wheeler B. C., Corey J. M., Brewer G. J., and Branch D. W., Microcontact printing for precise control of nerve cell growth in culture. *J. Biomech. Eng.*, 121(1), 73–78, 1999.

71. Faid K., Voicu R., Bani-Yaghoub M., Tremblay R., Mealing G., Py C., and Bariovanu R., Rapid fabrication and chemical patterning of polymer microstructures and their applications as a platform for cell cultures. *Biomed. Microdevices*, 7(3), 179–184, 2005.

72. Schmalenberg K. E. and Uhrich K. E., Micropatterned polymer substrates control alignment of proliferating Schwann cells to direct neuronal regeneration. *Biomaterials*, 26(12), 1423–1430, 2005.

73. Heller D. A., Garga V., Kelleher K. J., Lee T. C., Mahbubani S., Sigworth L. A., Lee T. R., and Rea M. A., Patterned networks of mouse hippocampal neurons on peptide-coated gold surfaces. *Biomaterials*, 26(8), 883–889, 2005.

74. Thiébaud P., Lauer L., Knoll W., and Offenhäusser A., PDMS device for patterned application of microfluids to neuronal cells arranged by microcontact printing. *Biosens. Bioelectron.*, 17(1/2), 87–93, 2002.

75. Turcu F., Tratsk-Nitz K., Thanos S., Schuhmann W., and Heiduschka P., Ink-jet printing for micropattern generation of laminin for neuronal adhesion. *J. Neurosci. Methods*, 131(1/2), 141–148, 2003.

76. Chen Q. Z., Thompson I. D., and Boccaccini A. R., 45S5 Bioglass®-derived glass-ceramic scaffolds for bone tissue engineering. *Biomaterials*, 27(11), 2414–2425, 2006.

77. Gerhardt L. C. and Boccaccini A. R., Bioactive glass and glass-ceramic scaffolds for bone tissue engineering. *Materials*, 3(7), 3867–3910, 2010.

78. Rezwan K., Chen Q. Z., Blaker J. J., and Boccaccini A. R., Biodegradable and bio-active porous polymer/inorganic composite scaffolds for bone tissue engineering. *Biomaterials*, 27(18), 3413–3431, 2006.

79. Guarino V., Causa F., and Ambrosio L., Bioactive scaffolds for bone and ligament tissue. *Expert Rev. Med. Devices*, 4(3), 405–418, 2007.

80. Kim H. W., Lee E. J., Jun I. K., Kim H. E., and Knowles J. C., Degradation and drug release of phosphate glass/polycaprolactone biological composites for hard-tissue regeneration. *J. Biomed. Mater. Res. B Appl. Biomater.*, 75(1), 34–41, 2005.

81. Marcolongo M., Ducheyne P., and LaCourse W. C., Surface reaction layer formation in vitro on a bioactive glass fiber/polymeric composite. *J. Biomed. Mater. Res.*, 37(3), 440–448, 1997.

82. Marcolongo M., Ducheyne P., Garino J., and Schepers E., Bioactive glass fiber/poly-meric composites bond to bone tissue. *J. Biomed. Mater. Res.*, 39(1), 161–170, 1998.

83. Silva A. I., de Matos A. N., Brons I. G., and Mateus M., An overview on the develop-ment of a bio-artificial pancreas as a treatment of insulin-dependent diabetes mellitus. *Med. Res. Rev.*, 26(2), 181–222, 2006.

84. Petersen P., Lembert N., Stenglein S., Planck H., Ammon H. P., and Becker H. D., Insulin secretion from cultured islets encapsulated in immuno- and virus-protective capillaries. *Transplant. Proc.*, 33(7/8), 3520–3522, 2001.

85. Petersen P., Lembert N., Zschocke P., Stenglein S., Planck H., Ammon H. P., and Becker H. D., Hydroxymethylated polysulphone for islet macroencapsulation allows rapid diffusion of insulin but retains PERV. *Transplant. Proc.*, 34(1), 194–195, 2002.

86. Silva A. I. and Mateus M., Development of a polysulfone hollow fiber vascular bio-artificial pancreas device for in vitro studies. *J. Biotechnol.*, 139(3), 236–249, 2009.

87. Vilar G., Tulla-Puche J., and Albericio F., Polymers and drug delivery systems. *Curr. Drug Deliv.*, 9(4), 367–394, 2012.

88. Allen T. and Cullis P., Drug delivery systems: Entering the mainstream. *Science*, 303(5665), 1818–1822, 2004.

89. Peer D., Karp J. M., Hong S., Farokhzad O. C., Margalit R., and Langer R., Nanocarriers as an emerging platform for cancer therapy. *Nat. Nanotechnol.*, 2(12), 751–760, 2007.

90. Lewinski N., Colvin V., and Drezek R., Cytotoxicity of nanoparticles. *Small*, 4(1), 26–49, 2008.

91. Tao S. and Desai T., Microfabricated drug delivery systems: From particles to pores. *Adv. Drug Deliv. Rev.*, 55(3), 315–328, 2003.

92. Nelson B. J., Kaliakatsos I. K., and Abbott J. J., Microrobots for minimally invasive medicine. *Annu. Rev. Biomed. Eng.*, 12, 55–85, 2010.

93. Gastaldello K., Melot C., Kahn R. J., Vanherweghem J. L., Vincent J. L., and Tielemans C., Comparison of cellulose diacetate and polysulfone membranes in the outcome of acute renal failure. A prospective randomized study. *Nephrol. Dial. Transplant.*, 15(2), 224–230, 2001.

94. Rahimy M. P., Chin S., Golshani R., Aras C., Borhani H., and Thompson H., Polysulfone capillary fiber for intraocular drug delivery: In vitro and in vivo evaluations. *J. Drug Target.*, 2(4), 289–298, 1994.

95. Sivaraman K. M., Kellenberger C., Pané S., Ergeneman O., Lühmann T., Luechinger N. A., Hall H., Stark W. J., and Nelson B. J., Porous polysulfone coatings for enhanced drug delivery. *Biomed Microdevices*, 14(3), 603–612, 2012.

96. Kwatra D. and Mitra A. K., Drug delivery in ocular diseases: Barriers and strategies. *World J. Pharmacol.*, 2(4), 78–83, 2013.

97. Bourges J. L., Bloquel C., Thomas A., Froussart F., Bochot A., Azan F., Gurny R., BenEzra D., and Behar-Cohen F., Intraocular implants for extended drug delivery: Therapeutic applications. *Adv. Drug Deliv. Rev.*, 58(11), 1182–1202, 2006.

98. Meng Q., Zhang G., Shen C., and Qiu H., Sensitivities of gel entrapped hepatocytes in hollow fibers to hepatotoxic drug. *Toxicol. Lett.*, 166(1), 19–26, 2006.

99. Meng Q., Three-dimensional culture of hepatocytes for prediction of drug induced hepatotoxicity. *Expert Opin. Drug Metab. Toxicol.*, 6(6), 733–746, 2010.

100. Shen C., Zhang G., and Meng Q., Enhancement of the predicted drug hepatotoxicity in gel entrapped hepatocytes within polysulfone-g-poly (ethylene glycol) modified hollow fiber. *Toxicol. Appl. Pharmacol.*, 249(2), 140–147, 2010.

101. Tang M., Xue J. M., Yan K. L., Xiang T., Sun S. D., and Zhao C. S., Heparin-like surface modification of polyethersulfone membrane and its biocompatibility. *J. Colloid. Interface Sci.*, 386(1), 428–440, 2012.

102. Tamada Y., Murata M., Goto K., and Hayashi T., Anticoagulant mechanism of sulfonated polyisoprenes. *Biomaterials*, 23(5), 1375–1382, 2002.

103. Park J. Y., Acar M. H., Akthakul A., Kuhlman W., and Mayes A. M., Polysulfone-graft-poly(ethylene glycol) graft copolymers for surface modification of polysulfone membranes. *Biomaterials*, 27(6), 856–865, 2006.

104. Wang L. R., Qin H., Nie S. Q., Sun S. D., Ran F., and Zhao C. S., Direct synthesis of heparin-like poly(ether sulfone) polymer and its blood compatibility. *Acta Biomater.*, 9(11), 8851–8863, 2013.

105. Huang X. J., Guduru D., Xu Z. K., Vienken J., and Groth T., Immobilization of heparin on polysulfone surface for selective adsorption of low-density lipoprotein (LDL). *Acta Biomater.*, 6(3), 1099–1106, 2010.

106. Huang X. J., Guduru D., Xu Z. K., Vienken J., and Groth T., Blood compatibility and permeability of heparin-modified polysulfone as potential membrane for simultaneous hemodialysis and LDL removal. *Macromol. Biosci.*, 11(1), 131–140, 2011.

107. Bowry S. K., Gatti E., and Vienken J., Contribution of polysulfone membranes to the success of convective dialysis therapies. In: *High-Performance Membrane Dialyzers* (Contributions to Nephrology 173), eds. Saito A., Kawanishi H., Yamashita A. C., Mineshima M., Karger, Basel, Switzerland, 110–118, 2011.

108. Krieter D. H., and Lemke H. D., Polyethersulfone as a high-performance membrane. In: *High Performance Membrane Dialyzers* (Contributions to Nephrology 173), eds. Saito A., Kawanishi H., Yamashita A. C., Mineshima M., Karger, Basel, Switzerland, 130–136, 2011.

109. Sasaki M., Development of vitamin E-modified polysulfone membrane dialyzers. *J. Artif. Organs*, 9(1), 50–60, 2006.

110. Su B. H., Fu P., Li Q., Tao Y., Li Z., Zao H. S., and Zhao C. S., Evaluation of polyethersulfone high flux hemodialysis membrane in vitro and in vivo. *J. Mater. Sci. Mater. Med.*, 19(2), 745–751, 2008.

111. Wang H. T., Yu T., Zhao C. Y., and Du Q. Y., Improvement of hydrophilicity and blood compatibility on polyethersulfone membrane by adding polyvinylpyrrolidone. *Fibers Polym.*, 10(1), 1–5, 2009.

112. Wang Y. Q., Wang T., Su Y. L., Peng F. B., Wu H., and Jiang Z. Y., Protein-adsorption-resistance and permeation property of polyethersulfone and soybean phosphatidylcholine blend ultrafiltration membranes. *J. Membr. Sci.*, 270(1/2), 108–114, 2006.

113. Zhao W., Su Y., Li C., Shi Q., Ning X., and Jiang Z., Fabrication of antifouling polyethersulfone ultrafiltration membranes using Pluronic F127 as both surface modifier and pore-forming agent. *J. Membr. Sci.*, 318(1/2), 405–412, 2008.

114. Chen W., Peng J., Su Y., Zheng L., Wang L., and Jiang Z., Separation of oil/water emulsion using Pluronic F127 modified polyethersulfone ultrafiltration membranes. *Sep. Purif. Technol.*, 66(3), 591–597, 2009.

115. Erlenkötter A., Endres P., Nederlof B., Hornig C., and Vienken J., Score model for the evaluation of dialysis membrane hemocompatibility. *Artif. Organs*, 32(12), 962–969, 2008.

116. Arahman N., Maruyama T., Sotani T., and Matsuyama H., Fouling reduction of a poly(ether sulfone) hollow-fiber membrane with a hydrophilic surfactant prepared via non-solvent-induced phase separation. *J. Appl. Polym. Sci.*, 111(3), 1653–1658, 2009.

117. Zou W., Huang Y., Luo J., Liu J., and Zhao C., Poly (methyl methacrylate-acrylic acid-vinylpyrrolidone) terpolymer modified polyethersulfone hollow fiber membrane with pH-sensitivity and protein antifouling property. *J. Membr. Sci.*, 358(1/2), 76–84, 2010.

118. Torto N., Ohlrogge M., Gorton L., Van Alstine J. M., Laurell T., and Marko-Varga G., In situ poly(ethylene imine) coating of hollow fiber membranes used for microdialysis sampling. *Pure Appl. Chem.*, 76(4),879–888, 2004.

119. Goma-Bilongo T., Akbari A., Clifton M. J., and Remigy J. C., Numerical simulation of a UV photografting process for hollow-fiber membranes. *J. Membr. Sci.*, 278(1/2), 308–317, 2006.

120. Akbari A., Desclaux S., Rouch J. C., and Remigy J. C., Application of nanofiltration hollow fiber membranes, developed by photografting, to treatment of anionic dye solutions. *J. Membr. Sci.*, 297(1/2), 243–252, 2007.

121. Batsch A., Tyszler D., Brügger A., Panglisch S., and Melin T., Foulant analysis of modified and unmodified membranes for water and wastewater treatment with LC-OCD. *Desalination*, 178(1–3), 63–72, 2005.

Index

Note: Locators followed by "*f*" and "*t*" denote figures and tables in the text

Printed and bound by CPI Group (UK) Ltd, Croydon, CR0 4YY

22/10/2024

01777613-0011